ASSESSMENT AND TREATMENT OF MUSCLE IMBALANCE

The Janda Approach

Phil Page, PT, ATC

Baton Rouge, LA

Clare C. Frank, DPT

Movement Links, Inc. and Kaiser Permanente Movement
Science Fellowship, Los Angeles, CA

Robert Lardner, PT

Chicago, IL

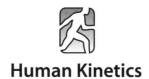

Human Kinetics

Library of Congress Cataloging-in-Publication Data

Page, Phillip, 1967-
  Assessment and treatment of muscle imbalance : the Janda approach / Phil Page, Clare Frank, Robert Lardner.
      p. cm.
  Includes bibliographical references and index.
  ISBN-13: 978-0-7360-7400-1 (hard cover)
  ISBN-10: 0-7360-7400-7 (hard cover)
  1. Janda, Vladimír, Doc. MUDr. 2. Myalgia--Patients--Rehabilitation. 3. Musculoskeletal system--Diseases--Patients--Rehabilitation. I. Frank, Clare, 1962- II. Lardner, Robert. III. Title.
  [DNLM: 1. Musculoskeletal Diseases--diagnosis. 2. Muscles--physiopathology. 3. Musculoskeletal Diseases--rehabilitation. 4. Neuromuscular Manifestations. WE 141 P142a 2010]
  RC935.M77P34 2010
  616.7'42--dc22
                                                2009026864

ISBN-10: 0-7360-7400-7 (print)
ISBN-13: 978-0-7360-7400-1 (print)

Copyright © 2010 by Benchmark Physical Therapy Inc., Clare C. Frank, and Robert Lardner

Acquisitions Editor: Loarn D. Robertson, PhD; **Developmental Editor:** Maggie Schwarzentraub; **Managing Editor:** Melissa J. Zavala; **Assistant Editors:** Nicole Gleeson, Casey A. Gentis, and Joanna Hatzopoulos Portman; **Copyeditor:** Jocelyn Engman; **Indexer:** Craig Brown; **Permission Manager:** Dalene Reeder; **Graphic Designer:** Fred Starbird; **Cover Designer:** Keith Blomberg; **Photographer (cover):** Neil Bernstein; **Photographers (interior):** Phil Page, Clare C. Frank, and Robert Lardner unless otherwise noted. Photos on pages 161 (Figure 11.2), 168 (Figure 11.12), 170 (Figure 11.15), 181-184, 201-202, 203 (Figures 13.9 & 13.10), 204 (Figures 13.12, 13.13, & 13.14), and 205 © Performance Health/Hygienic Corporation; **Photo Asset Manager:** Laura Fitch; **Visual Production Assistant:** Joyce Brumfield; **Photo Production Manager:** Jason Allen; **Art Manager:** Kelly Hendren; **Associate Art Manager:** Alan L. Wilborn; **Illustrator:** Jason M. McAlexander, MFA; **Printer:** Sheridan Books

Printed in the United States of America   20   19   18   17   16   15   14   13   12   11

The paper in this book is certified under a sustainable forestry program.

Human Kinetics
Website: www.HumanKinetics.com

United States: Human Kinetics
P.O. Box 5076
Champaign, IL 61825-5076
800-747-4457
e-mail: humank@hkusa.com

Canada: Human Kinetics
475 Devonshire Road, Unit 100
Windsor, ON N8Y 2L5
800-465-7301 (in Canada only)
e-mail: info@hkcanada.com

Europe: Human Kinetics
107 Bradford Road
Stanningley
Leeds LS28 6AT, United Kingdom
+44 (0)113 255 5665
e-mail: hk@hkeurope.com

Australia: Human Kinetics
57A Price Avenue
Lower Mitcham, South Australia 5062
08 8372 0999
e-mail: info@hkaustralia.com

New Zealand: Human Kinetics
P.O. Box 80
Torrens Park, South Australia 5062
0800 222 062
e-mail: info@hknewzealand.com

We dedicate this book to the memory of Vladimir Janda and to all those who have striven to learn more about his wonderful approach to helping patients. His knowledge and passion helped transform our own clinical practice and gave us the ability to share his teachings with others. This book is also dedicated to the researchers who have yet to prove many of Janda's theories.

We also would like to dedicate this book to promoting better understanding and cooperation among different disciplines, hoping to bridge the gaps among physiotherapy, chiropractic, and medicine.

Most importantly, we dedicate this book to our families, who endured our countless hours of research, writing, and revisions.

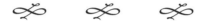

To Angela, Madison, Caitlin, Hannah, and Andrew Page, thank you for your understanding and support. I couldn't have done anything without the best wife in the world, my best friend Ange.

Phil Page

To Kirsten and Lauren Frank, thank you for your constant loving reminders to persevere. You are the best daughters any mother can ask for.

Clare Frank

I very humbly dedicate this book to Professor Karel Lewit, who has inspired me ever since I knew of him and his wonderful work.

Robert Lardner

CONTENTS

PREFACE

Vladimir Janda was a clinician, researcher, and educator well known not only in his native Prague but also around the world. His theories of muscle imbalance served as the basis for evaluation and treatment of patients throughout Europe, giving him the title *Father of Rehabilitation*. As he lectured in the United States and other parts of the world, he developed an interdisciplinary following of physiotherapists, chiropractors, and physicians.

Janda's approach provided a unique perspective on rehabilitation to many Western practitioners. In contrast to the traditional structural view of rehabilitation, Janda suggested a more functional approach by emphasizing the importance of the sensorimotor system in controlling movement and in chronic musculoskeletal pain syndromes. His theories were so revolutionary that he was often years ahead of science.

Janda once compared his approach to musculoskeletal pain to Mendeleev and the periodic table. Mendeleev created a system for classifying elements because he knew there was a systematic way of predicting their properties. At the time Mendeleev developed the table, he left blank spaces for elements that he knew must exist because they fit the pattern but that were not yet discovered by science. Using a similar philosophy, Janda created a systematic and predictable approach to chronic musculoskeletal pain that has yet to be fully discovered by science.

We were fortunate enough to spend time with Janda both in the United States and in Prague many times before his death in 2002. His philosophies were revolutionary and often contrasted the traditional theories taught in school and practiced daily in the United States. After implementing his approach in our clinical practice, we saw its practicality and results. His ideas revolutionized our approach to treating many patients with chronic pain, often the most difficult patients to treat. We knew we had to continue his legacy and protect his approach by teaching workshops to clinicians in the United States.

Janda's approach has been discussed in many textbooks, often in chapters that he authored. Despite his popularity around the world, there was no text to integrate his approach into evidence-based practice. It was likely difficult for the humble Janda to write a textbook devoted to himself and his methods; he always gave credit to others in framing his approach. Many years ago he published a muscle testing book in English but it is now out of print. His last text on muscle testing is not available in English. There are several collections of his articles in English, but they are often difficult to draw from in clinical application. We were frustrated by a lack of any definitive resources to guide clinicians, so we wrote this textbook to preserve and share Janda's teachings with a practical, evidence-based approach.

This book was written for health care providers treating patients with musculoskeletal complaints. Exercise experts may also find Janda's theory of muscle imbalance valuable in developing exercise programs. Our goal in writing this text was to provide a practical, systematic approach to implementing his theories in everyday clinical practice. We have provided a scientific basis for many of his theories, which often preceded the available evidence.

Chapters are divided into four parts filled with illustrations, photos, and step-by-step instructions. Part I provides the scientific

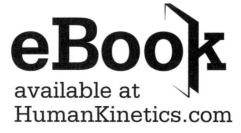

IX

basis for Janda's approach to muscle imbalance. The four chapters review the different paradigms of muscle imbalance, describe the role of the sensorimotor system in function and dysfunction, explain different chain reactions throughout the body, and introduce Janda's classification of muscle imbalance.

Part II describes the functional evaluation of muscle imbalance, outlining Janda's step-by-step system of evaluation. These chapters include analysis of posture, balance, and gait; evaluation of Janda's movement patterns; muscle length testing; and soft-tissue assessment.

Part III outlines Janda's approach to the treatment of musculoskeletal syndromes. Chapters include details on normalizing peripheral structures, restoring muscle balance, and sensorimotor training. Each chapter has many photographs and detailed descriptions of evaluation and treatment techniques.

Finally, part IV brings the theory, evidence, and practical applications together to apply Janda's approach to specific body regions. This helps clinicians easily implement Janda's approach in everyday practice when evaluating and treating cervical, upper-extremity, lumbar, and lower-extremity pain syndromes. Each chapter describes the practical implementation of Janda's system of evaluation and treatment outlined in parts II and III. Specific musculoskeletal conditions commonly seen in the clinic, such as chronic neck pain, chronic back pain, shoulder impingement, and anterior knee pain, are also discussed with emphasis on applying Janda's approach. Each chapter concludes with a case study that compares Janda's approach with the traditional approach to treatment.

In conclusion, we wanted to write a text that both preserves and supports Janda's teachings. This book is only a tool for everyday practitioners; it is not meant to address all chronic pain syndromes or even all muscle imbalance syndromes. Instead, it provides practical, relevant, and evidence-based information arranged into a systematic approach that can be implemented immediately and used along with other clinical techniques.

A TRIBUTE

Vladimir Janda was born in 1928. At the age of 15, he contracted polio. He was paralyzed as a quadriplegic and unable to walk for 2 years. He eventually recovered walking function, but he developed postpolio syndrome and had to use a walker until the end of his life in 2002.

As a physician, he focused on postpolio patients early on. One of his early influences was Sister Kinney, who introduced the treatment of polio in Czechoslovakia. In 1947 he served as an interpreter for Sister Kinney as a first-year medical student and decided to pursue an interest in physiotherapy after medical school. He received the Kinney Physiotherapist Certificate after graduation from medical school. He was one of the first physicians to combine therapy and medicine in a hands-on approach and one of the earliest to practice physical medicine and rehabilitation.

He became more interested in pain syndromes of the locomotor system. His first book, published in 1949 at the age of 21, was on muscle testing and function and was the first of its kind in Czech. He continued as a prolific researcher and writer; before his death, he published more than 16 books and 200 papers on muscle function.

At the age of 24, he was working in a rehabilitation center for postpolio patients. He was interested in evaluating the claims in muscle testing textbooks at the time. Using electromyography, he began studying the muscle activity of the hip joint in physiotherapy students. He found that muscles that weren't supposed to be activated actually were, noting the accessory roles of muscles outside of their primary movements. Specifically, he found that subjects without activity in the gluteus maximus during hip extension used an increased pelvic tilt to accomplish the extension. This led to his lifelong passion to study movement rather than individual muscles, as was common during the polio era. He recognized the importance of testing muscle function rather than strength. This was the beginning of thinking globally rather than locally in terms of muscle function.

In the 1960s, Freeman and Wyke published several papers on afferent input and mechanoreceptors. They described the use of wobble boards in the treatment of chronic ankle instability. Janda noted a connection between chronic ankle instability and chronic low back pain: proprioception. This led to Janda's development of sensorimotor training, a progressive exercise program using simple exercises and unstable surfaces. He rarely recommended strengthening exercises, instead focusing on balance and function. This was in contrast to the traditional rehabilitation approach in the 1960s and '70s, which emphasized strength training.

In 1964 Janda completed his thesis on patients with sacroiliac dysfunction, finding weakness and inhibition of the gluteus maximus even in the absence of pain. He recognized that certain other muscles were prone to weakness. Janda subsequently defined movement patterns to estimate the quality of movement. He discovered that muscle imbalance is systematic and predictable and involves the entire body.

In 1979, he defined his crossed syndromes: the upper-crossed, lower-crossed, and layer syndromes. He subsequently noted that his crossed syndromes were his only discovery; he always gave credit for his work to the others who influenced his approach. Janda had a wide range of influences that provided him with a comprehensive viewpoint:

- Berta Bobath, a physiotherapist, and her husband Karel, a neurophysiologist from London, who were leaders in neurodevelopmental principles and treatment in physiotherapy

- Hans Kraus, an Austrian physician who before World War II first described hypokinetic disease in low back pain, which was noted as a lack of movement
- Karel Lewit, a colleague and lifelong friend who practiced with Janda in Prague for many years and shared his expertise on manual therapy and the locomotor system
- Václav Vojta, a Czech physician who described the influence of developmental kinesiology in human movement and pathology
- Alois Brügger, a Swiss neurologist who described the neurological basis of muscle imbalance
- Florence Kendall, the person who first influenced Janda on the concept of muscle imbalance
- John Basmajian, a Canadian expert in electromyographic analysis who led Janda's postdoctoral studies
- David Simons, an expert in trigger points and muscle pain

Janda was an avid reader and collector of books and papers on muscles. His ability to speak five different languages allowed him to read and learn from work performed all over the world. His international influence continued to spread when he served as a consultant to the World Health Organization in the 1960s and '70s.

Janda founded the department of rehabilitation medicine and directed the physiotherapy school at the Charles University at Prague, where he continued to practice until his death on November 25, 2002. The authors of this text had the opportunity to be with him 3 months before on his last visit to North America. The Father of Rehabilitation will continue to be missed by many. For an excellent review of Janda's life and contributions, read the paper by Morris and colleagues (2006), *Vladimir Janda, MD, DSc: Tribute to a Master of Rehabilitation* (*Spine* 31[9]: 1060-4).

ACKNOWLEDGMENTS

We would like to thank Human Kinetics, in particular Loarn Robertson for recognizing the need for this text and everyone who helped push this book along. Special thanks to Maggie Schwarzentraub, who kept us all together and stayed on top of things for three very busy authors.

Thank you to everyone at the Hygenic Corporation for seeing the value of Janda's approach and the need to share it with the world. In particular, thank you to Ludwig Artzt, who first introduced Phil to Janda in Germany (we immediately became close friends). Thank you to Herm Rottinghaus and Mark Anderson, who both encouraged and supported the many workshops and lectures we presented around the world.

We would like to acknowledge several other individuals who helped us learn more about the entire Prague school, including Brügger's approach, dynamic neuromuscular stabilization, and the Vojta approach: Joanne Bullock-Saxton, Jurgen Foerester, Suzanne Lingitz, Pavel Kolář, and Dagmar Pavlu.

Thanks to Craig Liebenson and Craig Morris for helping to support Janda's approach in the United States. And thank you to our colleague Andre Labbe for helping to spread the word and provide the all-important clinical perspectives.

Special thanks to our families for supporting us not only in writing this book but also in all the time we spend traveling to learn more and teach others.

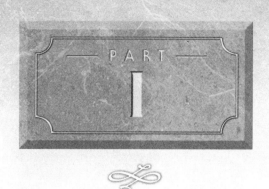

THE SCIENTIFIC BASIS OF MUSCLE IMBALANCE

There are several schools of thought regarding muscle imbalance. Each approach uses a different paradigm as its basis. Vladimir Janda's paradigm was based on his background as a neurologist and physiotherapist. Janda was a prolific researcher and writer as well as a clinician and educator. Well versed in the current literature, the humble Janda often cited the work of others as the scientific basis for an approach to musculoskeletal medicine he developed through clinical experience. Using his vast array of knowledge, Janda was able to create a paradigm shift from a more structural approach to a more functional approach.

Part I establishes the scientific basis for Janda's approach to muscle imbalance. He often referred to the work of Sister Kinney, the Bobaths, the Kendalls, Freeman and Wyke, Vojta, Brügger, and his longtime friend and colleague, Karel Lewit. Each chapter helps explain the scientific basis for Janda's approach to the neuromuscular system and his recognition of muscle imbalance syndromes. Chapter 1 describes the current philosophical approaches to muscle imbalance and how Janda's approach relates to these current schools of thought. Janda taught that muscle imbalance is based on neurophysiological principles of motor development and control. He believed that the sensorimotor system, composed of the sensory system and motor system, could not be functionally divided, and he emphasized the importance of proper proprioception. Chapter 2 describes the critical role of the sensorimotor system in controlling human movement as well as in mediating muscle imbalance syndromes. One of Janda's most important clinical contributions to evaluation and treatment was the recognition of muscular chains and their influence on pathology and function. Chapter 3 reviews the concept of chain reactions in the human body, describing articular, muscular, and neurological chains, while chapter 4 introduces Janda's classification of muscle imbalance through pathology and pathomechanics. By combining research with clinical experience, Janda developed his own classification system for muscle imbalance syndromes. This system was the only aspect of his approach that he really took credit for, often citing the work of others rather than his own.

STRUCTURAL AND FUNCTIONAL APPROACHES TO MUSCLE IMBALANCE

The late Dr. Vladimir Janda (1923-2002), a Czech neurologist, observed that there are two schools of thought in musculoskeletal medicine: structural and functional. The traditional structural approach is rooted in anatomy and biomechanics. Orthopedic medicine is influenced by a structural approach to pathology, relying heavily on visualization of structures through X-ray imaging, magnetic resonance imaging (MRI), or surgery. Structural lesions are damages to physical structures such as ligaments and bones that can be diagnosed by special clinical tests such as the anterior drawer sign in anterior cruciate ligament (ACL) dysfunction. These structural lesions are repaired through immobilization, surgery, or rehabilitation. The diagnosis and treatment of structural lesions such as ligament tears are well supported in the scientific literature. The structural approach is the foundation of medical education and practice.

In some patients, however, the diagnostic tests for structural lesions are inconclusive or the surgery does not cure the lesion, leaving the patient and clinician at a loss. More than likely, a functional lesion is the cause of the problem. Janda defined functional pathology as impairment in the ability of a structure or physiological system to perform its job; this impairment often manifests in the body through reflexive changes. Unfortunately, this type of lesion is less easy to diagnose and treat, requiring a new way of thinking and visualization. Functional lesions cannot be observed directly with structural tools such as MRI; rather, clinicians must visualize the dysfunction virtually by understanding the complex interactions of structures and systems. This is a paradigm shift from thinking only in terms of structure and not understanding true function. This functional approach allows us to better understand the cause of the pathology rather than focus on the pathology itself.

The traditional structural approach relies on visualizing static structures, focusing on their anatomical presence, and forms the basis of most medical education. When describing muscle function, clinicians often look at function from an origin and insertion point of view, meaning a muscle functions only to move the insertion closer to the origin. In contrast, the functional approach recognizes the true function of the muscle, which is based on coordinated movement in relation to other structures, and takes into account the stabilizing roles of muscle. For example, the primary function of the rotator cuff is not to rotate; rather, it is to adduct the humeral head and stabilize the glenohumeral joint. While understanding both the structural and the functional approach is necessary for clinical practice, the functional approach is the key to rehabilitating dysfunction syndromes.

This chapter first differentiates the two musculoskeletal approaches of structure and function and then discusses the role of muscle balance in function and pathology. Finally, two paradigms of muscle imbalance are described: a biomechanical approach and a neurological approach.

Intrinsic Versus Extrinsic Function

The term *functional* is used to describe an approach to exercise prescription that tries to reproduce the same movements used in a functional activity. For example, some may classify the movement of an overhead lifting exercise as a functional movement. This is only an extrinsic viewpoint of function; it's important to first remember intrinsic function, or the function of structures and systems. By understanding the underlying function of these intrinsic processes, clinicians can better understand the pathology of functional lesions. Three intrinsic views of function are physiological, biomechanical, and neuromuscular function.

- **Physiological** function is the response of tissue to dysfunction and damage as well as the healing process itself. Clinicians should be aware of these physiological processes so they can better understand the consequences of dysfunction and the process of rehabilitation.

- **Biomechanical** function encompasses the osteo- and arthrokinematics involved in human movement and the resulting force vectors imparted on human tissues. Recognizing the biomechanical functions of structures helps clinicians understand the concept of chain reactions and how the entire kinetic chain is involved in both movement and pathology.

- **Neuromuscular** function relates to the sensorimotor aspects of movement such as proprioception and reflexes. Clinicians must also understand the processes of motor control and motor relearning for effective exercise prescription.

Extrinsic function is made up of the specific, purposeful, and synergistic movements that integrate the three intrinsic systems. Therefore, the three views of intrinsic function are not independent of each other; rather, they are interdependent in all human movement. For example, unbalanced biomechanical joint stresses that result from muscle imbalance may lead to joint damage, setting up a vicious cycle of pain and inflammation. The structural inflammation then affects the neuromuscular system of

Structural or Functional?

Chronic shoulder pain such as that due to subacromial (SA) impingement is a common complaint. There are two types of SA impingement: structural (primary) and functional (secondary). Traditional musculoskeletal medicine takes a structural approach to the injury, diagnosing the injury by examining structures with special tests and X rays. A structural abnormality such as a hooked acromion (type III) may lead to structural impingement by reducing the SA space. The structural approach to managing primary SA impingement is surgery. In contrast, functional impingement presents with normal X-ray findings, although pain and weakness are typically observed. Interestingly, this weakness is often pronounced in the scapular stabilizers, far from the point of pain. This type of pathology requires a different treatment approach: restoring muscle balance through specific exercises that work not just the glenohumeral joint but the entire shoulder complex.

As you can see, structural and functional shoulder pathology present differently and should be treated differently. If clinicians do not understand this concept and rely on only one type of approach, they are doomed to fail. To achieve optimal outcomes, clinicians should implement the appropriate approach at the appropriate time.

the joint, creating further dysfunction. Eventually, the body adapts the motor program for movement to compensate for the dysfunction. The functional cause of the problem is muscle imbalance, while the symptom is pain and inflammation resulting from a structural lesion. Therefore, it is possible to have both a structural and a functional lesion, but for accurate diagnosis and treatment, the clinician must decide which lesion is the actual cause of dysfunction.

Clinicians must learn to treat the cause of the pain rather than the pain itself, as is often done in a structural approach. By not understanding or recognizing the pathophysiology of a functional lesion, clinicians may worsen a patient's condition, creating a downward spiral. Perhaps this is one reason why so many patients experience failed back surgeries: Addressing the structures through surgery is not identifying and treating a functional dysfunction.

Muscle Balance in Function and Pathology

Muscle balance can be defined as a relative equality of muscle length or strength between an agonist and an antagonist; this balance is necessary for normal movement and function. Muscle balance may also refer to the strength of contralateral (right versus left) muscle groups. For example, Jacobs and colleagues (2005) reported significant differences in hip abductor strength between the dominant and the nondominant side in young adults. Muscle balance is necessary because of the reciprocal nature of human movement, which requires opposing muscle groups to be coordinated. Muscle imbalance occurs when the length or strength of agonist and antagonist muscles prevents normal function. For example, tightness of the hamstrings may limit the full range of motion (ROM) and force of knee extension.

Muscles may become unbalanced as a result of adaptation or dysfunction. Such muscle imbalances can be either functional or pathological (see table 1.1). These types of imbalances are most common in athletes and are necessary for function. Functional muscle imbalances occur in response to adaptation for complex movement patterns, including imbalances in strength or flexibility of antagonistic muscle groups. For example, Beukeboom and coworkers (2000) reported that indoor track athletes experience adaptive changes of the ankle invertors and evertors because of the incline of the track. Soccer athletes exhibit different patterns of strength and flexibility depending on the position they play (Oberg et al. 1984). Ekstrand and Gillquist (1982) found that soccer players are less flexible than age-matched nonplayers but did not find a relationship between tightness and injury. Volleyball players have greater internal rotation, elbow extension, and wrist extensor strength compared with nonplayers (Alfredson, Pietilä, and Lorentzon 1998; Wang et al. 1999; Wang and Cochrane 2001). Athletes who use a lot of overhead movements, such as swimmers (McMaster, Long, and Caiozzo; Ramsi et al. 2001; Rupp, Berninger, and Hopf 1995; Warner et al. 1990) and baseball players (Cook et al. 1987; Ellenbecker and Mattalino 1997; Hinton 1988; Wilk et al. 1993), also

Table 1.1 Functional and Pathological Muscle Imbalance

Functional imbalance	Pathological imbalance
Atraumatic	With or without trauma
Adaptive change	Adaptive change
Activity specific	Associated with dysfunction
No pain	With or without pain

exhibit greater internal rotation strength. Baseball players generally have significantly more external rotation ROM and less internal rotation ROM (Borsa et al. 2005, 2006; Donatelli et al. 2000; Tyler et al. 1999).

Because such imbalances are important for sports, they must be managed before they become pathological. Kugler and colleagues (1996) reported that the muscle imbalance that volleyball players exhibit in the shoulder is more pronounced in athletes with shoulder pain (Kugler et al. 1996). Clinicians must recognize when to treat muscle imbalances, given the pathology and the demands of the sport.

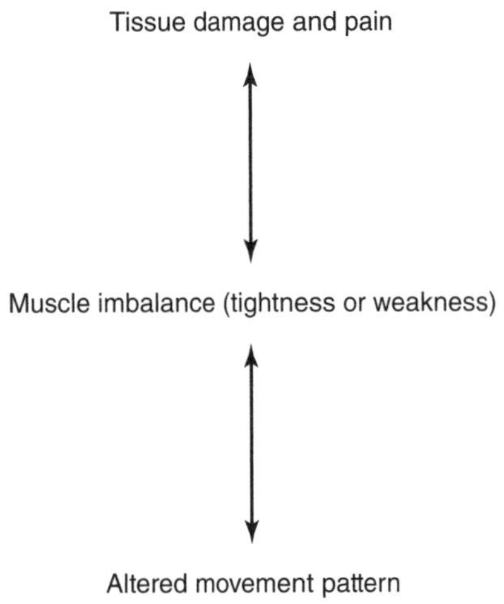

Tissue damage and pain

↕

Muscle imbalance (tightness or weakness)

↕

Altered movement pattern

Figure 1.1 The muscle imbalance continuum.

When muscle imbalance impairs function, it is considered to be pathological. Pathological muscle imbalance typically is associated with dysfunction and pain, although its cause may or may not result from an initial traumatic event. Pathological imbalance may also be insidious; many people have these muscle imbalances without pain. Ultimately, however, pathological muscle imbalance leads to joint dysfunction and altered movement patterns, which in turn lead to pain (figure 1.1). Note that this muscle imbalance continuum may progress in either direction; muscle imbalance may lead to altered movement patterns and vice versa.

Some injuries cause muscle imbalance, while others may result from muscle imbalance. Shoulder impingement is associated with muscle imbalances of the rotator cuff (Burnham et al. 1993; Leroux et al. 1994; McClure, Michener, and Karduna 2006; Myers et al. 1999; Warner et al. 1990) and scapular stabilizers (Cools et al. 2003, 2004, 2005; Ludewig and Cook 2000; Moraes, Faria, and Teixeira-Salmela 2008; Wadsworth and Bullock-Saxton 1997). Shoulder instability is also associated with muscle imbalances (Barden et al. 2005; Belling Sørensen and Jørgensen 2000; Wuelker, Korell, and Thren 1998).

Sometimes pathological imbalances are a functional compensation for an injury. For example, Page (2001) found that 87% of ACL-reconstructed athletes with anterior knee pain had weak hip abductors and tight iliotibial (IT) bands and postulated that hip weakness resulting from surgery is compensated for by a shortened IT band. Runners with IT band syndrome also exhibit weakness of hip abductors (Fredericson et al. 2000).

Poor hip strength has been associated with anterior knee pain. Robinson and Nee (2007) reported that subjects with knee pain demonstrated significant decreases in hip extension (–52%), abduction (–27%), and external rotation (–30%) when compared with a control group without knee pain. Piva and colleagues (2005) found that hip abduction strength and soleus length could distinguish between patients with patellofemoral pain syndrome and controls.

Page and Stewart (2000) reported that patients with anterior innominate rotation in sacroiliac (SI) joint dysfunction demonstrate hamstring weakness on the involved side. Low back pain has also been associated with decreased ROM in hip extension (Van Dillen et al. 2000) and internal rotation (Ellison et al. 1990).

Prospective studies have reported that muscle imbalance is associated with pathological conditions, although specific pathologies may relate to a muscle length imbalance, a strength imbalance, or both. For example, athletes with muscle imbalance in the shoulder are more likely to experience shoulder injury (Wang and Cochrane 2001). Prospective studies on muscle imbalances and sport injuries may help clinicians screen athletes before they begin their sport and implement preventive exercise programs to restore muscle balance in athletes.

Researchers have shown that low back pain and lower-extremity injury are associated with hip extensor weakness in females but not in males (Nadler et al. 2001). Lower-extremity injuries have been associated with muscle weakness and tightness (Knapik et al. 1991), while knee tendinitis has been associated with muscle tightness rather than weakness (Witvrouw et al. 2001). Witvrouw and colleagues (2003) found that professional soccer players with tight hamstrings or quadriceps are at higher risk for lower-extremity injuries. They did not find any injury risk associated with tightness of the plantar flexors or hip adductors.

Strength ratios are used to quantify muscle imbalance between agonists and antagonists in the study of sport injuries. Tyler and colleagues (2001) found that groin muscle strains occurring among hockey players are more prevalent in athletes with a ratio of hip abduction and adduction strength that is less than 80%, reporting a 17-fold increase in risk in athletes with low ratios. Baumhauer and coworkers (1995) reported that athletes with a high ratio of eversion strength to inversion strength, as well as athletes with a low ratio of dorsiflexor strength to plantar flexor strength, were more likely to experience inversion ankle sprains.

Muscle Imbalance Paradigms

There are two schools of thought on muscle imbalance: one that believes in a biomechanical cause of muscle imbalance resulting from repetitive movements and posture and one that believes in a neurological predisposition to muscle imbalance. Both biomechanical and neurological muscle imbalance are seen clinically, so clinicians must understand both in order to make a more accurate diagnosis and treatment. Patients may also exhibit hybrid muscle imbalance syndromes consisting of factors from each paradigm, further challenging clinicians as they work to prescribe the appropriate treatment.

Biomechanical Paradigm

The traditional view of muscle imbalance relates to biomechanics. The biomechanical cause of muscle imbalance is the constant stress that muscles experience due to prolonged postures and repetitive movements. The biomechanical muscle imbalance paradigms are covered extensively in texts by Kendall and colleagues (1993) and Sahrmann (2002a) and will be mentioned only briefly here.

Sahrmann suggests that repeated movements or sustained postures can lead to adaptations in muscle length, strength, and stiffness; in turn, these adaptations may lead to movement impairments. Muscles grow longer or shorter as the number of sarcomeres in series increases or decreases, respectively. These muscle adaptations can result from everyday activities that alter the relative participation of synergists and antagonists and eventually affect movement patterns. The precision of joint motion changes when a particular synergist becomes dominant at the expense of the other synergists; this change may lead to abnormal stresses in the joint. For example, if the hamstring muscle is dominant and the gluteus muscle is weak, the result may be a repeated hamstring strain and a variety of painful hip joint dysfunctions. Hence, careful monitoring of the precision of joint motion as indicated by the path of the instantaneous center of rotation is imperative to identify the muscles that display dominance. Treatment is directed toward restoring the precise joint motion by shortening the longer muscles and strengthening the weaker muscles.

Recently, Bergmark (1989) introduced a classification scheme that divides the muscle systems equilibrating the lumbar spine into global and local. Global muscles are superficial, fast-twitch muscles. They have a tendency to shorten and tighten.

Local muscles, on the other hand, are slow-twitch, deep stabilizers that are prone to weakness. Bergmark (1989) described the local system as muscles inserting or originating at lumbar vertebrae and the global system as muscles originating on the pelvis and ribs. There is some overlap between the two systems, with portions of individual muscles exhibiting characteristics of both systems. While mostly structurally based, Bergmark's classification scheme also has some functional (neurological) components related to motor control, lending itself to the control model of lumbar stability (Hodges 2005).

Neurological Paradigm

Although Janda is considered the father of the neurological paradigm of muscle imbalance, he did also recognize that muscle imbalances may result from biomechanical mechanisms (Janda 1978). He felt that muscle imbalance in today's society is compounded by a lack of movement through regular physical activity as well as a lack of variety of movement, most notably in repetitive movement disorders.

The neurological approach to muscle imbalance recognizes that muscles are predisposed to become imbalanced because of their role in motor function. The neural control unit may alter the muscle recruitment strategy to stabilize joints temporarily in dysfunction. This change in recruitment alters muscle balance, movement patterns, and ultimately the motor program.

Janda considered muscle imbalance to be an impaired relationship between muscles prone to tightness or shortness and muscles prone to inhibition. More specifically, he noted that predominantly static or postural muscles have a tendency to tighten. In various movements, they are activated more than the muscles that are predominantly dynamic and phasic in function, which have a tendency to grow weak (Janda 1978). He found these characteristic patterns of muscle imbalance in children as young as 8 , noting that the pattern does not differ among individuals—rather, only the degree of the imbalance differs. Janda believed these patterns of muscle imbalance to be systematic and predictable because of the innate function of the sensorimotor system (see chapter 2).

Janda described functional pathology as impaired function of the motor system in the pathogenesis of common pain conditions. He noted that all systems in the human body function automatically except for the motor system. He recognized that muscles are very vulnerable and labile structures and believed that muscles, being the most exposed part of the neuromuscular system, provide an excellent window into the function of the sensorimotor system. He often stated that muscles are at a functional crossroads because they must respond to stimuli from the central nervous system (CNS) as well as react to changes in the peripheral joints (see figure 1.2).

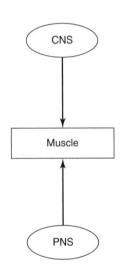

Figure 1.2 Muscles are at a functional crossroads between the central nervous system (CNS) and the peripheral nervous system (PNS).

Janda noted how natural reflexes influence muscle balance and function, leading to adaptation throughout the body through chain reactions. Recognizing the interaction of joint structure, muscle function, and CNS control in function, he believed that changes in one system are reflected by adaptive changes elsewhere in the body. Janda asserted that many chronic musculoskeletal pain conditions result from defective motor learning that prevents the motor system from properly reacting or adapting to different changes within the body. This abnormal recovery of the motor system is then reflected in poor mechanical and reflexive motor performance.

From Janda's viewpoint, chronic musculoskeletal pain and muscle imbalance are a functional pathology mediated by the CNS (see figure 1.3). He based his approach on his observations that patients with chronic low back pain exhibit the same patterns of muscle tightness and weakness that patients with upper motor neuron lesions such as cerebral palsy exhibit, albeit to a much smaller degree. Muscle imbalance often begins after injury or pathology leads to pain and inflammation. Imbalance may also develop insidiously from alterations in proprioceptive input resulting from abnormal joint position or motion. These two conditions lead muscles to either tighten (hypertonicity) or weaken (inhibition), creating localized muscle imbalance. This imbalance is a characteristic response of the motor system to maintain homeostasis. Over time, this imbalance becomes centralized in the CNS as a new motor pattern, thus continuing a cycle of pain and dysfunction. Janda believed that muscle imbalance is an expression of impaired regulation of the neuromuscular system that is manifested as a systemic response often involving the whole body.

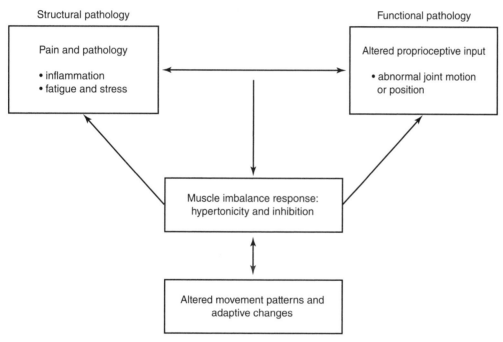

Figure 1.3 Janda's neurological paradigm of muscle imbalance.

Janda's neurological paradigm was further strengthened by his findings of minimal brain dysfunction in patients with chronic low back pain (Janda 1978). He found a lack of coordinated behavior in all areas of function, including psychological (intellectual and stress adaptation) as well as neuromuscular (motor and sensory deficits) dysfunction. He concluded that the presence of minimal brain dysfunction symptoms in 80% of patients with chronic low back pain supports the theory of an organic lesion of the CNS with maladaptation of the system as a functional pathology (Janda 1978). In doing so, he became one of the first to support a biopsychosocial approach to low back pain.

Clearly, Janda's approach was influenced by his clinical observations as a neurologist, while Sahrmann's approach suggests a more biomechanical influence. We see both types of muscle imbalance clinically. While evaluating patients with muscle imbalance, clinicians must be able to determine if the imbalance is due to neurological or biomechanical etiology. Table 1.2 compares the two approaches.

Table 1.2 Comparison of Janda's and Sahrmann's Approaches to Muscle Imbalance

	Sahrmann's biomechanical approach	**Janda's neuromuscular approach**
Basic concept	Repeated movements and sustained postures cause tissue changes and movement patterns. A joint develops a directional susceptibility to movement (DSM) in a specific direction. The DSM becomes the cause of pain because of the microtrauma caused by stress or movement in the specific direction. A deviation of the path of instantaneous center of rotation (PICR) from the kinesiological standard is the result of impairments in the movement system. The purpose of the examination is to identify the DSM and the contributing factors for diagnosis.	All structures from both the CNS and the musculoskeletal system are interdependent. The muscular system is at a functional crossroads since it is influenced by stimuli from both systems. Proper proprioceptive information is integral to motor regulation.
Etiology of imbalance	Muscles maintained in a lengthened position add sarcomeres. This shifts the length–tension curve to the right and increases their tension generation capacity ("stretch weakness"). On the other hand, muscles maintained in a shortened position lose sarcomeres and become weak and infiltrated with connective tissue. The length–tension curve shifts to the left ("active insufficiency"). Dissociated length–tension changes occur in synergistic muscles. One of the synergistic pair becomes short and the other maintains a normal length or is excessively long. The more dominant muscle becomes short and the compensatory motion is often rotation.	There are characteristic patterns of muscle tightness and weakness to pain and pathology at peripheral joints. These muscle reactions are not random but are consistent throughout the whole muscular system. Muscle responses to joint dysfunction are similar to those of spastic muscles seen in structural lesions of the CNS (e.g., hemiplegia and cerebral palsy). Systemic response of the muscular system is due to both extrinsic and intrinsic factors. These factors are a result of a reflex (neurological) nature as well as a result of adaptation due to lifestyle. Muscle imbalance is considered as one of the perpetuating factors for recurrences and chronic pain syndromes.
Movement impairment	In a multijoint system, movement occurs at the joint with least resistance. This is associated with a compensatory site of movement. The compensatory movement is usually in a specific direction at a joint. The stabilizing structures (muscles, ligaments, capsule) become more flexible than those at the primary joint.	Muscles prone to tightness are approximately one-third stronger than those prone to inhibition. Tight muscles are readily activated during various movements. Characteristic patterns of impaired movement provide clues to presence of imbalance (six tests).
Evaluation	Evaluation involves identifying all impairments and their contributions to the pain syndrome. Identifying the mechanical cause is more important than identifying the painful tissues in correcting the problem and alleviating the pain, unless the tissue degeneration or strain is severe.	Muscle evaluation includes posture analysis, gait analysis, muscle length assessment, and movement coordination. Evaluation of movement patterns is more important than evaluating the strength of individual muscles. It evaluates the timing (sequencing) of the firing pattern and the degree of the activity of the synergists.
Treatment	Address muscular component by shortening long muscles, reducing load on weak or long muscles, and supporting weakened or strained muscles. Utilize specific muscles to train patient to activate specific muscles in a precise manner. Emphasize correct use of muscles in postural positioning activity and functional activity.	Normalize function of all peripheral structures. Restore muscle balance of tight and weak muscles. Improve CNS control and programming by increasing proprioceptive flow from the periphery and activate systems that regulate coordination, posture, and equilibrium . Improve endurance in coordinated movement patterns.

Summary

Functional pathology of the motor system describes impaired function of structures rather than damage to structures. Traditionally, clinicians have taken a more structural approach, relying on their knowledge of anatomy and biomechanics in a purely orthopedic approach to chronic musculoskeletal pain. In contrast, the functional approach recognizes unseen mechanisms related to the function of the neuromuscular system. Muscle imbalance is an example of a functional pathology in which opposing muscle groups are imbalanced in length or strength, creating abnormal joint function. There are several muscle imbalance paradigms, most notably biomechanical and neurological perspectives, each with clear clinical evidence. Dr. Vladimir Janda was a pioneer in neurological muscle imbalance leading to chronic musculoskeletal pain. He suggested that the nervous system plays a key role in pain pathogenesis and maintenance.

THE SENSORIMOTOR SYSTEM

Janda believed that the joints, muscles, and nervous system are functionally integrated, and the premise of his approach to muscle imbalance was the integration of the sensory system and the motor system. Janda noted that these two systems, while anatomically separate, must function together as one: the sensorimotor system. The sensorimotor system is global; it regulates function throughout the body and is interconnected. Sensory information is connected to motor response through the CNS and peripheral nervous system (PNS). This creates a looped system in which afferent information from the environment is processed in the CNS, which then sends efferent information back to the motor system; the subsequent motor activity then provides more afferent feedback to continue the cycle (see figure 2.1). Because of this interconnectivity, any changes in the sensorimotor system are reflected elsewhere in the system.

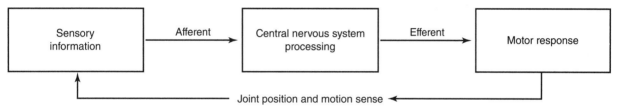

Figure 2.1 The sensorimotor system.

Panjabi (1992a) described a model of spinal stabilization similar to Janda's philosophy. Panjabi's model consists of three subsystems: the skeletal system, the muscular system, and the CNS. A dysfunction in any component within the subsystem can lead to one of three conditions:

1. Successful compensations from another system, or normal adaptation
2. Long-term adaptation by one or more subsystems
3. Injury to one or more components of any subsystem, or pathological adaptation

This chapter begins by using a computer analogy to describe the software and hardware that make up the sensorimotor system and to discuss the input of information through sensory receptors, the processing of that information, and the output that signals the movement of muscle fibers. Next, the chapter looks at the postural and joint stabilizing mechanisms that are the neuromuscular results of the sensorimotor system. Then it concludes with a discussion of the role that the sensorimotor system plays in joint pathology and the local and global effects of that pathology.

Sensorimotor Hardware and Software

Motor control can be described in terms of hardware and software and input and output on a computer. Information from various sources (keyboard, mouse, and so on) is inputted to the central processing unit (CPU) of the computer, which then processes that information with various types of software. Finally, information is outputted via the screen or printer.

Sensory Receptors

Sensory input into the CNS is referred to as *afferent information.* Sherrington (1906) first defined proprioception as the sense of position, posture, and movement. Although the specialized afferent receptors had not been identified at the time, Sherrington knew the human body had some system of information to control movement from proprioceptors (Sherrington 1906). Nearly a century later, Lephart and Fu (2000) redefined proprioception as the "acquisition of stimuli by peripheral receptors, as well as the conversion of these mechanical stimuli to a neural signal that is transmitted along afferent pathways to the CNS for processing" (Lephart and Fu 2000, xvii-xix). Note that the definition of proprioception does not include the processing or response from sensory information, as many clinicians and researchers often mistake when measuring proprioception through joint position sense or detection of motion. These two measurements are indirect measures of the processing of proprioceptive information rather than direct measures of proprioception itself.

Afferent information sent from sensory receptors plays several roles in creating motor responses (Holm, Inhahl, and Solomonow 2002). These include (a) directly triggering the reflex response; (b) determining the parameter of programmed, voluntary responses; and (c) integrating feedback and feed-forward mechanisms for automatic motor output for maintaining balance during standing and walking.

Cohen and Cohen (1956) described an arthrokinematic reflex in which afferent information from joint receptors coordinates the activity of the muscles around the joint. Proprioceptive input includes information on position sense from muscle and joint afferents as well as information on movement from exteroceptors in the skin (Grigg 1994). In the computer analogy, sensory receptors can be considered to be the hardware used to input information into the CNS. The hardware structures involved in sensory input are specialized afferent receptors that include the mechanoreceptors, muscular receptors, and exteroceptors.

Mechanoreceptors

Wyke (1967) identified four types of mechanoreceptors in joint capsules. Capsular afferents are activated at the limits of motion and provide information on joint position. The different types occur in different areas of the joint and demonstrate different stimulation thresholds and adaptations to stimuli. Each type provides specific afferent information regarding joint position (Grigg 1994). These are summarized in table 2.1.

Wyke and Polacek (1975) noted that all articular mechanoreceptors exhibit powerful facilitatory or inhibitory reflexive influence on the muscles involved in maintaining gait, posture, and respiration. In particular, type I receptors contribute

Table 2.1 Articular Mechanoreceptors

Type	Location	Characteristics	Information
Type I, Ruffini	Superficial layers of capsule	Static and dynamic, low threshold, slow adapting	Stretch, particularly in limits of rotation
Type II, Paciniform	Deeper layers of capsule and articular fat pads	Dynamic, low threshold, rapid adapting	Compression
Type III, Golgi tendon organ	Joint ligaments	Dynamic, high threshold, slow adapting	Active tension (not passive tension)
Type IV, free nerve endings	Fibrous capsule and fat pads	Nociceptive, high threshold, nonadapting	Pain and inflammation (not directional)

significantly to postural and kinesthetic sensations. Wyke and Polacek went on to note that damage to mechanoreceptors caused by disease or trauma results in reflexive abnormalities in posture and movement as well as disrupts postural and joint position awareness.

Muscular Receptors

There are two types of muscular receptors that provide proprioceptive information: muscle spindles and Golgi tendon organs (GTOs). Muscle spindles (intrafusal fibers) are located within the muscles and run parallel to the muscle fibers (extrafusal fibers). Muscle spindles detect the length and the rate of change of the extrafusal fibers, thus providing information for conscious perception of limb position and movement (Fitzpatrick, Rogers, and McCloskey 1994). GTO receptors are located within the tendons of muscles as well as within their fascial coverings. These receptors are sensitive to muscle contraction.

Exteroceptors

Specialized receptors in the skin that sense touch are referred to as *exteroceptors*. These receptors provide proprioceptive information on movement as the skin is stretched at various points along the ROM (Grigg 1994). For example, if the knee is fully extended, the skin behind the knee becomes taut, signaling knee extension. Other receptors in the skin such as thermoreceptors and pain receptors provide afferent information though not proprioceptive information per se. These receptors do, however, generate signals that stimulate the motor responses of the flexor reflex and crossed extensor reflex. These reflexes are also called *withdrawal reflexes* since they create a reflexive motor reaction to remove a body part from a dangerous stimulus. They are spinal-level reflexes designed to protect the body from nociceptive stimuli such as heat or pain.

During both of these withdrawal reflexes, the flexors of the extremity are activated while the extensors are relaxed. In the flexor reflex, only the involved side is active, while the crossed extensor reflex involves both limbs. The crossed extensor reflex flexes the involved limb and relaxes the extensors while concomitantly extending the opposite limb and relaxing the flexors. An example of this reflex is the reaction to stepping on a tack; the hip and knee on the involved side flex while the contralateral extensors activate to support the limb.

Key Areas of Proprioception

Articular receptors contribute significantly to postural reflexes, joint stabilization, and motor control (Freeman and Wyke 1966, 1967a). Three key areas of proprioceptive input for the maintenance of posture are the sole of the foot, the SI joint, and the cervical spine.

Sole of the Foot

Afferent input from the sole of the foot affects postural awareness (Kavounaodias et al. 2001; Roll, Kavounoudias, and Roll 2002). Cutaneous reflexes from the foot are important to posture and gait (Aniss, Gandevia, and Burke 1992; Freeman and Wyke 1966; Haridas, Zehr, and Misiaszek 2005; Horak, Nashner, and Diener 1990; Knikou, Kay, and Schmit 2007; Meyer, Oddsson, and De Luca 2004; Sayenko et al. 2007). Lower-limb afferents alone provide enough information to maintain upright stance and are critical in perceiving postural sway (Fitzpatrick, Rogers, and McCloskey 1994; Fitzpatrick and McCloskey 1994; Tropp and Odenrick 1988). In addition, movement discrimination in the ankle is better barefoot when compared with wearing shoes (Waddington and Adams 2003b). Stimulation of the sole of the foot improves kinesthesia and postural sway (Maki et al. 1999; Watanabe and Okubo 1981; Waddington 2003). Altered feedback from cutaneous receptors alters gait and patterns of muscle activation (Freeman and Wyke 1967a; Nurse and Nigg 2001). Visual input often substitutes for a loss of plantar sensory information in healthy patients (Meyer, Oddsson, and De Luca 2004; McKeon and Hertel 2007) and lumbar discectomy patients (Bouche et al. 2006).

The position and posture of the foot and ankle may also play an important role in proprioceptive input. Individuals with supinated or pronated feet exhibit less postural control than people with neutral feet exhibit (Tsai et al. 2006). Also, Hertel, Gay, and Denegar (2002) showed increased postural sway in subjects with cavus feet compared with subjects with neutral feet. This increase is likely due to the hypomobility of a supinated foot or the decreased afferent sensory input resulting from reduced plantar contact.

Sacroiliac Joint

Lumbar proprioception is needed for proper gait (Fukushima and Hinoki 1984). The SI joint helps transmit forces between the lower extremity and the trunk. Vilensky and colleagues (2002) showed that proprioceptive input from the mechanoreceptors in the SI joint is important for maintaining upright posture. Because of its influence in proprioception, gait, and posture, the SI joint is often a source of dysfunction in patients with chronic low back pain. Although the SI joint itself is arguably hypomobile, proprioceptive dysfunction may well be the main factor in SI joint dysfunction.

Cervical Spine

Cervical spine afferents from cervical facets contribute to postural stability (Abrahams 1977) and play a role in cervical pain (McLain 1994). In infants, primitive reflexes related to the position of the neck, such as the tonic neck reflexes, directly influence the position of the trunk, as is demonstrated in stereotypical patterns. Also, patients with chronic cervical dysfunction often exhibit balance deficits (Karlberg, Persson, and Magnusson 1995; Madeleine et al. 2004; McPartland, Brodeur, and Hallgren 1997; Sjostrom et al. 2003; Treleaven, Jull, and Sterling 2003, 2005).

Proprioceptive information travels upward in the spinal cord along specific tracts that depend on the type of information being transmitted. Unfortunately, there is no way to measure isolated proprioceptive input. Current methods to evaluate proprioception involve conscious awareness and include joint position sense and time to detect passive movement (TTDPM). Other indirect methods of studying proprioception include measuring reflexive latency using electromyography (EMG), postural stability, and somatosensory evoked potentials (SSEPs). Proprioception from several areas has been investigated with SSEPs. Tibone, Fechter, and Kao (1997) found that shoulder ligaments and tendons produce similar SSEPs, while articular cartilage and the humeral head do not produce SSEPs. The ACL demonstrates SSEPs (Pitman et al. 1992) that can be restored after ACL rupture through ACL reconstruction (Ochi et al. 2002).

Conscious proprioception travels up the dorsolateral tracts, while unconscious proprioception travels at much higher velocities along the spinocerebellar tract. Regardless of the tract used, specific proprioceptive information terminates at various levels within the CNS for processing.

Central Processing

The software involved in motor control includes information from several levels. In the computer analogy, the background operating system is the collection of basic movement patterns that humans are born with for motor control. These include primitive reflexes and balance and righting reactions. Programs that run on the operating system are the functional movements and skills needed for daily life.

The sensorimotor system is controlled on three levels: the spinal, subcortical, and cortical levels (see table 2.2). The processing at the three levels differs in speed, control, and awareness.

Table 2.2   Three Levels of Control for the Sensorimotor System

Location	Speed	Control	Awareness
Spinal	Fastest	Involuntary	Unconscious
Subcortical	Intermediate	Automatic	Subconscious
Cortical	Slowest	Greatest	Conscious

Spinal Level

Control at the spinal level involves isolated spinal cord reflexes that are influenced directly by afferent information from joint receptors. These reflexes are very fast, involuntary, and unconscious and are coordinated between agonist and antagonist muscles. Sherrington (1906) identified this coordination as the law of reciprocal inhibition: When an agonist contracts, its antagonist automatically relaxes.

An example of this law is the stretch reflex, commonly seen as the knee jerk resulting from a patellar tendon tap. Figure 2.2 shows how the patellar tendon tap elongates the quadriceps fibers, sending afferent signals via muscle spindle afferents. These signals are then processed within the spinal cord segment to facilitate the quadriceps to restore tendon length (shorten) and at the same time inhibit the antagonist hamstrings to allow for knee extension. This inhibition occurs through an inhibitory interneuron within the spinal cord and is referred to as *reciprocal inhibition.*

The opposite of the spinal-level muscle spindle reflex is the GTO reflex. When GTO receptors become stretched, their afferent signals inhibit the motor neuron innervating the agonist while facilitating the motor neuron of the antagonist. Therefore, this reflex is also known as an *autogenic inhibitory reflex.* In this situation, overstretched muscle reflexively relaxes in order to avoid injury.

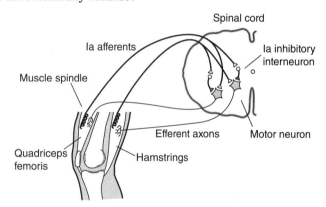

Figure 2.2   Neural circuits of the stretch reflex.

Reprinted, by permission, from R.M. Enoka, 2008, *Neuromechanics of human movement,* 4th ed. (Champaign, IL: Human Kinetics), 262.

Subcortical Level

The next level of neuromuscular control is the subcortical level. This level, which includes the brain stem, thalamus, hypothalamus, vestibular system, and cerebellum, is responsible for equilibrium as well as for automatic postural, righting, and balance reactions. The thalamus is an important relay station for information passing through the CNS. This region gives meaning to perceptions and is involved in temperature sensation through the spinothalamic tract. The vestibular system plays a critical role in maintaining upright posture through its intricate arrangement of semicircular canals. These canals are oriented in three planes and allow for the sensation of head position. The cerebellum is involved in coordinating movement as well as equilibrium.

The subcortical region involves multiple levels of activation rather than isolated segmental reflexes, although its responses are subconscious and automatic. Proprioceptive information can pass through the subcortical area via the spinocerebellar tracts or proceed directly into the cortical level via dorsolateral tracts.

Cortical Level

The highest level of neuromuscular control is the cortical level. The cortex allows us to initiate and control complex and voluntary movements. The cortical region is the phylogenetically youngest portion of the CNS and is probably the most fragile component of the system. The cortical level is the summation of processing from the lower-level input. Conscious motor control at the cortical level is slowest but most variable. This also provides the ability to improve conscious motor control with training.

The three key regions of the cortex are the primary motor cortex, premotor area, and supplemental motor area. The primary motor cortex receives proprioceptive information, the premotor area organizes and prepares movement, and the supplemental motor area programs groups of muscles for complex movements.

Feedback and feed-forward mechanisms are also controlled centrally. These two mechanisms are vital for motor learning and motor control to maintain posture and joint stability. Both feedback and feed-forward mechanisms rely on afferent information, but they differ in their regulation related to sensory detection of movement. Feedback mechanisms regulate motor control by correcting movement *after* sensory detection. They use closed reflex loops of mechanoreceptors and muscles across joints such as the shoulder (Guanche et al. 1995), lumbar spine (Solomonow et al. 1998), and knee (Tsuda et al. 2001). Cutaneous receptors in the foot connect directly to motor neurons controlling the ankle joint (Aniss, Gandevia, and Burke 1992).

Open-loop feed-forward mechanisms anticipate movement *before* sensory detection, in particular providing postural stabilization before limb movement in both the neck (Falla, Jull, and Hodges 2004) and the trunk (Hodges and Richardson 1997a, 1997b). Feed-forward function usually is quantified as EMG onset longer than 20 ms before motion (Aruin and Latash 1995; Hodges and Richardson 1997b).

Motor Output

The hardware for motor control output includes the alpha and gamma motor neurons innervating muscle fibers. Alpha motor neurons relay voluntary motor commands, while gamma motor neurons regulate unconscious length. The gamma motor neurons are controlled by the intrafusal muscle spindle afferents and are not responsible for extrafusal muscle contraction.

Motor units are groups of muscle fibers innervated by a single motor neuron. Motor units with larger numbers of muscle fibers are responsible for gross movements and often are located in proximal postural muscles. Motor units with smaller numbers of muscle fibers are involved in fine movements. Descending signals that initiate muscle action are modified by the sensory input from proprioceptive nerve endings (Holm, Inhahl, and Solomonow 2002). Proprioceptive feedback is essential to proper recruitment to specific fiber types (Drury 2000). Generally muscle fibers are classified into two types based on their contraction times and metabolism: slow-twitch (Type I) fibers and fast-twitch (Type II) fibers. Type I or slow-twitch fibers are aerobic and fatigue resistant, while Type II or fast-twitch fibers are anaerobic and fatigable.

Efferent signals to muscle fibers are either facilitatory or inhibitory. Both facilitatory and inhibitory signals are summated to determine the ultimate efferent response of facilitation or inhibition. Muscle contracts when it reaches an activation threshold as a result of alpha motor neuron signaling at the motor end plate. All fibers within a motor unit either contract or relax as a result of an efferent signal. This phenomenon is known as the *all or none principle*. As mentioned earlier, when a motor unit is facilitated the antagonist receives an inhibitory signal to relax, as described by Sherrington's law of reciprocal inhibition. Table 2.3 summarizes the structural and functional components of the sensorimotor system.

Table 2.3 Structural and Functional Components of the Sensorimotor System

STRUCTURAL		
Afferent	**Central**	**Efferent**
Mechanoreceptors Muscular receptors Exteroceptors	Spinal tracts Subcortical (brain stem) Cortical	Peripheral nerves (alpha and gamma motor neurons) Muscle
FUNCTIONAL		
Proprioception	Processing Motor programming	Stabilization (postural stability and joint stabilization) Movement

Neuromuscular Aspects of Postural Stability and Joint Stabilization

The commonly used term *neuromuscular* refers to the interdependence of the sensory and motor systems, especially regarding the effects of the CNS on the muscular system, which controls the skeletal system. Muscles often act as movers as well as stabilizers during functional movement; therefore, neuromuscular control can be defined as the unconscious activation of muscular stabilizers to prepare for and respond to joint movement and loading for functional joint stability (Riemann and Lephart 2002a). These stabilizing mechanisms occur both globally through postural stabilization and locally through functional joint stabilization.

Postural Stabilization

Postural stability (commonly referred to as *balance)* is defined as the ability of the body to maintain its center of gravity (COG) within its base of support (BOS) within the limits of stability (LOS). This arrangement is referred to as an *inverted cone* (see figure 2.3). When the COG is aligned within the BOS, the body is stable; as the COG and BOS lose alignment, postural stability decreases.

Postural stability is the result of the input, processing, and output of information from the PNS and CNS. In particular, the information involved in postural stability includes visual, vestibular, and somatosensory information. The visual system provides information on the surrounding environment and the relationship of the eyes to the horizon. The vestibular system provides information on head and body position as well as provides feedback from a moving BOS. Somatosensation encompasses all input from the periphery, including proprioception, thermoreception, and pain. Attention and

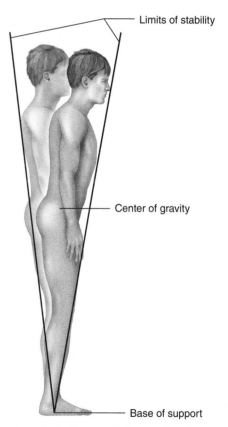

Limits of stability

Center of gravity

Base of support

Figure 2.3 The inverted cone of postural stability.

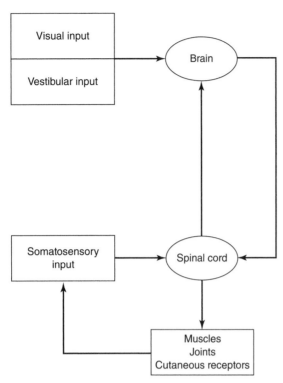

Figure 2.4 The postural stability loop.

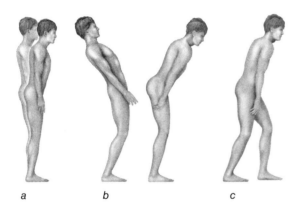

Figure 2.5 Balance strategies: *(a)* ankle, *(b)* hip, and *(c)* step.

cognition can also affect postural stability (Shumway-Cook and Woolacott 2000; Shumway-Cook et al. 1997). Because postural stability requires cognitive resources to process somatosensory input, any additional process that uses those resources can reduce a person's ability to maintain postural stability. All of this information is evaluated and processed in the CNS to create the necessary motor output commands to maintain postural stability. This entire process occurs constantly and automatically in a loop (figure 2.4).

The responses of the motor system to maintain postural stability are known as *automatic postural responses* (APRs; Cordo and Nashner 1982; Horak and Nashner 1986). These responses are mediated on a subcortical level, mainly in the cerebellum. They occur on the subconscious level before voluntary movement and are not modifiable by conscious effort (Cordo and Nasnher 1982). These automatic postural reactions are divided into three characteristic balance strategies: the ankle, hip, and step strategies (Horak and Nashner 1986). These three strategies are activated progressively to restore the alignment of the COG and BOS.

• **Ankle Strategy** (figure 2.5*a*). The ankle plays a central role in postural correction (Tropp and Odenrick 1988). Small changes to the COG are corrected through the ankle to reposition the COG over the BOS. This strategy commonly occurs when a person stands on altered support surfaces such as foam pads. The correction occurs distally to proximally while the head and hips move synchronously. This response is also known as an *inverted pendulum*.

• **Hip Strategy** (figure 2.5*b*). Larger changes to the COG are corrected through a multisegmental strategy at the hips. The correction occurs proximally to distally as the head and hips move asynchronously. This strategy is used when standing on small support surfaces.

• **Step Strategy** (figure 2.5*c*). When unable to reposition the COG with the ankle or hip strategy, the body repositions the BOS under the COG by taking a step.

Through EMG analysis, Horak and Nashner (1986) quantified the stereotypical, specific, and directional responses to weight-shift perturbations at the ankle. These responses have very short latencies, occurring between 73 and 110 ms after perturbation (Horak and Nashner 1986). This indicates that these responses occur on an automatic rather than voluntary level. The body responds to an anterior weight shift (AWS) with a characteristic pattern of dorsal muscle activation that begins with the distal gastrocnemius muscle, which is followed by the hamstrings and the lumbar paravertebrals. The posterior weight shift (PWS) is countered by a ventral muscle response that begins distally with the tibialis anterior and then involves the quadriceps and finally the abdominal muscles. Therefore, the muscle group opposite the direction of the weight shift or perturbation is responsible for maintaining postural stability. A medial weight shift (MWS) activates lateral muscles for stabilization, while a lateral weight shift (LWS) activates medial muscles. Table 2.4 summarizes these patterns of automatic muscle activation. These directional weight shifts can be measured objectively using computerized posturography and can be quantified as postural sway, which is the deviation of the COG within the BOS.

Table 2.4 Muscle Activation in Response to Weight Shifts

Weight shift	Muscle activation for stabilization
Anterior	Gastrocnemius, hamstrings, lumbar paravertebrals
Posterior	Tibialis anterior, quadriceps, abdominal muscles
Medial	Peroneals, lateral hamstrings, hip abductors
Lateral	Tibialis posterior, medial hamstrings, hip adductors

Horak, Nashner, and Diener (1990) reported that subjects with vestibular deficits use less hip strategy, while subjects with somatosensory deficits use more hip strategy. Injury, as well as the natural aging process, can alter normal APR patterns. Patients with musculoskeletal injury exhibit different postural patterns. Researchers have reported that subjects with functional ankle instability (Tropp and Odenrick 1988) or chronic low back pain (Byl and Sinnott 1991) demonstrate an increase in the hip strategy (rather than the ankle strategy) to maintain postural stability. Researchers have also found that older adults use the hip strategy more than younger subjects do (Okada et al. 2001). Woolacott (1986) reported that up to 50% of older adults have lost the ankle strategy or reverse the order of the balance reactions to begin with the step strategy.

Researchers have also recorded a reflexive activation of muscles that helps the body maintain postural stability when moving the limbs. Aruin and Latash (1995) demonstrated through EMG analysis that perturbing the COG with arm movement activates a feed-forward mechanism involving the superficial postural muscles to maintain stability in the opposite direction of the arm movement; thus these researchers noted a direction-specific response. In contrast, Hodges and Richardson (1997a, 1997b) demonstrated that in response to limb movement, the deeper transversus abdominis functions as a feed-forward postural stabilizer regardless of movement direction. Other trunk muscles (such as the obliques, multifidus, and rectus abdominis) vary in activation specific to the direction of the extremity motion, being activated in the opposite direction of motion.

Functional Joint Stabilization

Balance of agonists and antagonists is necessary to aid ligaments in providing joint stability and to equalize pressure distribution at the articular surface (Baratta et al. 1988). Joint stability results from both static and dynamic mechanisms. Static stability comes from passive structures such as bony congruity, ligaments, and joint capsules. Dynamic stability is created by muscular contraction and is referred to as *functional joint stabilization*. Cholewicki, Panjabi, and Khachatryan (1997) demonstrated a co-contraction of the trunk flexors and extensors around a neutral spine in healthy individuals. Locally, neuromuscular control of the sensorimotor system is responsible for functional joint stabilization.

Functional joint stabilization relies on the same automatic mechanisms that global stabilization uses to stabilize localized joints throughout the body. Often stabilization is required before movement, as is seen in the concept of proximal stability before distal mobility. Proprioceptive information is critical to functional stability and often relies on the feedback and feed-forward mechanisms described previously. Proprioceptive deficits can predict ankle injury (Payne, Berg et al. 1997). Functional joint stabilization is an automatic, fast, and unconscious process rather than a slow, deliberate, and voluntary action.

Closed-loop reflexes have been implicated in the functional stabilization of several joints, including the shoulder rotator cuff and glenohumeral ligaments (Guanche et al. 1995) and the knee stabilized by the ACL, quadriceps, and hamstrings (Solomonow et al. 1987; Tsuda et al. 2001). Muscles around the knee have been shown to stabilize joints reflexively in response to both perturbation (Buchanan, Kim, and Lloyd 1996) and electrical stimulation (Kim et al. 1995) of the collateral ligaments. Buchanan, Kim, and Lloyd (1996) demonstrated that perturbations at the knee evoke characteristic and predictable automatic responses of stabilizing muscles; these responses are independent of the muscles' roles as flexors or extensors. Mechanoreceptors of the sole of the foot have reflexive connections with muscles surrounding the ankle (Aniss, Gandevia, and Burke 1992; Nakajima et al. 2006). Stimulation of plantar cutaneous afferents at the heel elicits a reflex contraction of the soleus, which may help to control balance (Sayenko et al. 2007).

The transversus abdominis contracts to maintain intra-abdominal pressure during trunk movement and stabilization (Cresswell, Grundstrom, and Thorstensson 2002). Holm, Inhahl, and Solomonow (2002) reported that stimulation of lumbar afferents from the discs, capsules, and ligaments activates the multifidus and longissimus muscles 1 to 2 levels above and below the stimulated segments for reflexive stabilization. Similarly, Solomonow and colleagues (1998) showed that stress to the lumbar supraspinous ligament causes the multifidus muscle to stiffen from 1 to 3 lumbar segments away from the stimulation in order to prevent instability.

Fatigue may play an important role in proprioception. Janda believed that fatigue impedes feedback from the muscle spindle, thus affecting proprioception and posture. Lee and coworkers (2003) noted that muscle mechanoreceptors are responsible for decreased proprioception after fatigue. While some researchers have shown that muscle fatigue affects proprioception in the shoulder (Lee et al. 2003; Myers et al. 1999) and the trunk extensors (Vuillerme, Anziani, and Rougier 2007), others have shown little effect of fatigue on proprioception in the knee (Bayramoglu, Toprak, and Sozay 2007) and ankle (Shields, Madhavan, and Cole 2005).

Only 25% of a maximum voluntary isometric contraction (MVIC) is needed to provide articular joint stiffness (Hoffer and Andreassen 1981), and as little as 1% to 3% MVIC is required in the lumbar spine (Cholewicki, Panjabi, and Khachatryan 1997); therefore, absolute muscle strength is not the most important variable in pathology or rehabilitation of functional instability. Instead, the proper timing and automatic activation of dynamic stabilizers are more important than strength for functional stability, a finding that redirects our focus from strength to reflexive activation in both evaluation and treatment of chronic instability.

Pathology in Proprioception

The sensory system is the key to proper function of the motor system. Kurtz (1939) was the first to describe joint instability caused by proprioceptive dysfunction rather than ligamentous laxity. Freeman, Dean, and Hanham (1965) first described functional instability as a repetitive joint instability in the presence of normal strength and structure. They postulated that this instability was due to deafferentation, or the loss of afferent information into the CNS because of damage to joint mechanoreceptors in the injured ankle ligaments.

Tropp (2002) updated the definition of functional instability as a sensation of instability or recurrent sprains (or both) due to proprioceptive and neuromuscular deficits. Clinically, we see functional instability in diagnoses such as chronic sprain, microinstability, or chronic subluxation. Functional instability likely is present in patients with chronic pain in the ankle, shoulder, knee, back, and neck.

O'Connor and colleagues (1992) used an animal model to demonstrate the importance of afferent proprioceptive information in maintaining joint integrity. They evaluated the amount of knee joint degeneration in three groups of dogs: afferent denervation but ligamentous intact, ACL deficient (ACL-D), and ACL-D with denervation. The investigators noted no arthritic change in the denervated group, some changes in the ACL-D group, and significant arthritis in the unstable and denervated group. They concluded that the dogs in the denervated group were able to adapt their movement strategies and minimize stress and damage, whereas dogs in the unstable group experienced joint damage, particularly with the loss of afferent input. They termed this process *neurogenic acceleration of osteoarthrosis* (O'Connor et al. 1992). Barrett, Cobb, and Bentley (1991) noted that reduced proprioception in older adults may be responsible for the initiation or advancement of knee degeneration.

Proprioceptive deficits can create dysfunction throughout the sensorimotor system. Wojtys and Huston (1994) suggested that a lack of proprioception delays the protective muscular responses of reflexive joint stabilization. SSEPs that indirectly measure proprioception have shown abnormal levels in patients with knee instability (Pitman et al. 1992) and shoulder instability (Tibone, Fechter, and Kao 2002) compared with individuals without instability.

Ultimately, proprioceptive deficits lead to both local and global dysfunction. Insufficient or improper afferent information affects CNS processing, which in turn affects motor output and joint function. Therefore, clinicians must consider the whole body in sensorimotor dysfunction rather than focus on localized symptoms. Both muscle activation and balance strategies can change with joint pathology, suggesting both local and global effects.

Local Effects

Patients with low back pain (Gill and Callaghan 1998; Parkhurst and Burnett 1994; Taimela, Kankaanpaa, and Luoto 1999) and chronic neck pain (Heikkila and Astrom 1996; Revel et al. 1994) exhibit decreased proprioception. Joint effusion commonly causes reflexive inhibition of local muscles at the knee (Morrissey 1989; Stokes and Young 1984) and ankle (Hopkins and Palmieri 2004), likely through spinal reflex pathways (Iles, Stokes, and Young 1990). The degree of muscle inhibition is related to the amount of joint damage (Hurley 1997). Muscle atrophy has also been found in the suboccipitals of patients with chronic neck pain (McPartland, Brodeur, and Hallgren 1997), in the multifidus of patients with chronic low back pain (Hides et al. 1994), and in the vastus medialis of patients with ACL injuries (Edstrom 1970). Because this atrophy persists after the acute pain and injury, selective atrophy of Type II muscle fibers probably results from instability rather than pain (Edstrom 1970). Joint damage decreases the excitability of the alpha motor neuron (Hurley 1997), even when pain is not present (Shakespeare et al. 1985), implying that afferent information may play a more important role than pain in inhibition.

Changes in local muscle firing patterns have been found in many chronic musculoskeletal pathologies, suggesting a sensorimotor dysfunction. For example, patients with shoulder impingement demonstrate delayed activation of the lower trapezius

(Cools et al. 2003), subscapularis (Hess et al. 2005), and serratus anterior (Wadsworth and Bullock-Saxton 1997). Chu and colleagues (2003) demonstrated unbalanced muscle activation after elongating the ACL. They found increases in quadriceps EMG but no change in hamstring activation. Voight and Weider (1991) found a reversal in the normal firing pattern of the extensor mechanism in patients with anterior knee pain. Compared with pain-free subjects, patients with anterior knee pain had a faster onset of the vastus lateralis and a delayed onset of the vastus medialis. Patients with functional ankle instability demonstrate arthrogenic inhibition and prolonged reaction times of the peroneals (Konradsen and Ravn 1990; McVey et al. 2005; Santilli et al. 2005). Similarly, patients with chronic low back pain exhibit poor postural control and altered muscle responses (Oddson et al. 1999; Newcomer et al. 2002; Radebold et al. 2000; Taimela et al. 1993; Wilder et al. 1996). Other researchers have demonstrated delayed activation of the trunk muscles (particularly the transversus abdominis) in patients with chronic low back pain (Hodges and Richardson 1998; Radebold et al. 2001) and groin pain (Cowan et al. 2004).

Global Effects

Global effects of joint pathology are being discovered now, suggesting the entire motor system compensates for a loss of local stabilization through altered movement patterns. Proximal hip weakness has been implicated in female patients with anterior knee pain (Ireland et al. 2003). Bullock-Saxton (1994) found both local and global changes in patients with unilateral ankle sprains, noting local decreases in vibratory sensation at the ankle and significant alterations in proximal hip muscle recruitment. Hip weakness is also associated with functional ankle instability (Friel et al. 2006). Global postural stability deficits have been associated with ankle instability (Bullock-Saxton 1995; Cornwall and Murrell 1991; Goldie, Evans, and Bach 1994; Lentell, Katzman, and Walters 1990; Perrin et al. 1997; Ryan 1994; Tropp and Odenrick 1988; Wikstrom et al. 2007), knee instability (Zatterstrom et al. 1994), knee osteoarthritis (Hassan, Mockett, and Doherty 2001; Wegener, Kisner, and Nichols 1997), chronic neck pain (Karlberg, Persson, and Magnusson 1995; McPartland, Brodeur, and Hallgren 1995; Sjostrom et al. 2003), and chronic low back pain (Alexander and Lapier 1998; Byl and Sinnott 1991; Luoto et al. 1998; Mientjes and Frank 1999; Radebold et al. 2001). McPartland, Brodeur, and Hallgren (1997) concluded that reduced proprioceptive input from atrophied muscles results in chronic pain and poor postural stability because of a lack of proprioceptive inhibition of nociceptors at the dorsal horn in the spinal cord.

Higher motor system functions compensate for functional instability. Edgerton and colleagues (1996) proposed that decreased muscle recruitment (such as inhibited muscle) can result in increased recruitment from compensating motor neuron pools, possibly leading to further injury. Patients with ACL deficiency (Alkjaer et al. 2002; Chmielewski, Hurd, and Snyder-Mackler 2005; Gauffin and Tropp 1992; McNair and Marshall 1994), chronic back pain (Byl and Sinnott 1991), or ankle instability (Beckman and Buchanan 1995; Bullock-Saxton et al. 1994; Brunt et al. 1992; Delahunt, Monaghan, and Caulfield 2006; Monaghan, Delahunt, and Caulfield 2006; Tropp and Odenrick 1988) exhibit altered muscle activation and movement patterns in areas remote from the primary pathology. Delahunt, Monaghan, and Caulfield (2006) reported that patients with functional ankle instability exhibit altered kinematics during gait that are most likely due to compensatory changes in the feed-forward control of the motor program.

Compensatory movements for pain or dysfunction eventually become ingrained in the motor cortex, essentially reprogramming normal movement patterns. Some individuals with chronic instability such as ACL deficiency compensate well for their physical and functional limitations globally through the sensorimotor system; such patients are known as *copers*. ACL-D copers exhibit different patterns of muscle activation than noncopers exhibit (Alkjaer et al. 2002; Alkjaer et al. 2003; Chmielewski, Hurd, and Snyder-Mackler 2005). Copers exhibit increased co-contraction of the hamstrings and quadriceps during functional activities, while noncopers exhibit a decreased knee extension moment to reduce anterior shear. Therefore, global compensatory copers change their muscle firing patterns, while local compensatory noncopers change their biomechanics around the joint.

An interesting finding in some chronic musculoskeletal pathology is bilateral dysfunction in unilateral injury (Bullock-Saxton, Janda, and Bullock 1994; Cools et al. 2003; Røe et al. 2000; Wadsworth and Bullock-Saxton 1997; Wojtys and Hutson 1994). Bullock-Saxton, Janda, and Bullock (1994) found that subjects with chronic ankle sprain exhibit altered muscle activation patterns on both the injured and the uninjured sides. This supports the view that chronic pain is mediated by the CNS and suggests that clinicians should remember to consider the areas beyond the pain when addressing chronic joint pain.

Further evidence of the whole-body influence of the sensorimotor system is seen in studies of the crossover training effect. Unilateral strength training has been shown to increase neural activity and strength in the contralateral extremity by 10% to 30%, suggesting a strong CNS influence on the muscular system (Evetovich et al. 2001; Housh and Housh 1993; Moore 1975; Moritani and deVries 1979; Pink 1981; Ray and Mark 1995; Uh et al. 2000). Also, eccentric training of agonist muscles has been shown to increase strength in antagonists by 16% to 31% (Singh and Karpovich 1967).

Summary

The sensorimotor system is a complex integration of afferent and efferent information. Specialized receptors provide proprioceptive information that is processed at multiple levels. Efferent output provides stabilization globally through postural stability or locally through functional joint stabilization. Proprioception undoubtedly plays a key role in functional stabilization. The role of the sensorimotor system in pathology is well established. Clinicians addressing chronic pathology should remember to evaluate and treat the entire system.

CHAIN REACTIONS

In patients with chronic musculoskeletal pain, the source of the pain is rarely the actual cause of the pain. In fact, Czech physician Karel Lewit noted, "He who treats the site of pain is often lost." Lewit's colleague Vladimir Janda conceptualized of musculoskeletal pathology as a chain reaction. He was a strong proponent of looking elsewhere for the source of pain syndromes, often finding symptoms distant from the site of the primary complaint.

Janda noted that due to the interactions of the skeletal system, muscular system, and CNS (described in chapter 1), dysfunction of any joint or muscle is reflected in the quality and function of others, not just locally but also globally. Janda recognized that muscle and fascia are common to several joint segments; therefore, movement and musculoskeletal pathology are never isolated. He often spoke of muscle slings, groups of functionally interrelated muscles. Because muscles must disperse load among joints and provide proximal stabilization for distal movements, no movement is truly isolated. For example, trunk muscle stabilizers are activated before movement of upper or lower limbs begins (Hodges and Richardson 1997a, 1997b); therefore, it might be possible that shoulder pathology is related to trunk stabilization or trunk pathology is related to shoulder movement.

The human body possesses the biomechanical characteristic of *tensegrity* defined as the inherent stability of structures based on synergy between tension and compression forces. This means that the structure of the body provides it with inherent stability as it rearranges itself in response to changes in load. Increased tension in one area is accompanied by a change in tension in another, allowing constant stability with changing structure. For example, the body can change from standing to squatting while maintaining stability of the lumbar spine by increasing tension around the trunk.

Janda also acknowledged the importance of the entire sensorimotor system as a neurological chain (as suggested in chapter 2), noting that pathology in the sensorimotor system is reflected by adaptive changes elsewhere in the system. Further, Janda recognized two distinct systems of muscles that are linked neurodevelopmentally, the phasic and tonic systems. This recognition eventually led to his muscle imbalance paradigm.

In general, chain reactions can be classified as articular, muscular, or neurological; however, remember that no system functions independently. The type of chain reaction that develops depends on the functional demands, and its success depends on the interaction of these three systems (table 3.1). Pathology within a primary chain may be linked to dysfunction in a secondary chain, or vice versa.

Table 3.1 Interactions of Three Systems for Chain Reactions

Primary chain	Secondary chains	Types of chains
Articular	Muscular Neurological	Postural Kinetic
Muscular	Articular Neurological	Synergists Muscle slings Myofascial chains
Neurological	Articular Muscular	Primitive reflexive chains Sensorimotor system Neurodevelopmental locomotor chains

This chapter reviews the three types of chains, beginning with articular chains. The articular chains maintain posture and movement throughout the skeletal system. Next, the chapter describes the muscular chains, which provide movement and stabilization through muscular synergists, slings, and fascial chains. Finally, it explains how neurological chains provide movement control through protective reflexes, neuro-developmental motor progression, and the sensorimotor system. Collectively, these three chains form a neuromusculoskeletal model of functional movement.

Articular Chains

Articular chains result from the biomechanical interactions of different joints through-out a movement pattern. There are two types of articular chains: postural and kinetic.

Postural Chains

Postural chains are the position of one joint in relation to another when the body is in an upright posture. Postural chains influence positioning and movement through structural and functional mechanisms. Structural mechanisms describe the influence of static skeletal positioning on adjacent structures, while functional mechanisms describe the dynamic influence that the position of keystone structures (the pelvis and scapulae) has on muscles attaching to those structures. Structural chains are influenced by static joint position, while functional chains are influenced by muscle activity around joint structures.

Structural Postural Chains

The positioning of skeletal structures directly influences adjacent structures. The most recognized postural chain occurs throughout the spine. The postural position of the cervical, thoracic, and lumbar spine is often assessed in patients with musculoskeletal pain. Proper positioning in these regions is also emphasized during exercise to promote normal and safe movement.

Because the regions of the spinal column are interconnected through the vertebral system, changes in one region may affect another region through a chain reaction. Poor posture is a chain reaction occurring throughout the spine, from the position of the pelvis to the position of the head. Alois Brügger, a Swiss neurologist, used a cogwheel mechanism to describe this postural chain reaction in the spine (figure 3.1; Brügger 2000); this description became known as *Brügger sitting posture*. Poor sitting posture

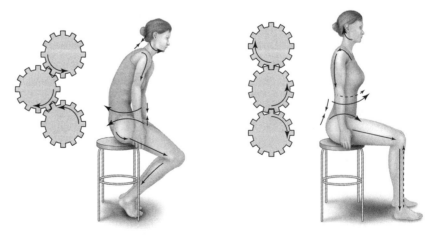

Figure 3.1 Cogwheel chain mechanism of poor posture.

Adapted from A. Brügger, 2000, *Lehrbuch der Funktionellen Störungen des Bewegungssystems* [Textbook of the functional disturbances of the movement system] (Brügger-Verlag GmbH, Zollikon & Benglen), 197.

encourages a posterior pelvic tilt (a counterclockwise cogwheel) that reduces the normal lordosis of the lumbar spine. This reverses the normal kyphosis of the thoracic spine through a counterclockwise cogwheel that then creates a counterclockwise cogwheel within the cervical spine. This final cogwheel influences the forward position of the head in typical poor posture.

Brügger used his cogwheel illustration as a teaching aid for patients. He encouraged them to assume proper posture by using the lower cogwheel to move the pelvis forward, which in turn moves the chest upward through the middle cogwheel and then stretches the neck to reposition the head through the uppermost cogwheel.

The rib cage is also an important skeletal structure to consider in the assessment of posture because of its direct influence on the position of the thoracolumbar spine. Patients with weakness of the diaphragm or deep spinal stabilizers often elevate the lower rib cage during inspiration as a compensation for breathing

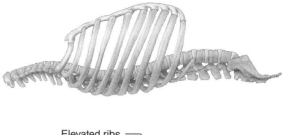
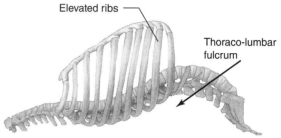

Elevated ribs

Thoraco-lumbar fulcrum

Figure 3.2 The influence of rib position on thoracolumbar position.

(see figure 3.2). This creates a localized hyperextension of the thoracolumbar junction that leads to segmental instability and subsequent dysfunction. The repetitive and continuous elevation of the ribs relative to the fixation point on the spinal vertebrae leads to posterior rotation of the ribs on the vertebrae at the costovertebral joint and to relative anterior rotation of the vertebrae on the ribs. Often this situation is complicated by loss of segmental thoracic spinal extension and hyperkyphosis.

The intercostal soft tissue and fascia can further limit rib cage mobility and promote the strategically necessary but pathological posture. Ideal posture is sacrificed in favor of maintaining respiratory integrity. As noted with Brügger's cogwheel concept of movement between spinal sections, the change of thoracic mobility and posture results in or can be caused by pathological postural compensations in the remaining sections. When correcting postural faults, mobility must be restored to the costovertebral joints and the intercostalis tissue and fascia so that the patient can integrate the ideal spinal and rib position into training a proper respiratory stereotype that serves both breathing and spinal stability.

Functional Postural Chains

The postural position of keystone structures contributes to pathology and dysfunction. Keystone structures include skeletal structures that serve as attachment points for groups of postural muscles, most notably the pelvis, ribs, and scapulae. These attachments may serve as either origins or insertions of muscle. Muscle tightness or weakness may be caused by or may be the cause of altered postural positioning. The position of these structures is considered a key in the assessment of posture and in the role these structures play in dysfunction (see chapter 5).

As stated previously, the pelvis can influence the position of the adjacent lumbosacral spine. It can also influence the length–tension relationship of muscles originating from the pelvis, such as the hip flexors and hamstrings. Anterior positioning of the pelvis is associated with tightness of the hip flexors, while posterior positioning of the pelvis is associated with tightness of the hamstrings (see figure 3.3).

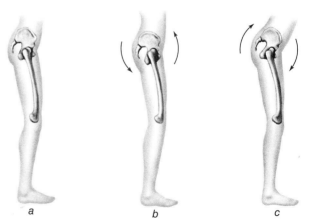

a   *b*   *c*

Figure 3.3 The influence of pelvic tilt on muscle length and tension. *(a)* Neutral position. *(b)* Posterior tilt, which results in tight hamstrings. *(c)* Anterior tilt, which results in tight hip flexors.

Reprinted from R.S. Behnke, 2006, *Kinetic Anatomy*, 2nd ed. (Champaign: Human Kinetics), 140.

Seventeen muscles either originate or insert on the scapula, influencing the position and movement of the shoulder girdle as well as the spine. For example, tightness of the upper trapezius from the cervical region influences shoulder joint movement by positioning the scapula upward and downwardly rotated. These functional postural chains can also influence movement patterns globally throughout the body via kinetic chains.

Kinetic Chains

Kinetic chains are most commonly recognized as the concepts of open kinetic chain and closed kinetic chain activities, in which focus is on movement of the joints. These kinetic chains are easily identified through biomechanical assessments such as gait assessment. The chain reaction of the lower extremity during gait is well known by its obligatory and sometimes compensatory movements. For example, foot pronation causes tibial internal rotation, which causes knee valgus and hip internal rotation. During gait, the neuromuscular system must control these linked kinetic motions. Often, pathology is related to a dysfunction in compensation in the kinetic chain: Through the kinetic chain, foot pronation may cause faulty lumbar positioning, requiring additional trunk stabilization. Therefore, clinicians must look away from the site of pain for possible biomechanical contributions.

For example, orthopedic surgeon Ben Kibler (1998a) used kinetic chains to describe both function and pathology of the shoulder. He noted that in the overhead throwing motion, force is summated throughout the kinetic chain via force production at various joints from the lower body to the hand (see figure 3.4). Kibler recognized that any change in timing or force generation may result in poor performance or pathology at another level within the chain. This demonstrates the principle that the kinetic chain is only as strong as its weakest link.

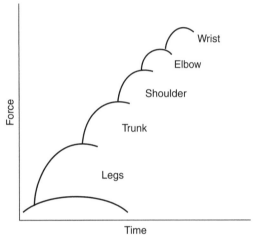

Figure 3.4 Kinetic chain dysfunction in overhead throwing.

Adapted from W.B. Kibler, 1998, Determining the extent of the functional deficit. In *Functional rehabilitation of sports and musculoskeletal injuries*, edited by W.B. Kibler et al. (Gaithersburg, MD: Aspen Publishers), 16-19.

Muscular Chains

Muscular chains are groups of muscles that work together or influence each other through movement patterns. There are three subtypes of muscular chains: synergists, muscle slings, and myofascial chains. Each type of muscular chain interdepends on both the articular and the neurological systems.

Synergists

A synergistic muscle works with another muscle (agonist) to produce movement or stabilization around a joint. Synergists may include secondary movers, stabilizers, or neutralizers. For example, during shoulder rotation, the rotator cuff is active. However, the rhomboids, serratus anterior, and trapezius must work as stabilizers of the scapula to ensure a stable origin for the rotator cuff. Therefore, pseudoweakness of the rotator cuff may be caused by poor stabilization of the scapula; if the scapula is stabilized manually, the patient demonstrates normal strength of the rotator cuff.

Synergists work together for isolated joint motion. Synergistic muscular chains are also recognized in force coupling. Force couples are two equal and opposite muscle forces that produce pure rotation around a center of motion. For example, the rotator cuff and deltoid provide a force couple for shoulder abduction. Clinicians must evaluate force coupling within a muscular chain for movement dysfunction.

Muscle Slings

In contrast to synergists that work together locally for isolated joint motion, muscle slings are global, providing movement and stabilization across multiple joints. Muscle slings (also referred to as *muscle loops*) have been recognized in European anatomy and medicine since the 1930s. Benninghof (1994), Tittel (2000), Brügger (2000), and Myers (2001) described how chains of muscles that are linked together, often in loops, influence the quality of the entire movement. Muscle slings are thought to facilitate rotation and to transfer forces through the trunk, particularly from the lower body to the upper body (Vleeming et al. 1995). Muscle slings also provide stabilization and movement in reciprocal and contralateral movements such locomotion. Typically, muscle slings are interconnected, as one muscle insertion is connected to the next muscle's origin via a common keystone structure (see table 3.2). These keystone structures act as fixation points from which the entire chain of muscles can stabilize. Myers (2001) referred to these muscular chains as *anatomy trains* and based his patterns on *fascial* connections throughout the body. Europeans, however, recognized the *functional* connections of muscles in their description of muscle slings and chains. Janda recognized both fascial and functional factors in muscular chains.

Several major muscle slings have been identified. Muscles within these slings work together to produce functional movement rather than isolated muscle contraction; therefore, we cannot think of muscle strength solely in terms of origin and insertion. Interestingly, Bergmark's classification (Bergmark 1989) generally considers the muscles involved in these slings to be global muscles due to their origins on the pelvis and thoracic cage.

Table 3.2 Muscle Slings and Their Anatomical Keystones

Muscle sling	Keystone
Rhomboid, serratus anterior	Scapula
Rhomboid, triceps	Scapula
Trapezius, biceps	Scapula
Biceps, pectoralis minor	Scapula
Biceps, pectoralis major	Humerus
Latissimus dorsi, triceps	Humerus
Serratus anterior, external oblique	Ribs
Pectoralis major, internal oblique	Ribs
Internal oblique, external oblique	Linea alba
Internal oblique, gluteus medius	Pelvis
Internal oblique, sartorius	Pelvis
External oblique, adductors	Pelvis
Hamstrings, gluteus maximus	Pelvis
Gluteus maximus, contralateral latissimus dorsi	Pelvis, thoracolumbar fascia
Gluteus maximus, quadriceps	Femur
Hamstrings, hip flexors	Femur
Hamstrings, tibialis anterior	Tibia
Quadriceps, plantar flexors	Tibia

Extremity Flexor and Extensor Slings

Extremity slings are designed for simultaneous compound movements of the limbs. In the lower extremity, the extensor sling consists of the gluteus maximus, rectus femoris, and gastrocnemius for hip extension, knee extension, and ankle plantar flexion, respectively (see figure 3.5). The iliopsoas, hamstrings, and tibialis anterior combine for hip flexion, knee flexion, and ankle dorsiflexion, respectively. During gait, for example, the swing phase activates the flexor chain with simultaneous hip flexion, knee flexion, and ankle dorsiflexion. During stance, the extensor chain propels the lower extremity with hip extension, knee extension, and plantar flexion. Throughout the gait cycle, these two chains alternate between facilitation and inhibition and reciprocate between the left and right limbs—in other words, the flexor chain is activated in the swinging leg while the extensor chain is activated in the stance leg. When both slings are activated simultaneously, the lower extremity is stabilized.

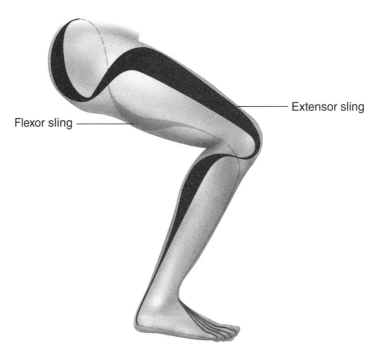

Figure 3.5 Flexor and extensor muscle slings in the lower extremity.

Based on T. Myers, 2001, *Anatomy trains* (Edinburgh, Scotland: Churchill Livingstone).

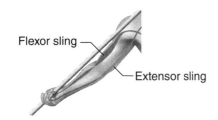

Figure 3.6 Flexor and extensor muscle slings in the upper extremity.

Based on T. Myers, 2001, *Anatomy trains* (Edinburgh, Scotland: Churchill Livingstone).

The upper-extremity flexor sling includes the pectoralis major, anterior deltoid, trapezius, biceps, and hand flexors, while the upper-extremity extensor sling consists of the rhomboids, posterior deltoid, triceps, and hand extensors (see figure 3.6). These extremity slings are activated along with the lower-extremity slings for reciprocal gait. During the swing phase, activation of the right upper-extremity flexor sling is coupled with activation of the left lower-extremity flexor sling, and vice versa. The functionality of these upper- and lower-extremity slings is well demonstrated in reciprocal gait.

Trunk Muscle Slings

Muscle slings in the trunk are necessary for facilitating reciprocal gait patterns between the upper and lower extremity as well as for rotational trunk stabilization. Three slings have been identified: the anterior, spiral, and posterior slings. The biceps, pectoralis major, internal oblique, contralateral hip abductors, and sartorius comprise the anterior sling (see figure 3.7). Wrapping from the posterior to the anterior, the rhomboids, serratus anterior, external oblique, contralateral internal oblique, and contralateral hip adductors create a spiral sling (see figure 3.8).

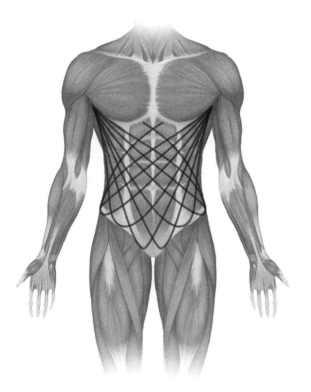 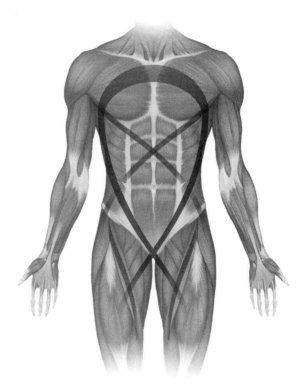

Figure 3.7   Anterior trunk muscle sling.

Adapted, by permission, from NSCA, 2008, Biomechanics of resistance exercise, by E. Harman. In *Essentials of strength training and conditioning*, 3rd ed., edited by T.R. Baechle and R.W. Earle (Champaign, IL: Human Kinetics), 68.

Figure 3.8   Spiral trunk muscle sling.

Adapted, by permission, from NSCA, 2008, Biomechanics of resistance exercise, by E. Harman. In *Essentials of strength training and conditioning*, 3rd ed., edited by T.R. Baechle and R.W. Earle (Champaign, IL: Human Kinetics), 68.

The hamstrings, gluteus maximus, thoracolumbar fascia, contralateral latissimus dorsi, and triceps create a posterior sling for extension during reciprocal gait, for trunk stabilization, and for force transmission from the lower to upper body (see figure 3.9). Vleeming and colleagues (1995) suggested that this posterior dynamic stabilizing muscular chain provides a stabilizing force for the ipsilateral SI joint. They noted that the ipsilateral gluteus maximus and the contralateral latissimus dorsi are connected functionally via the thoracolumbar fascia. Further, the gluteus maximus and latissimus dorsi are coactivated contralaterally during gait and trunk rotation (Mooney et al. 2001) as well as during running (Montgomery, Pink, and Perry 1994).

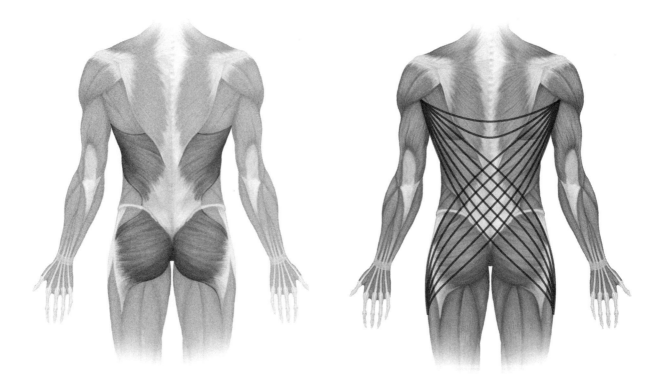

Figure 3.9   The figure on the left illustrates the superficial anatomy of the latissimus dorsi, gluteus maximus, and thoracolumbar fascia, while the figure on the right depicts the interconnectivity of these muscles through the thoracolumbar fascia (solid line), and the influence of the posterior chain on the upper and lower extremities.

Adapted, by permission, from NSCA, 2008, Biomechanics of resistance exercise, by E. Harman. In *Essentials of strength training and conditioning*, 3rd ed., edited by T.R. Baechle and R.W. Earle (Champaign, IL: Human Kinetics), 68.

The posterior chain can be a key indicator of dysfunction in the gluteus maximus and SI joint. Janda first noticed this in 1964 (Janda 1964), when he found that patients with an inhibited gluteus maximus (often due to SI dysfunction) activate the contralateral latissimus dorsi during active hip extension, thus demonstrating the compensation of this posterior chain.

The posterior chain was extended further through the discovery of the connection of the hamstrings to the ipsilateral gluteus maximus and erector spinae via the sacrotuberous ligament (figure 3.10). This finding supports the interconnectivity of the legs and the trunk through the posterior chain via the lumbar spine (Gracovetsky 1997). This chain can continue ipsilaterally or contralaterally (figure 3.11) from the sacrotuberous ligament. During gait, the body often compensates for weakness of the gluteus maximus with a reverse action of the erector spinae to extend the hip; this compensatory chain reaction is facilitated by the sacrotuberous ligament link. Hungerford, Gilleard, and Hodges (2003) found that patients with SI joint pain exhibit early activation of the biceps femoris and delayed activation of the gluteus maximus during single-leg stance; this finding suggests the biceps femoris helps stabilize the SI joint through the sacrotuberous ligament.

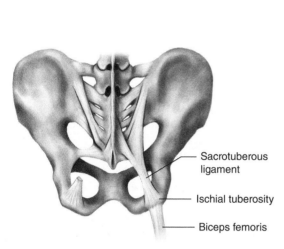

Figure 3.10 The role of the sacrotuberous ligament in the posterior chain.

Adapted from R.S. Behnke, *Kinetic Anatomy*, 2nd ed. (Champaign, IL: Human Kinetics), 174.

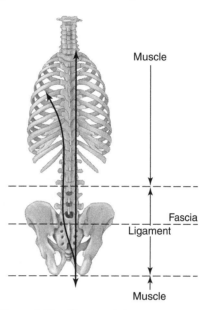

Figure 3.11 The sacrotuberous ligament facilitates either an ipsilateral or a contralateral posterior muscle sling.

Adapted from S. Gracovetsky, 1997. Linking the spinal engine with the legs: a theory of human gait. In *Movement, stability, and low back pain*, edited by V.A. Mooney et al. (Edinburgh: Churchill Livingstone), 243.

Brügger described a long, diagonal muscle loop used for maintenance of posture (Brügger 2000). He thought that normal posture requires coordination of the muscles within this functional grouping and that any muscle within the group may be involved in maintaining poor posture. Brügger's diagonal loop includes muscles that lift the chest, externally rotate the shoulder, retract the scapula, support the abdomen, anteriorly tilt the pelvis, and functionally support the leg. These muscles are the pectoralis major, infraspinatus, lower trapezius, sternocleidomastoid (SCM), scalene, TrA, diaphragm, sartorius, tensor fascia lata (TFL), peroneals, tibialis anterior, and posterior tibialis.

Often neuromuscular pathology is found within the same sling. By understanding the function and paths of these slings, clinicians may become better at diagnosing challenging musculoskeletal pain syndromes. For example, right shoulder pain may be related to left hip dysfunction and vice versa. These dysfunctions may present clinically as pain, muscle imbalances, or trigger points (TrPs) within the sling.

Patients with chronic musculoskeletal pain nearly always exhibit TrPs or tender points. These are areas that are painful to palpation and that often represent focal areas of hyperirritability in the muscle fibers. Lewit (2007) described a nociceptive chain related to postural balance. This nociceptive chain is seen clinically through tender points or TrPs. While this chain often occurs on only one side of the body, it may cross the body into the contralateral side. Common areas for this crossover include the SI joint and the spinal joints L5-S1, T12-L1, T4-T5, and C7-T1. These areas coincide with transitional zones within the spine.

Hong and Simons (1992) described how specific key TrPs facilitate satellite triggers along a chain. Often it is difficult to differentiate TrPs from tender points. In general, TrPs exhibit characteristic patterns of referred pain upon palpation, while tender points typically do not refer pain. For the purpose of evaluating chronic musculoskeletal pain, the clinician should determine if a chain of TrPs or tender points is present. This chain can then be used as an indicator of treatment effectiveness. If the chain improves after treatment, it is involved in maintaining pain. For more information on assessing TrPs and tender points, see chapter 8.

Myofascial Chains

Fascia is critical to integrated joint motion. It can exert tensile force via its attachments between muscle and bone, or it can produce an outward force via muscles contracting within fascial envelopes. It often forms aponeurotic attachments for muscles, particularly in the thoracolumbar fascia and abdominal fascia of the trunk. Fascia serves as a vital link to multiple muscles acting together for movement as well as connects the extremities through the trunk. For example, the thoracolumbar fascia links the lower extremity (gluteus maximus) and the contralateral upper extremity (latissimus dorsi; Vleeming et al. 1995), transferring load across the midline to control limb extension and trunk rotation (Snijders, Vleeming, and Stoeckart 1993). These fascial layers help connect muscle throughout the region, creating myofascial chains.

Abdominal Fascia

The abdominal fascia attaches to the external oblique, internal oblique, TrA, pectoralis major, and serratus anterior. It contains the links that form the diagonal muscle sling among the external oblique, pectoralis major, and serratus anterior.

Thoracolumbar Fascia

The thoracolumbar fascia attaches to the external oblique, internal oblique, TrA, latissimus dorsi, and gluteus maximus. It consists of three distinct layers: the anterior, middle, and posterior layers. The anterior fibers envelop the psoas and quadratus lumborum. The middle layer is continuous with the TrA and attaches to the obliques and latissimus dorsi. The posterior layer is probably the most important layer. It is designed to transmit forces among the shoulder girdle, lumbar spine, pelvis, and lower extremity (Vleeming et al. 1995; Barker and Briggs 1999). Interestingly, the posterior layer also attaches to the lower border of the rhomboid major and splenius cervicis to link the lumbar region and upper quarter (Barker and Briggs 1999).

The thoracolumbar fascia may play an important role in proprioception. Yahia and colleagues (1992) found that the thoracolumbar fascia contains mechanoreceptors; this finding suggests that it may contribute to sensorimotor control of the lumbar spine. These mechanoreceptors likely send information on tension to modify muscle activation.

Fascia has been viewed clinically as a potential source of dysfunction. The thoracolumbar fascia exhibits microscopic pathological changes in patients with chronic low back pain (Bednar et al. 1995). Because several muscles are connected through the same fascia, myofascial chains may contain restrictions and dysfunction in one area that influence a remote area. Because of its lack of extensibility and its intimate relationship with the muscular system, fascia may limit free movement of joints, facilitating further dysfunction (Lewit 2007). Clinicians should always consider the influence of fascia when evaluating chain reactions.

Neurological Chains

Obviously, the body is well linked neurologically through the PNS and CNS. These neurological chains are seen in protective reflexive movements, the sensorimotor system, and neurodevelopmental movement patterns.

Protective Reflexives

Arguably, the most important neuromuscular chains in the human body provide critical reflexes for function and protection. Two fundamental protective reflexes are the crossed extensor and withdrawal reflexes. These reflexes are triggered by sensory receptors. In the withdrawal reflex, a noxious stimulus such as excessive heat causes a limb to pull away from the stimulus; this reflex activates the flexors and inhibits the extensors on that side. In the crossed extensor reflex, a cutaneous noxious stimulus facilitates the flexors on the same side while facilitating the extensors on the contralateral side, causing the contralateral limb to extend and provide support.

Janda described four additional reflex chains (Janda 1986b) that are critical for the basic life skills of gait, prehension, eating, and breathing:

1. **Locomotion.** In the lower extremity, the combination of extension, adduction, and rotation provide the basis for gait patterns used to escape danger.
2. **Prehension.** In the upper extremity, flexion, adduction, and internal rotation are combined to bring food to the mouth.
3. **Mastication.** Adduction of the jaw (closing the mouth) is necessary to chew food.
4. **Breathing.** The breathing mechanism is highly automatized and is not easily influenced voluntarily for long durations.

These primitive reflexes serve as the basis for all human movement patterns. Under extreme or pathological conditions (stress, fatigue, or structural lesions), these reflexes tend to dominate (Janda 1986b).

Sensorimotor Chains

The sensorimotor system is linked neurologically through the afferent and efferent systems described in chapter 2. In controlling movement, feedback and feed-forward mechanisms provide a chain reaction of neuromuscular events. This provides both local and global dynamic stabilization of joints through muscular chains. These sensorimotor chains are affected by afferent input, controlled by the CNS, and realized through efferent motor output. Essentially, groups of muscles are linked together neurologically for function. Sensorimotor chains include reflexive stabilization chains and adaptation chains.

Reflexive Stabilization

Reflexive stabilization is an example of a functional neurological chain reaction. As discussed in chapter 2, reflexive stabilization occurs subconsciously through the sensorimotor system. Muscles contract to provide stabilization either locally or globally. In studying global stabilization, Horak and Nashner (1986) demonstrated chain reactions of muscle activation traveling from distal to proximal in response to perturbations; these reactions are the APRs (see chapter 2). These responses are characteristic of the direction of the shift, as demonstrated by a chain reaction of muscle activation on the opposite side: An anterior weight shift activates posterior dorsal muscles, while a posterior shift activates anterior ventral muscles. Davey and colleagues (2002) found that the contralateral erector spinae are activated during ipsilateral shoulder abduction, regardless of the influence of gravity. This observation suggests sensorimotor influence for spinal muscle stabilization during extremity movement.

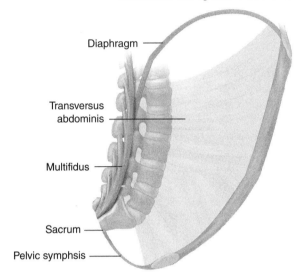

Diaphragm

Transversus abdominis

Multifidus

Sacrum

Pelvic symphsis

Figure 3.12 The pelvic chain.

The most important stabilizing sensorimotor chain is the pelvic chain, consisting of the TrA, multifidus, diaphragm, and pelvic floor (figure 3.12; Lewit 2007). These four muscles are coactivated for trunk stability and force transmission. The pelvic chain is the cornerstone of stability for the rest of the body; each muscle is linked intimately through the sensorimotor system. Because of this link, the pelvic region often shows the earliest signs of dysfunction occurring elsewhere in the sensorimotor chain. Pelvic weakness has been associated with both proximal and distal pathologies such as low back pain (Nadler, Malanga, and DePrince et al. 2000, 2002; Nadler, Malanga, and Bartoli 2002), groin strains (Tyler et al. 2001), IT band syndrome (Fredericson 2000), anterior knee pain (Cichanowski et al. 2007), ACL tears (Ireland et al. 2003), and ankle sprains (Bullock-Saxton 1994).

When initiating arm or leg movements, the body reflexively activates the TrA in a feed-forward mechanism that is independent of the speed and direction of the limb movements (Hodges and Richardson 1997a, 1997b). Howev85er, in patients with low back pain, the TrA is delayed, suggesting a sensorimotor dysfunction (Hodges and Richardson 1996, 1998). Janda was one of the first to note weakness of the TrA in patients with chronic low back pain (Janda 1987). Similarly, the TrA is delayed in subjects with groin pain (Cowan et al. 2004).

The pelvic floor and abdominal muscles each contract in response to the other, suggesting a pattern of coactivation (Sapsford et al. 2001). Researchers have shown that the diaphragm and TrA are activated with arm movement both in sitting and in standing (Hodges and Gandevia 2000a, 2000b). This finding suggests the diaphragm has both respiratory and postural function. Expiration activates all abdominal muscles (Hodges, Gandevia, and Richardson 1997), demonstrating a functional relationship between respiration and sensorimotor function that has implications for chronic low back pain.

The sensorimotor chain depends on proprioception; joint dysfunction often disrupts the dynamic stabilization of sensorimotor chains. For example, in evaluating the sensorimotor function of the cervical spine in patients with chronic whiplash disorders, researchers found delayed activation of the deep neck flexors with upper-extremity tasks (Falla 2004; Falla, Jull, and Hodges 2004). Poor proprioception resulting from injury to neck proprioceptors is thought to contribute to this sensorimotor dysfunction.

Similar pathologies are noted in the shoulder and result from joint pathology; these include delayed activation of the middle and lower trapezius in subjects with shoulder impingement (Cools et al. 2003) as well as delayed activation of the serratus anterior in swimmers with impingement (Wadsworth and Bullock-Saxton 1997). Patients with functional ankle instability change their postural stabilization by using a hip strategy, while subjects without instability favor an ankle strategy (Tropp and Odenrick 1988).

Sensorimotor Adaptation Chains

Janda described chain reactions to dysfunction within the sensorimotor system (Janda 1984). He noted that any change in the sensorimotor system due to pain or pathology is reflected by compensations throughout the system that lead to systemic and predictable patterns. Many signs and symptoms of impaired function of the musculoskeletal system may have a hidden cause in an unrecognized dysfunction located elsewhere (Janda 1993). Understanding these adaptation chains helps clinicians comprehend and predict the development of functional impairments and thus provide appropriate evaluation and treatment. Janda identified two chains of adaptation (or generalization) in the sensorimotor system: horizontal (anatomic) adaptation and vertical (neurological) activation.

1. **Horizontal adaptation.** Horizontal adaptation occurs when impaired function in one joint or muscle creates reaction and adaptation in other joint segments. It is most commonly seen in the spine; for example, low back pain often leads to cervical syndromes. Horal (1969) reported that 50% of subjects with low back pain develop cervical symptoms an average of 6 y after the first onset of low back pain. Muscle imbalances conform to horizontal adaptation, creating predictable patterns (see chapter 4). Horizontal adaptation can be proximal to distal or distal to proximal; it has been described most often as distal to proximal in the case of ankle sprains. Several researchers have found weakness and changes in muscle activation in the hip in subjects with ankle instability (Bullock-Saxton et al. 1994; Beckman and Buchanan 1995; Nicholas, Strizak, and Veras 1976) and anterior knee pain (Robinson and Nee 2007). This finding points to the importance of assessing beyond the site of injury through sensorimotor chains.

2. **Vertical adaptation.** Vertical adaptation occurs between the PNS and the CNS: Adaptation of one part of the sensorimotor system impairs the function of the entire motor system. This adaptation may progress from the PNS to the CNS or from the CNS to the PNS. Vertical adaptation is seen as a change in the motor programming that is then reflected in abnormal movement patterns. Vertical adaptation has been demonstrated in several musculoskeletal conditions, most notably by changes in global movement patterns or postural control. For example, Delahunt, Monaghan, and Caulfield (2006) reported that patients with functional ankle instability exhibit altered kinematics during gait that are most likely due to compensatory changes in the feed-forward control of the motor program.

Neurodevelopmental Locomotor Patterns

There are two groups of muscles regulated throughout the body by the CNS: the tonic muscle system and the phasic muscle system. They are separated phylogenetically by their neurodevelopmental progression. Tonic system muscles are older phylogenetically and are dominant. They are involved in repetitive or rhythmic activities and in the withdrawal reflex in the upper and lower extremities. Their function is predominantly that of flexion. Phasic system muscles, on the other hand, are more predominant in extension movements. The phasic muscles are younger phylogenetically and typically work against gravity, acting as postural stabilizers.

Infants are born with several innate reflexes that serve as the basis for motor programs. The tonic and phasic systems are involved in several stereotypical movements and are influenced by body position and its relation to gravity. These include the tonic labyrinthine reflex, symmetrical tonic neck reflex (STNR), and asymmetrical tonic neck reflex (ATNR). These reflexes become integrated in normal human development but remain or reemerge in upper motor neuron pathologies such as cerebral palsy and stroke.

The study of movement in infants as they mature is known as *developmental kinesiology*. Neurodevelopmentally, the tonic and phasic systems progress as the infant motor system develops. Fetal posture is maintained by the tonic (flexor) muscle system, which creates reciprocal inhibition against activation of phasic extensors. At approximately 1 mo of age, the phasic and tonic systems of the neck coactivate, allowing the baby to raise the head for visual orientation, with the phasic system acting against the tonic system. By 4 mo, the sagittal plane motor program is in place, allowing the baby in the supine position to flex both the hips and knees with a stable pelvic chain. At 5 to 7 mo, trunk rotation is evident as the oblique muscular chains are activated. Finally, the tonic and phasic chains within the extremities progress until upright posture is functional at approximately 3 y.

Janda identified other characteristics in these two groups of muscle. Though there is a relationship between the neurological innervations of a motor unit and the physiological fiber type, Janda was very careful to mention that there is no strong correlation between the physiological muscle fiber type (Type I slow-twitch and Type II fast-twitch fibers) and the tonic–phasic classification system of muscles. This is often an area of confusion: Physiologically, tonic and phasic muscles refer to the predominant metabolic fiber type; while neurologically, tonic and phasic muscles refer to their classification in neurodevelopmental movement patterns. Therefore, neurodevelopmental descriptions of muscle refer to the tonic and phasic systems of muscles as opposed to the tonic and phasic characteristics of individual muscle fiber types. Note that the tonic–phasic classification system is not rigid because of each person's variability in neurological control.

The tonic and phasic muscle systems do not function individually; rather, they work together through coactivation for posture, gait, and coordinated movement. This is what is meant by the concept of muscle balance: an interaction of the tonic and phasic systems for optimal posture and movement. This interaction provides centration of joints during movement, creating a balance of muscular forces to maintain joint congruency through movement. Several European clinicians such as Vojta and Peters (1997), Kolář (2001), and Brügger (2000) have noted the importance of recognizing this coactivation and balance in movement and posture.

The tonic and phasic systems are coactivated in specific chains of movement. Each chain is made up of a series of synergistic movements that are combined into coordinated movement patterns. These chains of movement reflect primitive reflexes and movement patterns and serve as the default motor program on which humans base more complicated movements. Upper-quarter (cervical and upper-extremity) tonic–phasic coactivation patterns are used for prehension, grasping, and reaching, while lower-quarter (lumbar and lower-extremity) patterns are used for creeping, crawling, and gait. The upper quarter and the lower quarter demonstrate similar but distinctive patterns of movement in the tonic and phasic systems (see table 3.3).

Table 3.3 Tonic and Phasic Chains of the Upper and Lower Quarter

Coactivation chains	Upper quarter	Lower quarter
Functional movements	Prehension, grasping, reaching	Creeping, crawling, gait
Tonic chain	Flexion Internal rotation Adduction Pronation	Plantar flexion Inversion Flexion Internal rotation Adduction
Phasic chain	Extension External rotation Abduction Supination	Dorsiflexion Eversion Extension External rotation Abduction

The proper balance of these two systems is demonstrated in normal gait and posture. The integration of the tonic and phasic systems between the upper and lower body is responsible for reciprocal locomotion. Specifically, the coactivation of the contralateral upper- and lower-quarter systems throughout the body produces the characteristic patterns of reciprocal arm and leg movements. For example, during the swing phase (leg flexion, a tonic movement pattern) of the left lower extremity, the right upper extremity performs a tonic movement pattern (arm flexion). During the stance phase (leg extension), the opposite arm is also extended, reciprocally coactivating the phasic system throughout the body (figure 3.13). This coordination of the limbs remains consistent during various locomotor activities such as walking, creeping, and swimming (Wannier et al. 2001). There is a direct neurological link between the upper extremity and the lower extremity. In their review, Ferris, Huang, and Kao (2006) noted that recent studies indicate that upper-limb activation has an excitatory effect on lower-limb activation during locomotor tasks.

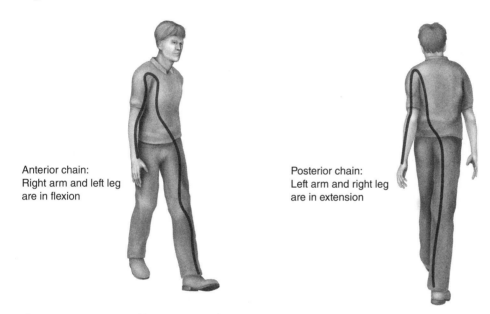

Anterior chain:
Right arm and left leg
are in flexion

Posterior chain:
Left arm and right leg
are in extension

Figure 3.13   Reciprocal locomotion and coactivation patterns.

Imbalance in one system can lead to postural compensation and adaptive changes in the opposing system, leading to muscle imbalance. These innate chains of movement allow clinicians to predict patterns of muscle imbalance and provide more effective assessment and treatment of musculoskeletal pain. It is not a coincidence that the muscles involved in these tonic and phasic chains respond characteristically in muscle imbalance syndromes. For example, the muscles that accomplish upper-quarter tonic movements (pectoralis major, subscapularis, forearm flexors, and pronators) are more prone to tightness, while the muscles involved in upper-quarter phasic movements (deltoid, posterior rotator cuff, forearm extensors, and supinators) are more prone to weakness. These are the observations Janda used to create his original classification of muscle imbalance (see chapter 4).

The ultimate function of a muscle relates directly to its functional demands at a specific moment; therefore, muscles can act both as flexors and as extensors. The neurological control of a muscle is the key factor in determining whether a muscle is a mover, stabilizer, or neutralizer at any point in time. What does not change is the predisposition of a muscle to function as a flexor or an extensor based on its phylogenetic classification and baseline neurological function.

Summary

Understanding chain reactions helps clinicians quickly identify and predict functional pathology. The concept of chain reactions emphasizes the clinical principle of looking beyond the site of pain and focusing on the cause of pain rather than the source of pain. There are three interdependent chains—the articular, muscular, and neurological chains—that should be considered in chronic neuromusculoskeletal pain. Adaptations within any chain in the body can be helpful or harmful; the clinician must decide if these adaptations are pathological or functional.

PATHOMECHANICS OF MUSCULOSKELETAL PAIN AND MUSCLE IMBALANCE

Janda believed that pain is the only way the musculoskeletal system can protect itself. As stated in previous chapters, functional pathology of the sensorimotor system points to the importance of examining dysfunction rather than structural lesions. Chronic musculoskeletal pain often arises from a functional pathology with resultant structural inflammation. Janda noted that structural lesions rarely cause pain themselves; rather, the inflammatory processes surrounding structural damage cause pain. Often, the site of pain is not the cause of the pain; unfortunately, some clinicians focus on the area of chronic pain (structure) rather than the cause of pain (function). An understanding of functional pathology forces clinicians to reevaluate their approach to the management of chronic musculoskeletal pain.

This chapter begins by reviewing the pathology of musculoskeletal pain. Next, the pathomechanics of muscle imbalance are presented with a discussion on tonic and phasic muscle systems and faulty movement patterns. The chapter then describes possible causes of muscle tightness and weakness and concludes with Janda's classification of muscle imbalance syndromes.

Pathology of Musculoskeletal Pain

Patients with chronic musculoskeletal pain continue to experience pain after a period of time that a peripheral pathology would normally resolve. This persistent pain suggests a persistent peripheral input. These patients also exhibit altered pain processing in the CNS. Evidence for the central influence of pain on the CNS is seen in the phenomenon of pain centralization, which often occurs in chronic pain patients. Pain stimuli can alter sensitivity to the central perception of pain and can alter the afferent signal at multiple levels. Curatolo and colleagues (2001) demonstrated centralized hypersensitivity to pain in patients with chronic neck pain resulting from whiplash. They found lowered pain thresholds in healthy regions throughout the body, regardless of the type of nociceptive input.

A simple algometer can be used to quantify a patient's response to painful pressure by measuring the pressure pain detection threshold (PPDT); a lower threshold means greater sensitivity to painful pressure. Changes in the PPDT both at the site of pain and elsewhere in the body indicate altered pain processing in the CNS. Patients with chronic musculoskeletal pain in fibromyalgia (FM; Gracely et al. 2002) and low back pain (Giesecke et al. 2004; Giesbrecht and Battié 2005) exhibit altered pain processing throughout the body.

Further evidence of CNS influence of chronic musculoskeletal pain comes from the finding that muscle dysfunction often occurs in both the symptomatic side and the contralateral side (Bullock-Saxton, Janda, and Bullock 1994; Cools et al. 2003; Røe et al.

2000; Wadsworth and Bullock Saxton 1997; Wojtys and Huston 1994). This finding has been confirmed by experimental pain studies demonstrating CNS mediation of chronic pain (Ervilha et al. 2005; Falla, Farina, and Graven-Nielsen 2007; Graven-Nielsen, Svensson, and Arendt-Nielsen 1997). Thus clinicians should evaluate and treat chronic muscle imbalance and chronic musculoskeletal pain as a global sensorimotor dysfunction.

Janda believed that muscles, as opposed to bones, joints, and ligaments, are most often the cause of chronic pain. Direct causes of muscle pain include muscle and connective tissue damage, muscle spasm and ischemia, and tender points or TrPs. Janda stated that most pain is associated with muscle spasm but is not the result of the spasm itself; rather, the pain is caused by ischemia from the prolonged muscle contraction. Prolonged muscle spasm leads to fatigue, which ultimately decreases the force available to meet postural and movement demands.

Indirect causes of muscle pain include altered joint forces due to muscle imbalance influencing movement patterns. Joint dysfunction without spasm usually is painless. For example, Janda (1986b) showed that subjects with SI joint distortion (faulty alignment) but no pain demonstrated significantly greater inhibition of the gluteus maximus and gluteus medius during hip extension and abduction when compared with subjects without faulty alignment.

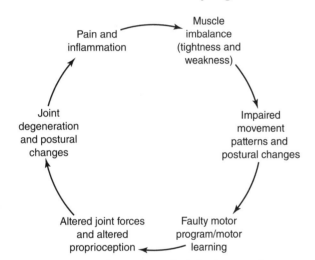

Figure 4.1 The chronic musculoskeletal pain cycle presented from a neurological perspective.

Muscle imbalance can develop after both acute pain and chronic pain. Acute pain leads to a localized muscle response that changes the movement pattern to protect or compensate for an injured area (Lund et al. 1991). Over time, this altered movement pattern becomes centralized in the CNS. While the theory of a vicious cycle of pain and spasm is indeed questionable (Lund et al. 1991), a vicious cycle of chronic pain involving the CNS and PNS seems plausible. These muscle imbalances often initiate the cycle shown in figure 4.1. Components of the cycle include the following:

• **Muscle imbalance.** Chronic pain is associated with a protective adaptive response in muscle in which agonists decrease in tone while antagonists increase in tone (Graven-Nielsen, Svensson, and Arendt-Nielsen 1997; Lund et al. 1991). This neurologically mediated response is seen in specific groups of muscles prone to tightness and weakness. The pattern of neurological imbalance is based on neurodevelopment of the tonic and phasic muscle systems (Janda 1978). Muscle imbalance presenting with facilitation of an agonist inhibits the antagonist (Baratta et al. 1988), possibly increasing risk of injury.

• **Impaired movement patterns and postural changes.** Postural responses to pain are common, facilitating the flexor response to protect the injured area. The protective adaptation to pain through compensatory movement results in decreased ROM and altered movement patterns (Lund et al. 1991). Tightness of antagonists subsequently inhibits agonists based on Sherrington's law of reciprocal inhibition (Sherrington 1906). This imbalance leads to further alterations in normal movement patterns. Impaired movement patterns may be compounded by the reemergence of primitive movement patterns and reflexes.

- **Faulty motor programming and motor learning.** Reemergence of primitive movement patterns and reflexes obviously affects normal movement patterns. Repetitive faulty movement patterns eventually supersede a normal motor program because of the effect of motor learning. The faulty program becomes ingrained in the motor cortex as the new normal program for a specific movement pattern, thus reinforcing the faulty movement.

- **Altered joint forces and altered proprioception.** Altered movement patterns change the normal patterns of joint stress. Muscle imbalance alters joint position, changing the distribution of stresses on the joint capsule and surfaces. Afferent input is essential in the modification of muscle activation to make movement well coordinated and functional (Holm, Inhahl, and Solomonow 2002).

- **Joint degeneration.** Poor proprioception ultimately may be responsible for joint degeneration (Barrett, Cobb, and Bentley 1991; O'Connor et al. 1992). The recently discovered central pattern generators (CPGs) in the spinal cord may provide some protection to joints (O'Connor and Vilensky 2003) by balancing the contraction of agonists and antagonists during gait. Janda believed that muscle imbalance presents a much greater danger for joints than muscular weakness alone presents (Janda 1993). Therefore, functional pathology may in fact cause structural pathology.

- **Chronic pain.** Inflammatory mediators such as histamine and bradykinins are known to cause pain. Joint pain and inflammation sensitize musculoskeletal afferent receptors (Guilbaud 1991; Schaible and Schmidt 1985; Sessle and Hu 1991). As stated earlier, pain causes an adaptive response of muscle imbalance and altered posture and movement patterns and thus facilitates the vicious cycle.

Pain does not necessarily precede inhibition or spasm; rather, altered proprioception is a more important factor (Janda 1986a). Muscle imbalance may cause pain or may be caused by pain. Altered muscle tension usually is the first response to nociception by the sensorimotor system; this change in tension leads to muscle imbalances. Changes in the motor system may occur before the onset of pain and may predispose the development of spinal pain (O'Sullivan et al. 1997). Patients with low back pain (especially those with sciatica) demonstrate significant decreases in lumbar extensor strength when compared with controls (McNeill et al. 1980).

Janda believed that pain is the strongest stimulus to central motor programming. Both experimental and clinical pain can alter EMG patterns in functional tasks (Madeleine et al. 1999). Throwing athletes with shoulder pain exhibit delayed activation of the subscapularis when compared with those without pain (Hess et al. 2005).

Johansson and Sojka (1991) proposed that prolonged static muscle contractions activate type III and IV afferents, activating the gamma motor neurons on the side of the contraction as well as the contralateral muscle. This activation influences the stretch sensitivity of muscles on both sides of the body, increasing muscle stiffness and creating a vicious cycle.

Painful stimuli seem to have an inhibitory effect on muscle activation. Matre and colleagues (1998) noted that experimental pain increases the stretch reflex, possibly leading to overactivation; however, pain stimulation does not increase activation of the alpha motor unit. This observation questions the validity of a peripheral vicious cycle of muscle spasm, as the pain itself does not cause muscle spasm—rather, spasm causes pain due to ischemia.

The pain adaptation model is used to describe acute pain from muscle (Lund et al. 1991) and is often used to refute the pain and spasm cycle. The pain adaptation model predicts a decrease in EMG activity of the agonist and an increase in EMG activity of the antagonist, as well as a decrease in strength, range, and velocity of movement. This adaptation is thought to be due to small-diameter muscle afferents, interneurons, and alpha motor neurons. Researchers have demonstrated less powerful and slower movement in experimental pain models (Graven-Nielsen, Svensson, and Arendt-Nielsen 1997), a finding that supports the pain adaptation model. Lund and coworkers (1991) defined dysfunction as a normal protective response to pain rather than a cause of pain.

Janda referred to *minimal brain dysfunction* as a congenital risk factor for developing chronic pain (Janda 1978), becoming one of the first to note the influence of biopsychosocial factors in chronic low back pain. Minimal brain dysfunction is a developmental syndrome with characteristics of choreoathetosis and microspasticity—identified through increased muscle tone and hyperreflexive tendon responses—and slight paretic signs, all of which are usually asymmetrical (Janda 1978). Minimal brain dysfunction results in an inefficient overflow of muscle activity with a subsequent decrease in the ability to perform and adjust fine movements. Janda found that 80% of 500 patients with chronic low back pain of early onset in adulthood had symptoms of minimal brain dysfunction (Janda 1984).

Pathomechanics of Muscle Imbalance

Janda thought that the muscular system lies at a functional crossroads since it is influenced by both the CNS and the PNS. Muscles must be able to respond to a variety of simultaneous factors such as gravity, repetitive movement, and upright posture. Muscles are influenced by both neurological reflexes and biomechanical demands; therefore, muscles can be considered to be a window into the function of the sensorimotor system. Postural defects resulting from muscular imbalance also provide clues to sensorimotor function.

While treating patients with upper motor neuron lesions such as cerebral palsy and cerebrovascular accident, Janda recognized the neurological manifestations of muscle imbalance. Cerebral palsy accompanies the loss of central inhibition against the constant peripheral afferent input of the force of gravity, which is augmented by activities of daily living (ADL). In 1964, Janda reported weakness of the gluteal muscles in patients with SI joint dysfunction (Janda 1964). He subsequently found that patients with chronic musculoskeletal pain (most notably chronic low back pain) exhibit the same patterns of muscle tightness and weakness as patients with CNS disorders exhibit, a finding that indicates a link between muscle imbalance and the CNS.

Tonic and Phasic Systems

As described in chapter 3, the tonic system is the first used by the human body, as it is responsible for maintaining the fetal posture in newborn infants. The phasic system soon is activated as the infant learns to lift her head for visual orientation. The development of normal movement patterns utilizes reflexive coactivation of the tonic and phasic systems. These reflexes (such as the Babinski reflex, ATNR, and so on) disappear in the normally developing child; however, in patients with upper motor neuron lesions, such as cerebral palsy or stroke, these default patterns reemerge or predominate. Specifically, muscles that are phylogenetically tonic demonstrate increased tone or spasticity, while muscles that are phylogenetically phasic demonstrate decreased tone or spasticity. In patients with chronic musculoskeletal pain, this pattern of muscle imbalance occurs at a much lower level, manifesting as tightness and weakness in the tonic and phasic muscles, respectively. This finding supports Janda's observation that chronic musculoskeletal pain is mediated by the CNS and reflected in the sensorimotor system throughout the body. It also allows us to predict typical muscle responses because of these neurodevelopmental chains.

Janda conceptualized muscle imbalance as an impaired relationship between muscles prone to tightness or shortness and muscles prone to inhibition (Janda 1964). More specifically, he believed that muscles predominantly static, tonic, or postural in function have a tendency to get tight and are readily activated in various movements—more so than muscles that are predominantly dynamic and phasic in function, which have a tendency to grow weak (Janda 1978). The fundamental differences between these two systems are the basis for Janda's functional approach to muscle imbalance (see table 4.1).

Table 4.1 Tonic and Phasic Muscle Systems

Tonic system	Phasic system
Phylogenetically older	Phylogenetically younger
Generally flexor or postural muscles	Generally extensor muscles
Tendency toward tightness, hypertonia, shortening, and contractures	Tendency toward weakness, hypotonia, and lengthening
Readily activated in movement, especially with fatigue or novel or complex movement patterns	Less readily activated in most movement patterns (delayed activation)
Less likely to atrophy	More likely to atrophy
Less fragile	More fragile
Typically one-joint muscles	Typically two-joint muscles

While some research shows a predominance of Type I muscle fibers in tonic muscles and more Type II fibers in phasic muscles (Johnson et al. 1973), Janda was careful to point out that it is not possible to differentiate phasic and tonic groups of muscles histologically (Janda 1978). He noted that fiber type doesn't always influence function: Rather, muscle performs based on functional demands and the sensorimotor system. Muscle fibers may also change histologically in response to functional demands. Uhlig and colleagues (1995) performed neck muscle biopsies on patients with whiplash and found significant transformation toward more Type II fibers, similar to the pattern seen in patients with rheumatoid arthritis.

Janda (1983) believed that muscle should not be considered as postural or anti-gravity muscle based on the two-leg stance. He preferred to consider the function of muscle in relation to a one-leg stance, noting that the muscles involved in maintaining upright posture during single-leg balancing show a tendency toward tightness. Janda's classification of muscles prone to tightness and weakness is shown in table 4.2.

Table 4.2   Janda's Classification of Muscles Prone to Tightness or Weakness

Tonic system muscles *prone to tightness*	Phasic system muscles *prone to weakness*
UPPER QUARTER	
Suboccipitals Pectorals (major and minor) Upper trapezius Levator scaplua SCM Scalenes* Latissimus dorsi Upper-extremity flexors and pronators Masticators	Middle and lower trapezius Rhomboids Serratus anterior Deep cervical flexors (longus colli and capitis) Scalenes* Upper-extremity extensors and supinators Digastricus
LOWER QUARTER	
Quadratus lumborum Thoracolumbar paraspinals Piriformis Iliopsoas Rectus femoris TFL-IT band Hamstrings Short hip adductors Triceps surae (particularly soleus) Tibialis posterior	Rectus abdominis TrA Gluteus maximus Gluteus medius, minimus Vastus medialis, lateralis Tibialis anterior Peroneals

*The scalenes may be tight or weak.

This classification is not rigid. Janda noted that no muscle is exclusively phasic or tonic; some muscles may exhibit both tonic and phasic characteristics. Muscles do, however, have a tendency to be either tight or weak in dysfunction. For example, the scalenes are phylogenetically classified as phasic muscles, but often they are prone to tightness due to overload resulting from poor posture and ergonomics. Muscles that are prone to tightness are sometimes found to be weak, while muscles prone to weakness are sometimes found to be tight. Simply put, these findings might suggest the presence of a localized structural lesion rather than a functional pathology of the sensorimotor system.

Czech physiotherapist Pavel Kolář expanded on Janda's original list of tonic and phasic muscles from a more neurodevelopmental perspective (Kolář 2001). He classified the following muscles as phasic: rectus capitis anterior, supraspinatus, infraspinatus, teres minor, and deltoid, and the following muscles as tonic: coracobrachialis, brachioradialis, subscapularis, and teres major. Kolář also noted that the latissimus dorsi may be either tonic or phasic. In contrast to Janda, Kolář categorized the piriformis and gastrocnemius as phasic muscles and suggested that the biceps, triceps, and hip adductors exhibit both tonic and phasic portions. Specifically, the long head of the triceps and short head of the biceps are tonic, while the medial and lateral triceps and long head of the biceps are phasic. The short adductors are tonic, while the long adductors are phasic.

Faulty Movement Patterns

As noted earlier in the chapter, Lund and colleagues' pain adaptation model (1991) supports Janda's theory of facilitation of antagonists (flexors) and inhibition of agonists (extensors) in response to pain. The subsequent muscle imbalances lead to changes in movement patterns. Altered recruitment patterns typically begin with a delayed activation of a primary mover or stabilizer, along with early facilitation of a synergist. Muscle tightness leads to overactivation of certain muscles, while muscles that should be activated are not, possibly due to inhibition or motor reprogramming (Janda 1987). Janda (1978) noted that altered peripheral input due to pain leads to these changes in muscle activation, causing faulty movement patterns that eventually become centralized in the motor program.

Janda found these characteristic patterns of muscle imbalance in children as young as 8 y (Janda 1989b). Muscle tightness increases between ages 8 and 16 and then remains constant. Janda found a correlation between body height and muscle tightness as well as poor fitness (Janda 1989b). He further noted that imbalances in children begin in the upper extremity as opposed to the lower extremity, as is seen in adults. He believed these patterns of muscle imbalance to be systematic and predictable because of the innate function of the sensorimotor system. Subsequently, adaptive changes within the sensorimotor system (either vertical or horizontal) affect the entire system, most often progressing proximally to distally. This muscular reaction is specific for each joint, suggesting a strong relationship between joint dysfunction and muscle imbalance (Janda 1986a).

Although Janda is considered the father of the neurological paradigm of muscle imbalance, he recognized that muscle imbalances also occur as a result of biomechanical mechanisms (Janda 1978). Lifestyle often contributes to muscle imbalance as well; Janda felt that muscle imbalance in today's society is compounded by stress, fatigue, and insufficient movement through regular physical activity as well as a lack of variety of movement (Jull and Janda 1987). This lack of variety contributes to repetitive movement disorders. Janda noted that most repetitive movements reinforce the postural system, neglecting the phasic system, and lead to imbalance.

Causes of Muscle Tightness and Weakness

Muscle tension (or tone) is the force with which a muscle resists being lengthened (Basmajian 1985). Muscle tension may also relate to a muscle's activation potential or excitability; thus, testing muscle tension has two components: viscoelastic and contractile (Mense and Simons 2001; Taylor, Brooks, and Ryan 1997). The viscoelastic component relates to the extensibility of structures, while the contractile component relates to the neurological input. Each of these components plays a role in the causes of muscle tightness and weakness (see table 4.3).

Table 4.3 Contractile and Noncontractile Components of Muscle Tightness and Weakness

	Muscle tightness	Muscle weakness
Contractile and neuroflexive components	Limbic system activation TrPs Muscle spasm	Reciprocal inhibition Arthrogenic weakness Deafferentation Pseudoweakness TrP weakness Fatigue
Viscoelastic and adaptive components	Adaptive shortening	Stretch weakness Tightness weakness

Muscle Tightness

Janda felt that muscle tightness is the key factor in muscle imbalance. In general, muscles prone to tightness are one third stronger than muscles prone to inhibition (Janda 1987). Muscle tightness creates a cascade of events that lead to injury. Tightness of a muscle reflexively inhibits its antagonist, creating muscle imbalance. This muscle imbalance leads to joint dysfunction because of unbalanced forces. Joint dysfunction creates poor movement patterns and compensations, leading to early fatigue. Finally, overstress of activated muscles and poor stabilization lead to injury.

Janda believed that there are three important factors in muscle tightness (Janda 1993): muscle length, irritability threshold, and altered recruitment. Muscles that are tight usually are shorter than normal and display an altered length–tension relationship. Muscle tightness leads to a lowered activation threshold or lowered irritability threshold, which means that the muscle is readily activated with movement (Janda 1993). Movement typically takes the path of least resistance, and so tight and facilitated muscles often are the first to be recruited in movement patterns. Tight muscles typically maintain their strength, but in extreme cases they can weaken.

Structurally, increased muscle tension is caused by a lesion of the CNS that results in spasticity or rigidity, as is seen in cerebral palsy or Parkinson's disease. Tight muscles are also described as *hypertonic* or *facilitated.* Functionally, increased muscle tension results from either neuroflexive or adaptive conditions. These two conditions are based on the contractile (neuroflexive factors) and viscoelastic (adaptive factors) components of muscle tension.

Neuroflexive Factors for Increased Tension

Factors from the contractile components of muscle that increase tension are limbic system activation, TrPs, and muscle spasm:

• **Limbic system activation** (Umphred 2001). Stress, fatigue, pain, and emotion contribute to increased muscle tightness through the limbic system. Muscle spasms due to limbic system activation usually are not painful but are tender to palpation. They are most frequently seen in the shoulders, neck, and low back and in tension headache.

• **TrPs** (Simons et al. 1999). TrPs are focal areas of hypertonicity that are not painful during movement but are painful with palpation. Essentially, they are localized, hyperirritable taut bands within muscle.

• **Muscle spasm** (Mense and Simons 2001). Muscle spasm causes ischemia or an altered movement pattern or joint position resulting from altered tension. The spasm itself does not cause pain because spasm is not associated with increased EMG activity (Mense and Simons 2001). Muscle spasm is a typical response to joint dysfunction or pain irritation due to an impairment of interneuron function at the spinal level (Janda 1991). Muscle spasm leads to a reflex arc of reciprocal inhibition for protection and subsequently impaired function of the motor system. These muscles are also tender to palpation.

Adaptive Factors for Increased Tension

Increased muscle tension also results from adaptive shortening (Kendall et al. 1993; Sahrmann 2001). Over time, muscle remains in a shortened position, causing a moderate decrease in muscle length and subsequent postural adaptation. Adaptive shortening is often considered overuse. These shortened muscles usually are not painful at rest but are tender to touch. They exhibit a lowered irritability threshold and are readily activated with movement. Over the long term, strength decreases as active fibers are replaced by noncontractile tissue. It is very important for the clinician to identify the cause of increased muscle tension in order to apply the appropriate treatment.

Causes of Muscle Weakness

Muscle tension can decrease as a result of a structural lesion in the CNS such as a spinal cord injury or stroke. A loss of tension leads to flaccidity or weakness. Weak muscles are also described as *hypotonic* or *inhibited*. Functionally, muscle can be weak as a result of neuroflexive or adaptive changes and may exhibit delayed activation in movement patterns.

Neuroflexive Factors for Decreased Tension

Many contractile factors can contribute to decreased muscle tension:

- **Reciprocal inhibition** (Sherrington 1907). Muscle becomes inhibited reflexively when its antagonist is activated. Weakness is often reflex-mediated inhibition secondary to increased tension of the antagonist.

- **Arthrogenic weakness** (Stokes and Young 1984; DeAndrade, Grant, and Dison. 1965). Muscle becomes inhibited via anterior horn cells due to joint swelling or dysfunction. This weakness also leads to selective atrophy of Type II fibers (Edstrom 1970).

- **Deafferentation** (Freeman, Dean, and Hanham 1965). Deafferentation is a decrease in afferent information from neuromuscular receptors. Damage to joint mechanoreceptors (as seen with ligamentous injury) with subsequent loss of articular reflexes can cause altered motor programs, often influencing many muscles remote from the injured area (Bullock-Saxton 1994). This loss of afferent information ultimately leads to de-efferentation, or the loss of efferent signals to alpha motor neurons, which results in decreased muscle strength.

- **Pseudoparesis** (Janda 1986a). Pseudoparesis is a clinical presentation of weakness of neuroflexive origin. Pseudoparesis has three clinical signs: hypotonia upon inspection and palpation, a score of 4 out of 5 on a manual muscle test, and a change in the muscle activation pattern that may include delayed onset with early synergist activation or decreased EMG levels. Facilitatory techniques often restore muscle strength and activation. Normally facilitatory input can be inhibitory to a pseudoparetic muscle (Janda 1986a).

- **TrP weakness** (Simons, Travell, and Simons 1999). Hyperirritable bands of muscle fiber decrease the stimulation threshold, leading to overuse, early fatigue, and ultimately weakness. Muscles with active TrPs fatigue more rapidly than normal muscles do (Mense and Simons 2001), and they exhibit a decreased number of firing motor units and poor synchronization (Janda 1993).

- **Fatigue.** Muscle fatigue can be caused by metabolic or neurological factors. Often during exercise muscles are fatigued before pain is experienced. Thus the patient develops compensatory and faulty movement patterns before experiencing pain.

Adaptive Factors for Decreased Tension

Noncontractile factors causing decreased muscle tension are stretch weakness and tightness weakness:

- **Stretch weakness** (Kendall, McCreary, and Provance 1993; Sahrmann 2002a, 2002b). Stretch weakness is a condition in which a muscle is elongated beyond physiological neutral but not beyond the normal ROM (Janda 1993). Prolonged muscle elongation causes muscle spindle inhibition and the creation of additional sarcomeres. The increased muscle length also changes the length–tension curve. Stretch weakness is also known as *positional weakness* and is often associated with overuse and postural changes.

- **Tightness weakness** (Janda 1993). This is the most severe form of muscle tightness. It is often overlooked clinically. Overused muscle shortens over time, changing the muscle's length–tension curve and becoming more readily activated and weaker after time. There is also an increase in the noncontractile tissue and a decrease in elasticity, leading to hypertrophy. Ultimately, overuse leads to ischemia and degeneration of muscle fibers, which further weakens the muscle.

When an inhibited and weak muscle is resisted, as is the aim of strengthening exercises, its activity tends to decrease rather than increase (Janda 1987). It is important to distinguish between neuroflexive weakness and structural weakness. Often, if the tight antagonist is stretched, the weak and inhibited muscle spontaneously increases in strength.

Janda's Classification of Muscle Imbalance Patterns

Through his observations of patients with neurological disorders and chronic musculoskeletal pain, Janda found that the typical muscle response to joint dysfunction is similar to the muscle patterns found in upper motor neuron lesions, concluding that muscle imbalances are controlled by the CNS (Janda 1987). Janda believed that muscle tightness or spasticity is predominant. Often, weakness from muscle imbalance results from reciprocal inhibition of the tight antagonist. The degree of tightness and weakness varies between individuals, but the pattern rarely does. These patterns lead to postural changes and joint dysfunction and degeneration.

Janda identified three stereotypical patterns associated with distinct chronic pain syndromes: the upper-crossed, lower-crossed, and layer syndromes. These syndromes are characterized by specific patterns of muscle weakness and tightness that cross between the dorsal and the ventral sides of the body.

Upper-Crossed Syndrome

Upper-crossed syndrome (UCS) is also referred to as *proximal* or *shoulder girdle crossed syndrome* (figure 4.2a; Janda 1988). In UCS, tightness of the upper trapezius and levator scapula on the dorsal side crosses with tightness of the pectoralis major and minor. Weakness of the deep cervical flexors ventrally crosses with weakness of the middle and lower trapezius. This pattern of imbalance creates joint dysfunction, particularly at the atlanto-occipital joint, C4-C5 segment, cervicothoracic joint, glenohumeral joint, and T4-T5 segment. Janda noted that these focal areas of stress within

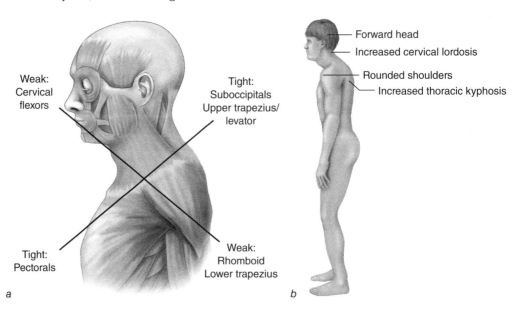

Figure 4.2 *(a)* UCS and *(b)* common posture in UCS.

the spine correspond to transitional zones in which neighboring vertebrae change in morphology. Specific postural changes are seen in UCS, including forward head posture, increased cervical lordosis and thoracic kyphosis, elevated and protracted shoulders, and rotation or abduction and winging of the scapulae (figure 4.2b). These postural changes decrease glenohumeral stability as the glenoid fossa becomes more vertical due to serratus anterior weakness leading to abduction, rotation, and winging of the scapulae. This loss of stability requires the levator scapula and upper trapezius to increase activation to maintain glenohumeral centration (Janda 1988).

Lower-Crossed Syndrome

Lower-crossed syndrome (LCS) is also referred to as *distal* or *pelvic crossed syndrome* (figure 4.3a; Janda 1987). In LCS, tightness of the thoracolumbar extensors on the dorsal side crosses with tightness of the iliopsoas and rectus femoris. Weakness of the deep abdominal muscles ventrally crosses with weakness of the gluteus maximus and medius.

This pattern of imbalance creates joint dysfunction, particularly at the L4-L5 and L5-S1 segments, SI joint, and hip joint. Specific postural changes seen in LCS include anterior pelvic tilt, increased lumbar lordosis, lateral lumbar shift, lateral leg rotation, and knee hyperextension. If the lordosis is deep and short, then imbalance is predominantly in the pelvic muscles; if the lordosis is shallow and extends into the thoracic area, then imbalance predominates in the trunk muscles (Janda 1987).

Janda identified two subtypes of LCS: A and B (see figure 4.3, b-c). Patients with LCS type A use more hip flexion and extension movement for mobility; their standing posture

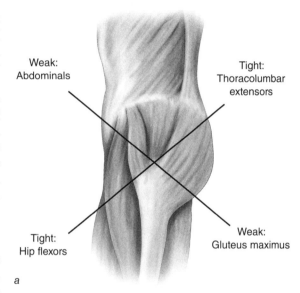

Weak: Abdominals

Tight: Thoracolumbar extensors

Tight: Hip flexors

Weak: Gluteus maximus

a

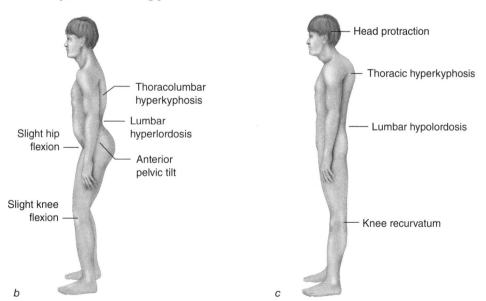

Thoracolumbar hyperkyphosis

Lumbar hyperlordosis

Slight hip flexion

Anterior pelvic tilt

Slight knee flexion

Head protraction

Thoracic hyperkyphosis

Lumbar hypolordosis

Knee recurvatum

b

c

Figure 4.3 *(a)* LCS and two types of posture in the LCS: *(b)* type A posture and *(c)* type B posture.

demonstrates an anterior pelvic tilt with slight hip flexion and knee flexion. These individuals compensate with a hyperlordosis limited to the lumbar spine and with a hyperkyphosis in the upper lumbar and thoracolumbar segments.

Janda's LCS type B involves more movement of the low back and abdominal area. There is minimal lumbar lordosis that extends into the thoracolumbar segments, compensatory kyphosis in the thoracic area, and head protraction. The COG is shifted backward with the shoulders behind the axis of the body, and the knees are in recurvatum.

Deep stabilizing muscles responsible for segmental spinal stability are inhibited and substituted by activation of the superficial muscles (Cholewicki, Panjabi, and Khachatryan 1997). Tight hamstrings may be compensating for anterior pelvic tilt or an inhibited gluteus maximus. LCS also affects dynamic movement patterns. If the hip loses its ability to extend in the terminal stance, there is a compensatory increase in anterior pelvic tilt and lumbar extension. This compensation creates a chain reaction to maintain equilibrium, in which the increased pelvic tilt and anterior lordosis increase the thoracic kyphosis and cervical lordosis (see chapter 3).

In adults, muscle imbalance begins distally in the pelvis and continues proximally to the shoulder and neck area. In children, this progression is reversed, and muscle imbalance begins proximally and moves distally.

Layer Syndrome

Janda's layer syndrome (also referred to as the *stratification syndrome*) is a combination of UCS and LCS (see figure 4.4). Patients display marked impairment of motor regulation that has increased over time and have a poorer prognosis than those with isolated UCS or LCS due to the long-standing dysfunction. Layer syndrome often is seen in older adults and in patients who underwent unsuccessful surgery for herniated nucleus pulposus.

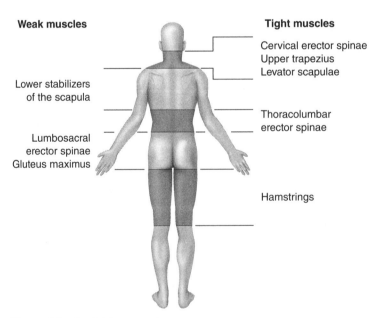

Weak muscles

Lower stabilizers of the scapula

Lumbosacral erector spinae
Gluteus maximus

Tight muscles

Cervical erector spinae
Upper trapezius
Levator scapulae

Thoracolumbar erector spinae

Hamstrings

Figure 4.4 Janda's layer syndrome.

Based on G. Jull and V. Janda, 1987, Muscles and motor control in low back pain. In *Physical therapy for the low back*, edited by L.T. Twomney and J.R. Taylor (Oxford, United Kingdom: Churchill Livingstone).

Summary

Chronic musculoskeletal pain can be caused by a number of pathologies, making it difficult for the clinician to provide a specific diagnosis. Janda recognized a relationship between muscle imbalance and chronic pain that is mediated by the sensorimotor system. He outlined the tonic and phasic groups of muscle as being prone to tightness and weakness, respectively. Further, he identified several factors from both contractile and noncontractile components causing changes in muscle tension. While chronic pain is difficult to treat, clinicians must be able to recognize Janda's UCS, LCS, or layer syndrome in order to provide appropriate treatment. A specific evaluation involving postural analysis and examination of movement patterns can diagnose these muscle imbalance syndromes. A specific treatment plan is then initiated to address the local and global changes associated with these syndromes.

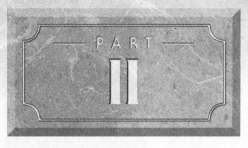

FUNCTIONAL EVALUATION OF MUSCLE IMBALANCE

The functional evaluation of muscle imbalance includes the patient's history and current complaints, orthopedic procedures, and, most importantly, visual and palpatory observations. The exam involves gathering little pieces of information and combining them, no matter how trivial they may seem, into a scenario describing the possible etiology and pathomechanism of the patient's complaints. The functional evaluation requires not only a variety of skills and a deep practical understanding of the topics discussed in part I but also a clear understanding and appreciation of functional anatomy and its kinesiology.

The four chapters of part II emphasize the visual and palpatory skills the clinician needs in order to critically assess and systematically organize faulty movement patterns to form a clinical framework for diagnosis and treatment. The skills required to integrate visual and palpatory subtleties into an orthopedic evaluation can be daunting but nevertheless feasible with careful practice. Great technical advances in posture and gait assessment in research laboratories have provided exciting new insights into and objective measures of the locomotor system, some of which prove or disprove previous empirical observation. However, visual observation and palpation, when skillfully practiced, provide the clinician with valuable and immediate feedback on the patient's adaptation, compensation, or decompensation. In short, functional examination of the muscular system provides a window into the patient's overall sensorimotor system.

POSTURE, BALANCE, AND GAIT ANALYSIS

A nalysis of standing posture provides a clinician with a wealth of information about the status of the muscular system. It also provides cues for subsequent clinical tests, such as muscle length or strength testing or evaluation of particular movement patterns, to confirm or refute what is observed. Adequate balance, timing, and recruitment of the musculature are imperative for smooth and efficient movement patterns. Imbalance or impairment in recruitment and coordination of muscles in any part of the kinetic chain manifests as faulty patterns and inefficient energy expenditure. Skilled observation of single-limb balance and gait provides important information about possible overstresses of critical segments or lack of muscular stability in the kinetic chain that may be causing or perpetuating musculoskeletal pain.

This chapter describes an assessment of static posture in standing and dynamic posture in balance and gait. Clinicians must always consider the entire body and sensorimotor system when evaluating chronic pain. A clinician can gather valuable information on the overall status of the sensorimotor system before even touching the patient. With experience, this assessment can be completed in several minutes. Although postural analysis is not diagnostic in and of itself, it provides a clinical guide for subsequent assessment and confirmatory tests.

Muscle Analysis of Standing Posture

Posture is a composite alignment of all the joints of the body at any given moment in time (Kendall, McCreary, and Provance 1993). Posture may also be described in terms of muscle imbalance, given that faulty alignment may cause undue stress and strain on bones, joints, ligaments, and muscles. From a biomechanical point of view, imbalance between opposing muscles in standing posture changes alignment and adversely affects the position of the parts of the body above or below the faulty area. Functionally, the neurological, muscular, and articular systems form an inseparable unit, which Janda termed the *sensorimotor system* (see chapter 2). Static posture provides a window into the overall status of the CNS, in that the muscular system lies at the functional crossroads between the CNS and the osteoarticular system. The muscular system exerts a strong influence on the articular system and CNS and vice versa. Hence, functional pathology in any part of the sensorimotor system is reflected by alterations in function elsewhere in the system. The primary functions of muscles to produce and control motion, to stabilize, and to protect joints are regulated by the CNS.

Dysfunction in muscles and the motor system as a result of injury, chronic overuse, pathology, and sedentary habits often leads to observable changes in muscle function. In addition, muscle function resulting from joint dysfunction usually displays characteristic patterns of inhibition or spasms, with subsequently poorer motor performance and postural control (Janda 1978, 1994, 1986a, 1987; Janda, Frank, and Liebenson 2007; Brumagne et al. 2000; Byl and Sinnot 1991; Gill and Callaghan 1998; Tuzun et al. 1999; Heikkila and Astrom 1996). Muscles may respond by developing TrPs, imbalances, or altered movement patterns. Muscle imbalance often leads to postural changes due to alterations in resting muscle tone. Thorough analysis of muscles is essential to provide a clearer understanding of the status of the motor system and its relevance to the patient's symptoms. Again, clinicians must always consider the entire body and sensorimotor system when evaluating chronic pain. As described previously, functional pathology is both local and global and may be influenced by any number of chain reactions.

During muscular analysis, the clinician observes the symmetry, contour, and tone of the muscles, as the muscles observed in static posture tend to respond through hyperactivity, hypertonicity, and hypertrophy or through atrophy, weakness, and inhibition. Careful and precise analysis of the shape, bulk, and tone of muscles may provide clues as to the amount of use or the contribution to a faulty movement pattern. Following is a description of a systematic postural and muscle analysis. Chapters 6 and 7 describe confirmatory tests of movement pattern and muscle length. Table 5.1 outlines an algorithm for systematic postural analysis.

Posterior View

Ideally, standing postural analysis is performed with the patient wearing minimal clothing and standing in good lighting. Patients are observed in three views: posterior, anterior, and lateral. Postural observation always begins at the pelvis regardless of the area of the primary complaint because most chronic musculoskeletal pain is first evident in postural asymmetries.

Position of the Pelvis

First the clinician makes an overall impression of postural alignment, taking note of the spinal curves, looking for any inadequacy or excessiveness, any structural or biomechanical variations such as scoliosis or leg-length discrepancy, and any other orthopedic deviations. Much attention is directed toward the position of the pelvis, as dysfunctions in the lumbar spine, SI joint, and lower limbs are often reflected in this region. Clinical and radiological studies (Levine and Whittle 1996; Dayet et al. 1984) have shown significant correlations between lumbar lordosis and pelvic tilt in that altering the pelvic tilt significantly changes the angle of lumbar lordosis. Pelvic tilt also tends to influence the orientation of the head and other parts of the body.

The position of the pelvis is observed for alignment in the sagittal, frontal, and transverse planes. The iliac crests are palpated for symmetry in height and rotation. The most common types of deviation that occur in the pelvis are anterior or posterior tilt in the sagittal plane, lateral tilt in the frontal plane, and rotation in the transverse plane (see figure 5.1). There are five key points to observe in the pelvis:

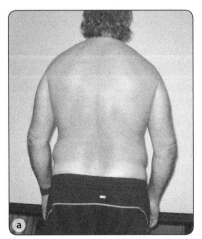 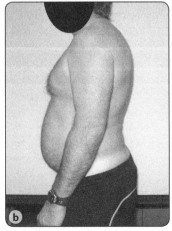

Figure 5.1   Pelvic position showing *(a)* lateral shift and pelvic rotation and *(b)* anterior tilt.

Table 5.1 Algorithm for Systematic Postural Assessment

Key point	Observation	Possible cause	Common clinical findings	Confirmatory tests
POSTERIOR VIEW				
1. Pelvis	Lateral tilt	Leg discrepancy Lumbar or SI pathology Shortness of quadratus lumborum or latissimus dorsi	Iliac crest height difference	Modified Thomas test Single-leg stance test Muscle length tests
	Lateral shift	Lumbar pathology Short hip adductors or weakened hip abductors	Pelvis shifted laterally relative to trunk	
	Rotation	Lumbar or SI pathology Shortness of TFL	ASIS anterior of the contralateral ASIS Hip medial rotation toward where pelvis is rotated	
	Anterior pelvic tilt	Gluteus medius or maximus inhibition or weakness Hip flexor hypertonicity or shortness	Increased lumbar lordosis	
	Posterior pelvic tilt	Tight hamstrings	Flat back or decreased lumbar lordosis	
2. Buttocks	Lower gluteal fold	SI joint dysfunction on ipsilateral side	Gluteus maximus inhibition Ipsilateral hamstring hypertrophy	Hip extension Palpation Muscle strength tests for gluteals
3. Hamstrings	Hypertrophy of lower two thirds of the belly of the hamstring	Gluteus maximus inhibition on ipsilateral side LCS	Hamstring hypertonicity, stiffness, or shortness	Palpation Hip extension Hamstring length test
4. Adductors	S shape in proximal groin area (adductor notch) Bulkier S shape that may be due to shortened pectineus Hypertonicity in obliques	Lumbar dysfunction Possible leg-length discrepancy Abductor weakness Abdominal wall weakness	Abductor weakness Abdominal weakness TrPs in adductors Rectus abdominis attachment on pubic symphysis	Palpation Hip adductor length test Hip abduction Muscle strength tests for gluteals
5. Calf and triceps surae	Broad and short Achilles tendon Prominence of soleus belly	Low back pain Use of improper shoes Poor posture that usually causes a larger gastrocnemius and soleus on dominant leg	Tight gastrocnemius or soleus Low back pain Plantar fasciitis Increased pronation of foot	Palpation Calf length test
6. Shape of heel	Rounded heel—normal Quadratic heel—central mass shifted to posterior Pointed heel—central mass shifted to anterior	Weakness of dorsiflexors Postural adaptation	Hypertonicity in gluteus maximus Tight hamstrings driven by pelvis Headaches	Palpation of cervical muscles, suboccipital Foot function test
7. Spinal extensors	Asymmetrical Thoracolumbar paraspinals Horizontal groove	Low back pain Segmental hypermobility Fascial tightness LCS	Abdominal weakness or incoordination Instability of lower spine Tight hip flexors	Schober's test Passive mobility testing Observation of abdominal function Breathing pattern

(continued)

Table 5.1 *(continued)*

Key point	Observation	Possible cause	Common clinical findings	Confirmatory tests
8. Scapula region	Winging medial to lateral Gothic shoulders (straightening of the shoulder and neckline)	UCS Tight pectorals C2 dysfunction	Weakness of dynamic scapular stabilizers Tight pectoral muscles, upper trapezius, or levator scapulae	Push-up Arm abduction Head flexion Muscle length tests for pectoral muscles, upper trapezius, levator scapulae Muscle strength tests for mid- and lower trapezius, serratus anterior, deep cervical flexors
ANTERIOR VIEW				
9. Abdominal wall	Breathing pattern	Excessive upper versus lower breathing	Tightness TrPs Weak abdominal muscles Lateral groove Low back pain Adductor spasm	Curl-up Breathing
	Hypertonic upper versus lower quadrant	Weak and inefficient diaphragm		
	Increased groove of rectus	Hypertonic accessory muscles of respiration Abdominal wall weakness or incoordination		
	Pseudohernia	Poor stability, weakened TrA		
10. Thigh	Bulk medial to lateral Vastus medialis bulk visible or prominent	Sport related Tight rectus femoris Forced knee hyperextension L4 lesions Lateral position of patella	Tendency to hyperextend knee, possible weakness Lateral deviation of patella Superior-lateral IT band TrP	Movement pattern tests (hip extension, abduction) Muscle length tests (hamstrings) Palpation Single-leg stance test
	Patella shifting	Foot dysfunction Proprioceptive deficits	Balance impairments	
11. Leg	Smaller tibialis anterior Flattening of L5	L5 dysfunction	Lumbar pain Gait impairments	Muscle tests Palpation
12. Upper extremity	Contour of deltoids Medial rotation of arms Arm position in sagittal plane Humeral head position	UCS Rule out Scheuermann's disease	Weakness of external rotators Insufficient dynamic scapular stabilization Tight or short latissimus dorsi, pectoral muscles	Muscle length tests of latissimus dorsi, pectoral muscles Muscle strength tests of mid- and lower trapezius, shoulder external rotators
13. Pectorals	Increased bulk Nipples face out superiorly or laterally	UCS	Tender points TrPs Medial rotation of arms Shoulder protraction Restricted rib mobility	Palpation Pectoral muscle length tests
14. Head	Forward head Groove anterior to SCM	UCS Scalene and deep cervical flexor weakness	Pain TrPs	Head flexion Cervical spine exam Mobility Palpation
	>90° angle between chin and neck	Hypertonic suprahyoid muscles	TMJ dysfunction	

1. An increased anterior pelvic tilt with an associated increase in lumbar lordosis leads to the pelvic crossed syndrome (Janda 1987; Janda, Frank, and Liebenson 2007). Contributing factors may include shortened or tight one- or two-joint hip flexors and lumbar extensors and weakness of the abdominal and gluteal muscles.

2. A posterior tilt usually is coupled with a flattened lumbar spine and may be associated with tight hamstrings (see figure 5.2; Kendall, McCreary, and Prvance 1993).

3. Pelvic lateral tilt in the frontal plane is noted if one iliac crest is higher than the other. Tightness of the quadratus lumborum or latissimus dorsi may cause a lateral pelvic tilt. Radiological findings or leg-length measurements can be used to rule out structural leg-length discrepancies. Nevertheless, lateral pelvic tilt usually is associated with the functional shortening of one leg secondary to muscle imbalances. Muscles that contribute to shortening of the leg are the one-joint hip adductors, iliopsoas, and quadratus lumborum. A shortened ipsilateral latissimus dorsi may also create a functional shortening of the leg via elevation of the pelvis from the trunk. On the other hand, a shortened piriformis may contribute to the functional lengthening of the leg (Janda 1995).

4. Lateral pelvic shift is detected when the pelvis is shifted laterally with respect to the trunk. A lateral pelvic shift may be caused by a lumbar pathology or by unilateral shortening of the hip adductors and associated hip abductor weakness or inhibition.

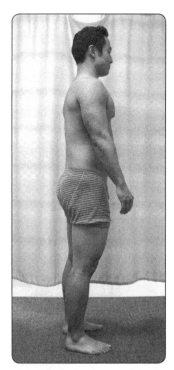

Figure 5.2 Posterior pelvic tilt.

5. Rotation of the pelvis in the transverse plane is detected when the anterior superior iliac spine (ASIS) is anterior to the contralateral ASIS. This is often associated with hip medial rotation on the side toward which the pelvis is rotated. The contributing factor is often a shortened TFL-IT band on the side toward which the pelvis is rotated (Sahrmann 2001).

Buttock Region

Observation of the gluteus maximus is directed toward the upper quadrant of the buttock region. The size, symmetry, and contour of the glutei are noted. The ideal glutei are well rounded; the gluteal line is horizontal. The left and right sides should be symmetrical. The glutei (maximus, medius, and minimus) are prone to hypotonia and are often inhibited early in chronic low back pain. Figure 5.3 illustrates asymmetrical gluteal muscles.

Flattening of the gluteal muscles in the upper quadrant of the buttocks or buttocks with a loosely hanging appearance may indicate weakness of the gluteus maximus or arthrogenic inhibition of the gluteus maximus due to dysfunction in the ipsilateral SI joint (Janda 1978; Janda, Frank, and Liebenson 2007; Hungerford, Gilleard, and Hodges 2003). Muscle changes associated with SI joint dysfunction include ipsilateral gluteus maximus inhibition or weakness; painful spasms in the ipsilateral iliacus, piriformis, and rectus abdominis; and contralateral gluteus medius inhibition or weakness (Janda 1978).

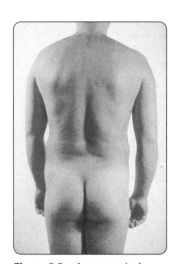

Figure 5.3 Asymmetrical gluteal muscles.

Hamstrings

The clinician observes the symmetry and contour of the hamstrings at the distal two thirds of the muscle belly of the posterior thigh (figure 5.4). Dominance or hypertrophy of the hamstrings usually is associated with hypotrophy or inhibition of the gluteus maximus on the ipsilateral side and hypertrophy of the thoracolumbar paraspinals. The hamstring muscles function synergistically with the gluteus maximus to produce hip extension. When there is gluteus maximus inhibition, the hamstrings substitute with hip extension during gait propulsion; therefore, gluteal atrophy often is associated with hypertrophy of the hamstrings on the ipsilateral side.

Adductors

The clinician observes the shape and contour of the proximal one third of the medial thigh muscles; normally this part of the thigh forms a very shallow S curve. A bulkier muscle belly or a deeper S curve in the upper medial thigh may indicate short or hypertonic one-joint adductors, namely the pectineus muscle. This is also known as an *adductor notch,* which can be seen in the upper part of the right thigh in figure 5.4. This area is often tender upon palpation in patients with painful hip joint dysfunctions. Tightness in the hip adductors may also be associated with leg-length discrepancy, lateral shift of the pelvis, or hip joint dysfunctions. Hip abductor weakness or inhibition is a common finding in hip joint dysfunction and tight or tender adductors.

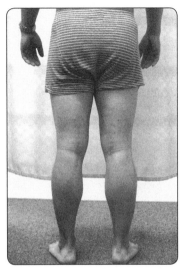

Figure 5.4 The hamstrings at the distal two thirds of the muscle belly of the posterior thigh. Note the adductor notch (increased bulk) seen in the upper part of the right thigh.

Triceps Surae

The clinician observes the bulk and shape of both the gastrocnemius and the soleus at the proximal and distal portions of the muscles, respectively (figure 5.5). If the entire triceps surae is short, the Achilles tendon appears shorter and broader. The lack of dorsiflexion range resulting from short and tight plantar flexors may prevent the patient from achieving a full heel strike during the gait cycle, forcing a compensatory hyperlordosis in the lumbar region for forward progression (Janda 1994; Janda, Frank, and Liebenson 2007). If the soleus is short and hypertrophied, the lower leg appears more cylindrical in shape, in contrast to the normal inverted bottleneck shape. Soleus tightness may be a hidden cause of back pain (Travell and Simons 1992) and may suggest an existing or a previous ankle or foot dysfunction (Janda 1994; Janda, Frank, and Liebenson 2007).

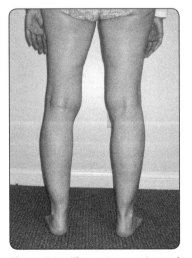

Figure 5.5 The gastrocnemius and soleus. When the entire triceps surae is short, the Achilles tendon appears shorter and broader (left side).

Shape of the Heel

The heel is rounded in shape during normal weight bearing on the heel and forefoot. (see figure 5.6). A quadratic or square shape indicates that the patient's center of mass is directed posteriorly; this may overstress the heel during gait. The lack of shock absorption at heel strike may attenuate forces up the kinetic chain to cause dysfunction in the knee, hip, and spine (Perry 1992; Powers 2003). On the other hand, a pointed heel suggests an anteriorly directed center of mass that possibly overstresses the forefoot during the gait cycle.

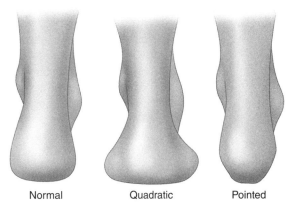

Normal   Quadratic   Pointed

Figure 5.6   Heel shapes.

Foot Posture

The foot plays an important role in weight bearing and propulsion, both of which require a high degree of stability. In addition, the foot must be flexible enough to adapt to uneven surfaces and absorb shock. The multiple bones and joints of the foot form an arch to serve the functions of both stability and flexibility. Inadequate muscular support of the foot leads to excessive stress on the various joints in the foot and on the proximal joints up the kinetic chain. Muscle imbalances in the lower kinetic chain can alter the precise balance of the foot and over time can cause tendon stresses or deformities such as hammertoes, claw toes, hallux valgus or bunions, curled toes, and so on. People with abnormally long toes, flat feet, or high arches have a greater tendency to develop toe deformities.

Spinal Extensors

Symmetry of the erector spinae muscle bulk at the lumbar and thoracolumbar regions is compared from side to side. In ideal postures, there are no significant differences between sides and regions of the spine. Hypertrophy of the thoracolumbar spinal extensors may indicate a compensatory overactivation of these muscles as a result of poor stabilization of the deep spinal stabilizers at the lumbar spine, a weak gluteus maximus, or tight hip flexors (see figure 5.7). In the presence of a weak and inhibited gluteus maximus, the ipsilateral thoracolumbar extensors help extend the trunk over the leg during the push-off phase of gait. This creates repetitive instability of the thoracolumbar spinal segments.

A horizontal groove may also be present. This groove indicates segmental hypermobility and is often the location where most lumbar motion is observed.

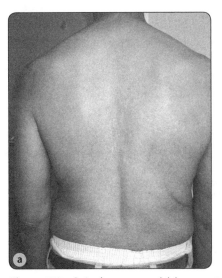 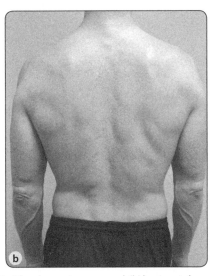

Figure 5.7   Spinal extensors. *(a)* Asymmetrical lumbar extensors and *(b)* horizontal grooves.

Scapular Region

The position of the scapula and the distance between the vertebral border of the scapula and the spine give valuable information about the quality of the musculature in this region. Normally the scapula is positioned between T2 and T7 and about 3 in. (7.6 cm) from the spine (Sahrmann 2001). The scapula should rest on the rib cage without observable winging. Any deviations from the normal position provide the clinician with valuable information on the quality and amount of shoulder girdle muscle activation. Flattening or hollowing of the interscapular area indicates inhibition and weakness of the rhomboids or middle trapezius (figure 5.8*a*). Similarly, flattening of the infraspinous or supraspinous fossa of the scapula indicates inhibition and weakness of the posterior rotator cuff (figure 5.8*b*).

If there is observable vertebral winging of the scapula (figure 5.8*c*), a weak serratus anterior or lower trapezius may be at fault. If the position of the scapula is abducted more than 3 in. (7.6 cm) from the spine (figure 5.9*d*), the imbalance may be reflected by weak dynamic scapular stabilizers (rhomboids and middle trapezius) and an overactive pectoralis major or minor or upper trapezius. In addition, overactive or dominant levator scapulae or rhomboids may cause the scapula to rotate downward, often contributing to impingement of the SA structures during arm elevation. All of these deviations contribute to the UCS described by Janda (see chapter 4).

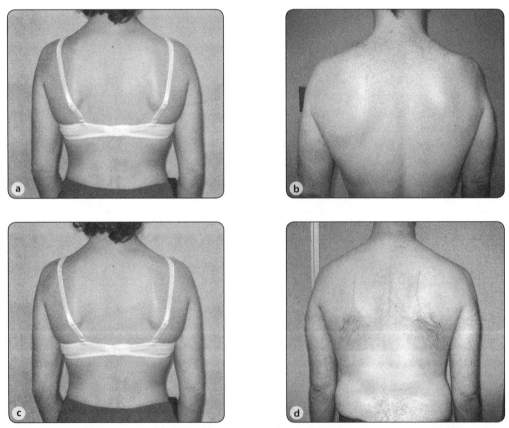

Figure 5.8 Scapular region. *(a)* Flat interscapular area with winging. *(b)* Infraspinatus atrophy (right side). *(c)* Scapular winging. *(d)* Scapular abduction. The left scapula is abducted more than 3 in. (7.6cm) from the spine.

Line of Neck and Shoulder

Tightness or shortness of the upper trapezius and levator scapulae can be observed at the line of the neck and shoulder. Straightening of this line indicates tightness of the upper trapezius. A gothic shoulder may also be observed when the upper trapezius is tight (figure 5.9*a*). The gothic shoulder is named after the Gothic-style church windows. If the levator scapulae is tight, a levator notch is observed (figure 5.9*b*) as an additional upward bulge in the area of the superior angle of the scapulae—in other words, at the insertion of the levator scapulae. Upper trapezius hyperactivity or dominance typically is associated with elevated and rounded shoulders, a forward head, and upper cervical extension, as found in Janda's UCS.

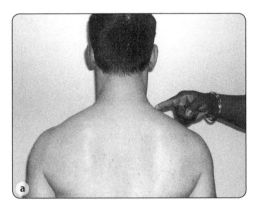 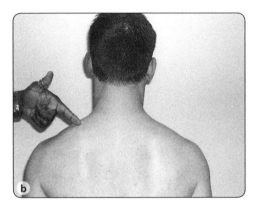

Figure 5.9 Line of the shoulder and neck. *(a)* Gothic shoulder on right. Note the increased slope of the line. *(b)* Levator notch, on left.

Anterior View

Once the posterior postural assessment is completed, the patient turns around. The clinician then assesses the anterior view, beginning again at the pelvic area.

Pelvic Tilt

The clinical observes the level of both ASISs. The findings here should confirm those of the pelvic position in the posterior view.

Abdominal Wall

The role of the abdominal muscles in the stabilization of the spine has been well established (Richardson et al. 2002; Richardson, Hodges, and Hides 2004; Hodges and Richardson 1996, 1998; McGill 2002). A sagging or protruding abdomen may reflect generalized weakness of the abdominal muscles and thus poor stabilization and protection of the low back from both normal and sudden movements. In addition, the upper and lower quadrants of the abdominal wall should be compared. An increased tone of the upper quadrants relative to the lower quadrants as well as a superiorly elevated rib cage suggests a faulty respiratory pattern (figure 5.10*a;* Lewit 1991; Kolář 2007). Overdominance of the obliques and a weak rectus abdominus may be observed as a distinct groove lateral to the rectus (figure 5.10*b*). This finding usually indicates decreased stabilization by the abdominal muscles in the anterior–posterior direction. Janda used the term *pseudohernia* to describe a lateral bulge in the abdomen, which indicates a weakness in the TrA (figure 5.10*b*).

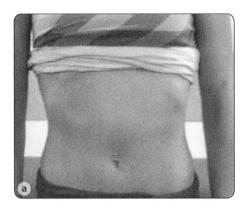 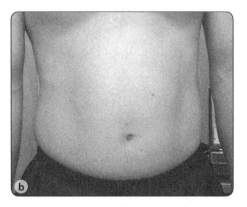

Figure 5.10 Abdominal wall. *(a)* Elevated position of rib cage. *(b)* Lateral abdominal groove (left side of the torso) and pseudohernia (right side of the torso).

Anterior Thigh Muscles

The quadriceps and TFL influence the lumbopelvic posture because of their insertions on the anterior ilium. Shortness or hypertonicity of these muscles contributes to the anterior pelvic tilt or rotated position in Janda's LCS (see chapter 4). Normally, the bulk of the TFL on the anterior proximal portion of the thigh is not visible in males and is rounded in females. However, a TFL that is distinct and coupled with the appearance of a groove on the lateral thigh usually indicates a short TFL that dominates over its synergist, namely the gluteus medius (figure 5.11). A tight tensor along with a weak gluteus medius and weak hip lateral rotators may result in a superior–lateral shift of the patella (Janda 1987; Janda, Frank, and Liebenson 2007). A short rectus femoris may contribute to a superior positioning of the patella in relation to the opposite knee.

A hypertrophied vastus medialis (figure 5.12) may indicate that the patient's sport requires repeated forced hyperextension of the knee joint, as is seen in soccer players

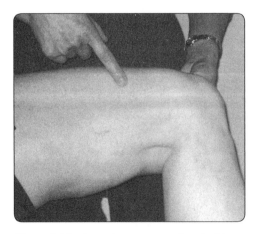 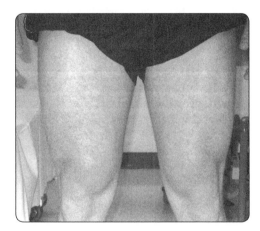

Figure 5.11 Lateral groove associated with tightness of the TFL.

Figure 5.12 Hypertrophy of the vastus medialis.

or cyclists. Genu recurvatum often accompanies vastus medialis hypertrophy. An atrophied medial quadriceps may indicate weakness of the entire muscle complex, as is commonly seen with arthrogenic inhibition of the knee.

Altered or inadequate proprioception from the knee joint may be detected by observing patella shifting in a superior–inferior direction. Such a shift is due to compensatory hyperactivity of the rectus femoris, typically the result of poor proprioception and neuromuscular control. Knee joint pathology often is responsible for such proprioceptive changes (Janda 1987 ; Janda, Frank, and Liebenson 2007).

Arm Position

Ideal shoulder alignment is less than one third of the humeral head protruding in front of the acromion (figure 5.13*a)* and neutral rotation with the antecubital fossa facing anteriorly and the olecranon process facing posteriorly. In addition, the proximal and distal ends of the humerus should lie in the same vertical plane. Any deviations from the ideal may indicate an imbalance of muscles about the shoulder joint complex. The most common deviation is medial rotation of the arms, which points to dominance of the medial shoulder rotators (see figure 5.13*b),* namely the pectoral and latissimus dorsi muscles over the lateral rotators. Internal rotation of the arms may also indicate a fixed thoracic kyphosis as in Scheuermann's disease or minimal brain dysfunction (Janda, 1978, 1994; Janda, Frank, and Liebenson 2007).

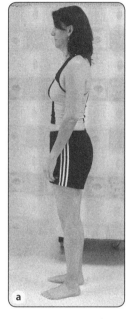
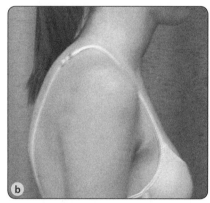

Figure 5.13 Position of the arms. *(a)* Ideal alignment of head and shoulders. *(b)* Medial rotation of the arm with anterior translation.

Pectoral Muscles

Tightness of the pectoralis major and minor usually results in a typical rounded and protracted shoulder position, as is often found in the UCS. A prominent muscle belly below the clavicle or a fuller thickness of the anterior axillary fold indicates a tight pectoralis major. The nipple line should be observed in males. Elevation of one nipple in relation to the other indicates tightness of the pectoral muscles on the elevated side (figure 5.14).

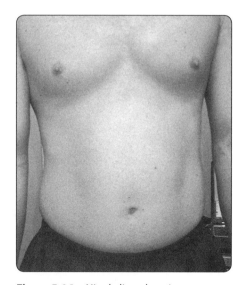

Figure 5.14 Nipple line elevation.

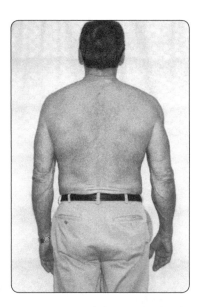

Figure 5.15 Left flattened deltoids with associated internal rotation of the arms.

Deltoids

Ideally, the deltoid muscles are rounded and symmetrical. Flattening of the deltoid muscle suggests a weakness or atrophy of the muscle (figure 5.15) and may be associated with a dysfunction at the C3-C4 segment. This is also an early sign of shoulder dysfunction.

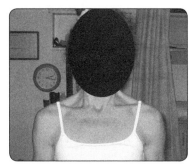

Figure 5.16 Overactive SCM and scalene muscles.

Sternocleidomastoid and Scalenes

In a patient with ideal posture, the SCM is slightly visible at the distal attachment at the sternum. Prominence of this muscle elsewhere with a groove along the medial border may indicate an overactive and tight SCM paired with weak deep cervical flexors (figure 5.16). Overactive SCM and scalene muscles may also result from an impaired respiratory pattern in which they act as accessory respiratory muscles due to diaphragm weakness or poor rib stabilization. In contrast, a groove anterior to the SCM indicates scalene weakness and often is noted in older adults.

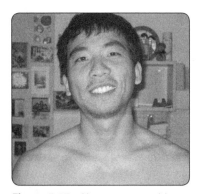

Figure 5.17 Uneven eye position, head compensation, and facial scoliosis.

Facial and Head Alignment

Visual position is the most important factor in orienting the head in the frontal plane (Zepa et al. 2003). The orientation of the eyes and other facial features in relationship to head position is an important diagnostic indicator for chronic musculoskeletal pain. Typically, the eyes should be parallel to the ear level, nose, and mouth. In some cases, the anatomical position of one eye is slightly higher than the position of the other (figure 5.17). During development the child compensates by orienting the head so that the eyes are parallel with the horizon. This changes the natural position of the head, which usually is slightly rotated to one side for compensation.

Janda described facial asymmetry, or facial scoliosis, in which the eyes, nose, and mouth are not parallel to each other, indicating a more severe alignment problem affecting the entire body (figure 5.17). He identified four points on the face to be aligned: the middle of the forehead, the bridge of the nose, the midmouth, and the midjaw. When present, facial scoliosis indicates possible total body asymmetry, which was also Janda's empirical observation of the various types of minimal brain dysfunction. Janda noted that persons with total body asymmetry have a poorer prognosis in chronic pain syndromes when compared with patients with isolated body asymmetries. Zepa and colleagues (2003) found that facial asymmetry is not affected by trunk asymmetry and hence concluded that facial scoliosis causes, rather than results from, body asymmetry.

Lateral View

The final postural view is the lateral view. With the patient in this position, the clinician first observes the general alignment of the head and spine, noting any excessive lordosis or kyphosis.

Chin and Neck Angle

The line of the throat is made by the angle between the chin and the throat. In the ideal posture, this angle is about 90°. Straightening of this line, which creates an angle greater than 90° (see figure 5.18), usually indicates an increased tone of the suprahyoid muscles; this may be the underlying cause of a temporomandibular joint (TMJ) dysfunction (Janda 1994).

Head Position

A forward head position is associated with an increased angular excursion at the upper and lower aspects of the cervical spine and is linked to weakness of the deep cervical flexors and dominance or tightness of the SCM, suboccipital, and scalene muscles. It is a classic sign of UCS. The faulty position of the head over the shoulders may overstress the atlanto-occipital, C3-C4, and T3-T4 joints. Poor endurance of the deep neck flexors has been associated with forward head posture in both healthy individuals (Grimmers and Trott 1998) and subjects experiencing headaches (Watson and Trott 1993).

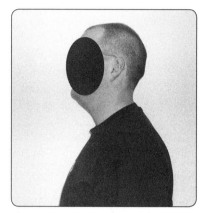

Figure 5.18 Excessive angle between the chin and the neck.

Evaluation of Balance

Janda noted that people rarely stand static on both legs. A majority of the gait cycle involves a single-leg stance, which requires lateral stabilization of the pelvis. The muscular lateral pelvic brace is provided by the gluteus medius, gluteus minimus, and TFL. As stated in chapter 2, poor postural stability is associated with several chronic musculoskeletal pain conditions such as neck and back pain. In addition, single-leg balance can discriminate patients with chronic back pain from those without pain (Luoto et al. 1998) and can be used to screen for risk of injury (McGuire et al. 2000; Tropp, Ekstrand, and Gillquist 1984).

A quick clinical test of these muscles is to have the patient stand on one leg. The patient is then asked to raise the opposite hip to 45° and knee to 90° while keeping the eyes open (see figure 5.19).

The single-leg stance test can be analyzed both qualitatively and quantitatively. Janda also described the following assessments of balance:

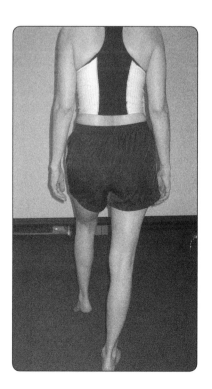

Figure 5.19 The single-leg stance test.

- **Static balance, qualitative assessment.** First, the clinician observes the quality of the movement as the patient attains and maintains single-leg balance, noting the amount of preshift to the stance leg and any unevenness of the pelvis or shoulders. Normally, preshift to the stance leg is no more than 1 in. (2.5 cm), and the patient should be able to maintain this single-leg stance for about 15 s without any compensatory movements. Excessive preshift of the pelvis, inability to hold 15 s of unilateral stance, elevation of the contralateral shoulder, or hip hiking indicates possible dysfunction. Inhibition or weakness of the lateral pelvic stabilizers is suspected if pelvic deviations are observed. These deviations include a lateral pelvic shift, contralateral hip drop (Trendelenburg sign), or medial rotation of the femur (secondary to the predominance of the TFL and hip medial rotators over the weaker or inhibited gluteus medius, gluteus minimus, and deep hip lateral rotators). The clinician also looks for excessive activity of the knee, tibialis anterior, or toes, which might indicate poor proprioception.

- **Static balance, quantitative assessment.** As in the qualitative test, the patient is asked to stand on one leg and, while keeping the eyes open, raise the opposite hip to 45° and flex the opposite knee to 90°. Next the patient is instructed to fix his gaze at a point directly in front of him and then close his eyes and attempt to balance himself on one leg for 30 s. The test is repeated up to five times per leg, and the best time is recorded for each leg. The test is discontinued if the patient opens his eyes, reaches with his arms, touches his non-weight-bearing foot onto the stance leg, hops, or puts his foot down. The following are the normative data for single-leg balance according to age (Bohannon et al. 1984):

Age	*Eyes Closed*
20-49 y	24-29 s
50-59 y	21 s
60-69 y	10 s
70-79 y	4 s

- **Dynamic balance testing (Janda's perturbation test).** Janda also described a more dynamic balance assessment in which he provided a small, unexpected displacement on the sacrum of patients during quiet standing. Patients were not aware of the perturbation and thus did not brace themselves. This test gave important information on the sensorimotor system processing for dynamic balance. Janda noted the dominant strategy the patient used to respond to the perturbation, studying the depth of forward displacement, the latency of attaining equilibrium, and the overall subjective quality of the response.

Evaluation of Gait

Gait mechanics have been discussed thoroughly in various texts (Perry 1992; Professional Staff Association of Rancho Los Amigos Medical Center 1989; Powers 2003; Inman 1966; Inman et al. 1981). The gait pattern is the most automatized movement; the basic reflexes for gait are regulated at the spinal cord level. However, the more complex reflexes are regulated on the subcortical or cortical levels. The gait pattern is highly individualized and deeply fixed in the CNS; it can be changed only with great difficulty. Walking involves a sequence of repetitious limb motions used to propel the body forward while maintaining stance stability. The gait cycle is defined as a single sequence of events for a single limb. Usually, the beginning is designated as the initial contact of the heel; the limb then progresses through midstance, terminal stance, and finally the swing phase. The gait cycle is 60% stance phase and 40% swing phase.

Phases of Gait and Associated Tasks

There are three distinct phases of the gait cycle. These are weight acceptance, single-limb support, and limb advancement.

- **Weight acceptance.** This phase is the most demanding task of the gait cycle because it requires an abrupt transfer of weight to a limb that has just completed the swing phase. Its two subphases include (1) initial contact, the point at which the foot touches the floor, typically at the heel, and (2) loading response, which covers the time from initial contact to contralateral toe-off. The three objectives of the weight acceptance phase are shock absorption, weight-bearing stability, and preservation of progression.

- **Single-limb support.** In this phase a person must support the body weight on one limb in addition to stabilizing the entire body while moving the body beyond the stationary foot. Its two subphases include (1) midstance (10%-30% of gait cycle), which is a single-limb stance used from contralateral toe-off to heel-off, and (2) terminal stance (30 %-50% of gait cycle), which is a single-limb stance used from heel-off to initial contact of the contralateral limb.

- **Limb advancement.** This phase involves completing limb advancement for forward progression as well as preparing the limb for stance. There are four main subphases of limb advancement: preswing, initial swing, midswing, and terminal swing. Table 5.2 summarizes the critical events in the gait cycle.

Table 5.2 Critical Events in the Gait Cycle by Phase

Weight acceptance (initial contact and loading response)	Single-limb support (midstance and terminal stance)	LIMB ADVANCEMENT	
		Preswing and initial swing	Midswing and terminal swing
Heel strike Knee flexion and ankle plantar flexion Heel rocker	Ankle dorsiflexion Heel rise Knee extension Hip hyperextension (trailing limb) Adequate pelvic stability Ankle rocker Forefoot rocker	Ankle dorsiflexion Adequate knee flexion (40°-60°) Adequate knee flexion	Ankle dorsiflexion Knee extension Adequate hip flexion (20- 30°) Adequate knee flexion (15°-25°)

Gait Pathology in Muscle Imbalance Syndromes

Adequate balance, timing, and recruitment of the musculature are imperative for smooth and efficient gait patterns. Any imbalance or any impaired recruitment and coordination of muscles in any part of the kinetic chain results in faulty patterns and inefficient energy expenditure. Skilled gait analysis provides important information to the clinician about possible overstresses of critical segments in the kinetic chain that may be causing or perpetuating a pain problem.

During the polio epidemic in the United States, several specific gait patterns were identified. These patterns corresponded to specific muscle weaknesses:

Muscle Weakness	*Gait Pattern*
Gluteus medius	Trendelenburg
Gluteus maximus	Lurch
Quadriceps	Knee hyperextension
Tibialis anterior	Foot slap

Not unsurprisingly, these muscles are the ones Janda classified as muscles prone to weakness. It is not uncommon to see these types of pathological gait to a very small degree in patients with LCS.

Janda described three specific types of gait. Each pattern relates to the mechanism used to propel the body forward.

• **Proximal gait pattern.** The body is propelled forward primarily through excessive hip and knee flexion, followed by hip extension past the midline. Greater overstress at the hip joints may result from this type of gait. The COG remains relatively level, and stresses on the ankle joint are minimal.

• **Distal gait pattern.** The body is propelled forward primarily through excessive plantar flexion with minimal motion at the hip and knee joints; the knee remains in extension. This gait pattern appears bouncy, as the COG is elevated with each step and the body simply falls forward. Overstress at the ankle and foot usually results from this type of gait.

• **Combined gait pattern.** Janda noted a combination of the proximal and distal gait patterns in some patients. These patients tend to have minimal hip flexion (as seen in the proximal gait pattern), as well as internal rotation, knee flexion, and foot eversion. The lower-extremity movement resembles that of the Charleston dance pattern.

Assessment and Observation of Gait

Gait assessment provides an overall picture of the dynamic function of the sensorimotor system. Patients are often instructed to walk distances of 20 ft (6.1 m) or more several times while the clinician observes the entire body both anteriorly and posteriorly. Much attention is directed toward the pelvis and trunk in the sagittal, frontal, and transverse planes.

Sagittal Plane

In the ideal gait pattern with adequate trunk stability, the pelvis and shoulders move forward in the same plane. However, if trunk stability is inadequate, the shoulders will lag behind the pelvis, causing overstress at the thoracolumbar or cervical joints.

During the terminal stance of gait, there should be an apparent hip hyperextension or trailing limb posture. However, if there is inadequate hip extension due to muscle imbalance or joint stiffness, the axis of motion may shift from the hip to the lumbar segments. The result is increased lumbar extension that overstresses these segments with each step the person takes. Overstress at the lumbar segments increases if the patient exhibits an existing anterior pelvic tilt.

The clinician should also study the movement of the upper extremities. The patient should demonstrate reciprocal flexion of the arm in tandem with movement of the contralateral hip (i.e., left swing phase equals left arm flexion). If there is no movement in the arms, the trunk often compensates with trunk rotation, which may place additional stress on spinal structures.

Frontal and Transverse Planes

Adequate lateral pelvic brace during the single-limb support in both the frontal and transverse planes is needed for efficient energy expenditure. The COG should stay relatively level when lateral pelvic and trunk stability is adequate. The primary muscles involved in supporting the lateral pelvic brace are the gluteal and abdominal muscles. The function of the gluteal muscles, in particular the gluteus medius, is necessary to counter the adduction moment and to control the femoral medial rotation during the early stance phase of the gait cycle. Excessive hip adduction during gait is the result of gluteus medius weakness (Reischl et al. 1999). Inadequate lateral pelvic and trunk stability and control often result in greater lateral pelvic shift on the stance leg, contra-lateral pelvic drop, or excessive pelvic rotation. In short, if pelvic motion is detected, it is usually excessive.

Janda also assessed backward walking to determine whether a gluteus maximus was simply inhibited or truly weak. If the gluteus maximus is weak, there will be a lack of hip extension that is compensated for by an increased lumbar lordosis or anterior pelvic tilt. If the gluteus maximus is only inhibited, the backward walk appears normal.

Summary

The sensorimotor system is functionally interdependent with the neurological and musculoskeletal systems. The muscular system lies at a functional crossroads because of its influence from both the CNS and the osteoarticular system. Dysfunction in any component of these systems is reflected by alterations in function elsewhere in the system, in the form of altered muscle balance, tone, contraction, coordination, and recruitment. Thorough analysis of posture, balance, and gait is essential to provide a clearer understanding of the status of the motor system and its relevance to the patient's symptoms.

EVALUATION OF MOVEMENT PATTERNS

Classic muscle strength testing involves providing a resistance against the characteristic movement of the tested muscle. Strength is tested along the structural lines of origin and insertion. Functional movement is never isolated because it is produced by several muscles acting as prime movers, synergists, or stabilizers that coordinate together. In addition, functional strength does not require maximal activation; rather, muscle onset and timing are more important. Hence, classic manual muscle strength testing does not provide sufficient or reliable information about the recruitment of all the muscles involved in functional movement.

While manual muscle testing (MMT) is an important tool, it gives clinicians little more than a quantification of weakness. Muscles that test strong during MMT may actually be inhibited when performing a coordinated movement pattern. On the other hand, muscles that test weak during MMT may only be inhibited. Janda described this as *pseudoparesis* (Janda 1989). He suggested that there are three characteristics of pseudoparesis: hypotonia, a score of 4 out of 5 during MMT, and delayed onset or absent EMG.

According to Janda, movement pattern analysis is more reliable than studying pain when assessing functional pathology because pain is very subjective. Movement patterns are examined immediately after the postural assessment so that touch or facilitation by the clinician does not influence any motor patterns. When observing movement patterns, the clinician should focus not only on the strength of the movement but also, and more importantly, on the sequencing and activation of all the synergists involved in the movement. In this respect, the initiation of the movement is more important than the final phase or completion of the movement. Understanding the quality and control of the movement pattern is imperative, as these characteristics may contribute to or perpetuate adverse stresses on the spine and other structures. Although movement and activation patterns are individualized due to variability in motor control, both typical and abnormal patterns can be observed. This chapter focuses on Janda's six basic movement patterns and their tests; these tests provide the clinician with valuable information regarding a patient's preferred movement strategy. Additional movement tests and selected MMT complementary to Janda's basic movement tests are also discussed.

Janda's Basic Movement Patterns

Janda identified six basic movement patterns that provide overall information about a particular patient's movement quality and control; these movements form the basis of the hip extension, hip abduction, curl-up, cervical flexion, push-up, and shoulder abduction movement pattern tests. Janda offered several important guidelines to follow when assessing these movements:

- The patient should disrobe as much as possible so that the clinician may visualize all parts of the body.

- The clinician should provide minimal verbal cues so that the patient's preferred movement pattern may be observed.
- The clinician should not touch the patient at all, as touch can be facilitatory.
- The patient should perform each movement slowly over three trials.

Each test has a typical motor response as well as clinical indicators of functional pathology. While Janda considered the firing order of these movements to be an important clinical sign, he also noted that the compensatory patterns observed during these movement tests are more valuable for diagnosis. The beginning of the movement is the most important for information on motor control (Janda 1984; Janda, Frank, and Liebenson 2007). The clinician should observe both the left and right sides for comparison. Muscle or limb trembling during these tests is considered a positive finding, indicating weakness or fatigue. Some patients do not need to perform all six tests at once; the clinician should decide which tests are indicated based on the postural analysis and history. Table 6.1 lists key indicators for the movement tests.

Table 6.1 Key Indicators for Janda's Movement Tests

Movement test	Key indicators
Hip extension	Decreased gluteus maximus bulk Increased hamstring bulk Observation of spinal horizontal grooves or creases Anterior pelvic tilt Increased or asymmetrical paraspinal bulk Decreased trailing limb posture at terminal stance during gait
Hip abduction	Lateral shift or rotation of pelvis Asymmetrical height of iliac crest Observation of adductor notch Adducted hips or varus position Increased lateral IT groove Positive result on single-leg stance test Trendelenburg sign or increased lateral pelvic shift during loading response during gait
Trunk curl-up	Decreased abdominal tone Lateral grooves in abdominal wall Impaired respiration Pseudohernia
Cervical flexion	Prominence of sternocleidomastoid at mid- to distal insertion Forward head posture Increased angle (>90°) between chin and neck Impaired respiration
Push-up	Forward head with protracted shoulders Increased internal rotation of arms Nipples that face out superiorly and laterally (in males) Scapula winging, tipping
Shoulder abduction	Forward head with protracted shoulders Gothic shoulder Levator notch Scapular winging, tipping

Hip Extension Movement Pattern Test

During the terminal stance of the normal gait cycle, the hip extends to the trailing limb posture of 10° of apparent hyperextension. There are 5° of backward pelvic rotation that contribute to these 10° of hyperextension. The functional significance of this trailing limb posture is that it allows the body to advance past the stable limb for forward progression (Perry 1992; Professional Staff Association of Rancho Los Amigos Medical Center 1989). Stiff or short hip flexors may reduce the available range in the hip and force the body to move the axis of rotation from the hip joint to a proximal point, namely the lumbar spine, in order to get the necessary forward progression.

The hip extension movement test is analyzed clinically to determine the patient's preferred recruitment pattern. The sequencing and degree of activation of the hamstrings, gluteus maximus, spinal extensors, and shoulder musculature are observed. To perform this test, the patient lies prone with the arms at the sides and the feet hanging over the table to allow for neutral leg rotation (see figure 6.1a). The patient's head should be placed in as neutral a position as possible. The patient is asked to lift the leg slowly toward the ceiling. Normally, the gluteus maximus as well as the contralateral lumbar erectors activate early in the movement. Janda suggested that a normal pattern of activation during prone hip extension is the hamstrings followed by the gluteus maximus followed by the contralateral erector spinae followed by the ipsilateral erector spinae.

The most common sign of a faulty movement pattern is over activation of the hamstrings and erector spinae and delayed or absent contraction of the gluteus maximus. The poorest pattern occurs when the thoracolumbar extensors or even the shoulder muscles initiate the movement delayed or absent the gluteus maximus contribution. Clinically, this pattern is observed as an anterior pelvic tilt with hyperlordosis in the lumbar spine as the patient lifts the leg into extension (figure 6.1b). Mechanical and compressive stresses in the lumbar spine are the result. An inability to maintain knee extension during the test should also be noted, as this observation may suggest hamstring dominance over the gluteus maximus (figure 6.1c). Positive findings during this test are associated with hypertrophy of the hamstrings and thoracolumbar extensors as well as atrophy of the gluteus maximus during postural analysis.

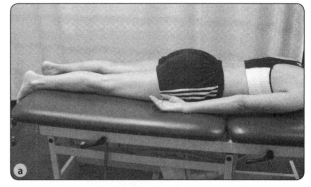

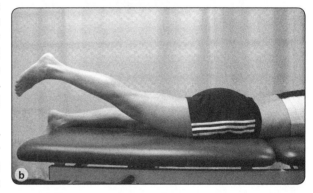

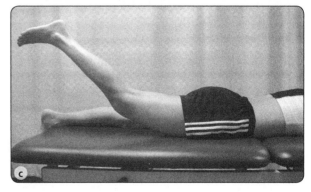

Figure 6.1 Prone hip extension test. *(a)* Starting position. *(b)* Lumbar extension and anterior pelvic tilt during hip extension. *(c)* Knee flexion during hip extension.

Occasionally, this faulty movement pattern overflows into the upper quarter and may be an underlying cause of neck pain. Clinicians should watch the contralateral insertion of the latissimus dorsi on the humerus for activation during hip extension. Such activation suggests poor spinal stabilization that is compensated for by a reverse action of the latissimus via the thoracolumbar fascia. Increased activity of the upper trapezius during the hip extension test is a sign of poor prognosis.

Studies of healthy human subjects (Bullock-Saxton, Janda, and Bullock 1994; Vogt and Banzer 1997; Pierce and Lee 1990; Hungerford, Gilleard, and Hodges 2003) have shown variations in the recruitment patterns and prime movers used for hip extension. Pierce and Lee (1990) found inconsistent patterns among healthy subjects; however, they began their hip extension test in 30° of hip flexion rather than in the neutral hip position used by Janda. Nevertheless, it is generally agreed that a delayed recruitment or a weak activation of the gluteus maximus induces compensatory overload stresses on the lumbar spine that are accompanied by simultaneous thoracolumbar erector spinae overactivity. Lewis and Sahrmann (2005) showed that patients with anterior hip pain have delayed onset of the gluteus maximus. Other studies (Hungerford, Gilleard, and Hodges 2003; Vogt and Banzer, 1997; Hodges and Richardson, 1996, 1998; McGill 2002; Radebold et al. 2001; Lee 1980) have shown the importance of the feed-forward mechanism (i.e., the anticipatory and stabilizing role of the abdominal muscles and lumbar erector spinae) in the premovement phase of hip extension for stabilizing the trunk to control the pelvis during limb movement.

Hip Abduction Movement Pattern Test

During the loading response phase of the gait cycle, the lower fibers of the gluteus maximus, hamstrings, and adductor magnus act eccentrically to counteract the hip flexion torque; thus, the hip joint is stabilized with minimal trunk flexion. In addition, the TFL, posterior gluteus medius and minimus, and upper fibers of the gluteus maximus contract eccentrically to stabilize the pelvis in the frontal plane. The result is that during midstance of the gait cycle, the pelvis is stabilized by the hip abductor group counteracting a strong varus (adductor) torque, thus preventing a hip drop or lateral shift of the pelvis.

The hip abduction test provides direct information about the quality of the lateral muscular pelvic brace and indirect information about the stabilization of the pelvis in the frontal plane during gait. This test is performed with the patient lying on her side with her bottom leg in a flexed position. The top leg is placed in a neutral position, in line with the trunk (figure 6.2a). The prime movers for hip abduction are the gluteus medius, gluteus minimus, and TFL, while the quadratus lumborum and abdominal muscles stabilize the pelvis during

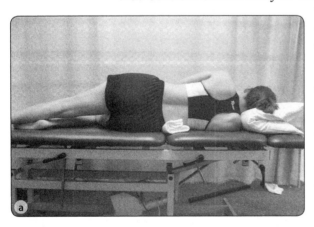

Figure 6.2a Hip abduction test. Start.

limb movement. The patient is instructed to lift the leg toward the ceiling (figure 6.2*b*). The normal pattern of hip abduction is abduction to about 20° without any hip flexion or internal or external rotation and with a stable trunk and pelvis—in other words, abduction without any hip elevation or trunk rotation.

Typically, the first sign of an altered movement pattern is the tensor mechanism of hip abduction facilitated by a tight TFL. Instead of pure hip abduction in the plane of the trunk, the movement is combined with hip flexion (figure 6.2*c*) due to the TFL's dual action as a hip flexor and abductor.

The poorest movement pattern is observed when the hip abduction is initiated by contraction

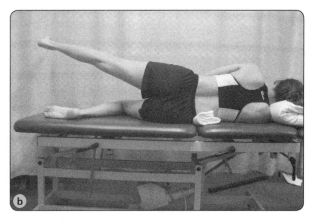

Figure 6.2b Hip abduction test. End.

of the quadratus lumborum before 20° of hip abduction, resulting in a lateral pelvic tilt or hip hike (figure 6.2*d*). In this case, the role of the quadratus lumborum changes from pelvic stabilizer to prime mover. Alterations observed in hip abduction can cause excessive stresses to the lumbosacral segments and hip during gait. Positive findings during the hip abduction test are associated with tightness of the IT band and atrophy of the gluteal muscles on the ipsilateral side during postural analysis and a failed single-limb stance test.

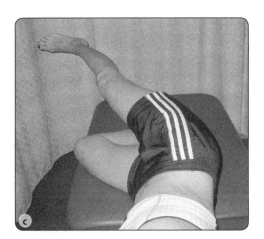
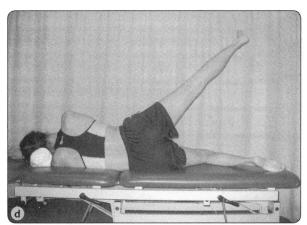

Figure 6.2 Hip abduction test. *(c)* Tensor mechanism. *(d)* Hip hike.

Trunk Curl-Up Movement Pattern Test

During the trunk curl-up, the abdominal muscles contract and shorten, thus flexing the spine. The upper trunk rounds, the lower back flattens, and the pelvis tilts posteriorly. The upward movement is completed when the scapulae clear the table. During this phase, the heels should remain in contact with the table. After the curl-up phase is completed, the hip flexors become dominant in further curling the spine into a sit-up position (Kendall, McCreary, and Provance 1993).

The trunk curl-up test estimates the interplay between the iliopsoas and the abdominal muscles. With the patient supine, the clinician analyzes the patient's preferred way of curling up. If the curl-up is performed with adequate abdominal contraction, a flexion or kyphosis of the upper trunk is observed. However, if the movement is performed primarily with the hip flexors, curling of the upper trunk is minimal and an associated anterior tilt of the pelvis may be observed.

The patient can also perform the curl-up test with the examiner placing his hands under the patient's heels to detect early loss of pressure (figure 6.3). If a loss of heel pressure is detected before the end of the curl-up, the test is positive, indicating the dominance of the hip flexors over the abdominal muscles (Jull and Janda 1987; Janda, Frank, and Liebenson 2007). This test has caused confusion and misinterpretation by some individuals describing a *Janda crunch* or *Janda sit-up* in which the patient performs the trunk curl while isometrically contracting the hamstrings. Janda suggested placing the hands under the patient's heels to detect heel elevation rather than provide resistance to knee flexion. Therefore, there is no such exercise as the Janda crunch, as some individuals have advocated.

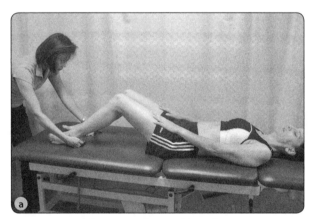 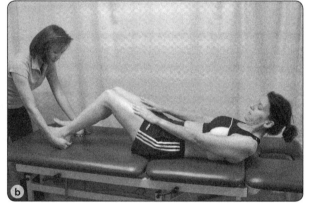

Figure 6.3 Curl-up test. *(a)* Start. *(b)* Finish.

Kendall has advocated using two separate tests to differentiate the upper- and lower-abdominal muscles because of their different attachments and respective lines of pull. The primary muscles involved in the trunk curl are the internal obliques and rectus abdominis; hence the term *upper-abdominal muscles.* The lower-abdominal muscles comprise the external obliques and the lower rectus abdominis, and these muscles are tested with the double-leg lowering test (Kendall, McCreary, and Provance 1993).

Lehman and McGill (2001) contend that a significant functional separation does not exist between the upper- and lower-abdominal muscles since the abdominal fascia contains the rectus abdominis and connects laterally to the aponeurosis of the three layers of the abdominal wall. Although regional differences do exist, all components of the abdominal muscles work both together and independently, resulting in spinal stability. The authors suggest the need for several exercise tests to challenge the various functioning divisions of the abdominal muscles (McGill 2002).

Cervical Flexion Movement Pattern Test

The primary deep flexors of the head and cervical spine are the longus capitis, longus colli, and rectus capitis anterior. Cervical spine and head flexion are also assisted by the SCM and anterior scalenes (Kendall, McCreary, and Provance 1993). A proper movement pattern would entail cervicocranial flexion throughout the test. The cervical flexion test estimates the interplay between the deep cervical flexors and the synergists, namely the SCM and anterior scalenes (see figure 6.4a). Surface EMG recordings of the SCM (Jull 2000) and direct recording of the deep neck flexor activity (Falla, Rainoldi, Merletti, and Jull 2003; Falla, Jull, Dall'Alba, Rainoldi, and Merletti 2003) have demonstrated a disturbance in synergistic movement in patients with idiopathic neck pain and patients with neck pain after whiplash injury. Impairments in the strength and endurance needed by the deep neck flexors for segmental control and support (Janda 1994; Jull 2000; Jull, Kristjansson, and Dall'Alba 2004) are compensated for by increased activity in the superficial SCM and anterior scalene. This finding is particularly true with patients experiencing recurrent headaches (Falla et al. 2003a,2003b; Falla, Jull, and Hodges 2004; Falla, Jull, and Hodges 2006; Jull, Barett, Magee, Ho 1999; Cibulka 2006).

This test is positive when the chin or jaw juts forward at the initiation of the movement (figure 6.4b). A jutting chin or jaw suggests a dominance of the SCM and scalenes over the weaker deep cervical flexors. A forward head posture indicates weak or inhibited deep cervical flexors. Observation of bulkiness at the middle of the SCM when the patient is at rest also suggests weakness of these flexors.

If the pattern is unclear, the clinician places 1 or 2 fingers against the patient's forehead to apply a slight resistance to the movement. This allows the clinician to detect any anterior translation of the cervical segments, which would confirm inadequate stabilization by the deep cervical flexors.

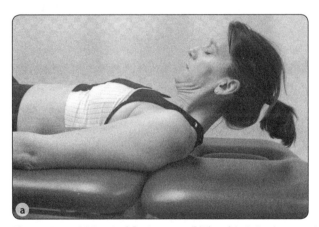 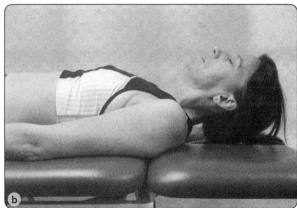

Figure 6.4 *(a)* Cervical flexion test. *(b)*The chin is jutting out, indicating a positive test.

Push-Up Movement Pattern Test

The push-up test examines the quality of dynamic scapular stabilization. When the patient performs the test properly, the scapula abducts and upwardly rotates as the trunk is lifted upward during the push-up. There is no associated scapular elevation. The force-coupling action of the serratus anterior and trapezius is imperative to provide the proper scapular movement, with the scapular synergists contributing to its stability (Cools et al. 2003). Weakness of the serratus anterior becomes evident when the patient displays winging of the scapula or excessive scapular adduction or is unable to complete the range of scapular motion in the direction of abduction. Dominance of the upper trapezius and levator scapulae is demonstrated by excessive shoulder elevation or shrug. The lowering of the body from the maximum push-up position is more sensitive in detecting excessive scapular rotation, elevation, tipping, winging, adduction, or abduction because of the eccentric loading on the muscles. The type of impaired scapular motion detected depends on the dominance of the associated synergists involved in the push-up movement pattern.

The push-up test is performed with the patient lying in a prone position with the legs extended in preparation for performing the push-up movement from the feet (see figure 6.5, *a-b)*. The clinician observes the quality of scapular and torso movements and notes any deviations from the ideal push-up movement (see figure 6.5, *c-d)*. This

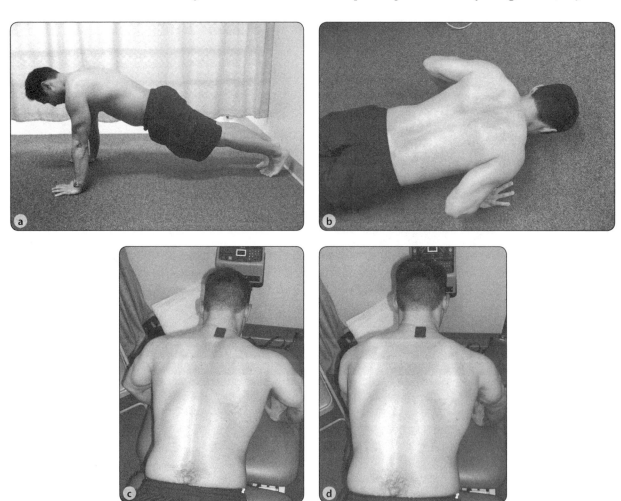

Figure 6.5   Push-up test. *(a)* Starting position. *(b)* Ending position. *(c)* Deviation. *(d)* Deviation.

test is quite challenging, as it requires adequate strength and endurance of the arm and torso muscles to maintain the erect posture of the body. If the patient is unable to perform this test with straight legs, she may perform the test with bent legs (figure 6.5*e*). Scapular winging, gothic shoulders, levator notch, and excessive bulk of the pectoral muscles observed during postural analysis indicate that the clinician should include the push-up test to confirm the muscular imbalances associated with the UCS described by Janda.

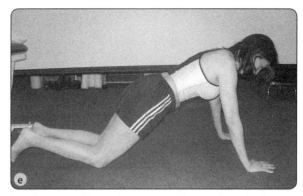

Figure 6.5e   The push-up test performed from the knees.

Shoulder Abduction Movement Pattern Test

The shoulder abduction test examines the coordination of the shoulder girdle muscles, namely the deltoids, rotator cuff muscles, upper trapezius, and levator scapula. Shoulder abduction in the frontal plane consists of synergistic abduction, scapular upward rotation, and scapular elevation.

The shoulder abduction test is performed with the patient in a seated position with the arms at the sides and the elbows flexed in order to control undesired rotation (figure 6.6*a*). Shoulder abduction comprises three major actions: abduction in the glenohumeral joint, upward rotation of the scapula, and elevation of the scapula. Activation of the contralateral upper trapezius is normal for stabilization. The decisive point of this movement pattern is at 60° of shoulder abduction, where there is an associated scapular elevation. Any noticeable elevation of the shoulder girdle before 60° of shoulder abduction is positive for incoordination and impairment of the force couples among the muscles involved in shoulder abduction (figure 6.6, *b-c*). Repeated or sustained shoulder girdle arm movements may overstress the spinal structures.

Possible causes of excessive scapular elevation during shoulder abduction are an overactive upper trapezius and levator scapulae. Initiation of shoulder abduction via shoulder girdle elevation, as is seen in patients with frozen shoulder syndrome, is also considered pathological. The worst scenario observed is contralateral lateral side bending of the trunk to initiate shoulder abduction. This movement pattern indicates severe weakness of the rotator cuff or deltoid and shortness or overactivity of the contralateral quadratus lumborum. Hypertrophy of the upper trapezius and atrophy of the deltoid and posterior rotator cuff are associated with positive findings. In addition, the shoulder abduction test commonly is associated with the observation of a gothic shoulder or levator notch during postural analysis.

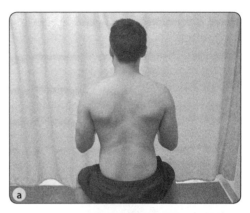

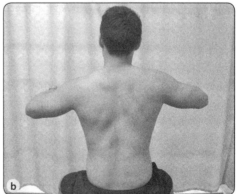

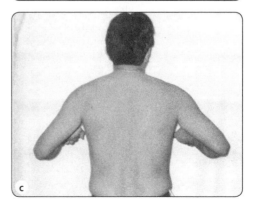

Figure 6.6   Shoulder abduction test. *(a)* Beginning position. *(b)* Faulty movement pattern. *(c)* Excessive right shoulder elevation before 60° of shoulder abduction. Note right cervical rotation, which indicates a dominance of the levator scapulae.

Additional Movement Tests Complementary to Janda's Tests

There are several other clinical tests of movement patterns that are complementary to Janda's basic movement tests. Some of these are tests for the deep cervical flexors, TrA, abdominal wall, and respiratory muscles.

Craniocervical Flexion Test

The craniocervical flexion (CCF) test assesses the strength and endurance of the deep neck flexors (Jull 2000). The patient is in a supine position with the knees bent and the feet flat (hook-lying position) to relax the lumbar spine. The head is in a neutral position; it should not be extended and the chin should not jut forward. If the patient is not able

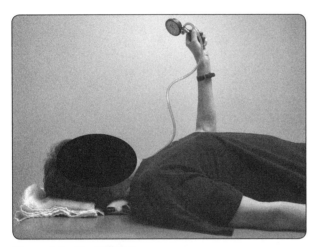

Figure 6.7 The CCF test.

to achieve this neutral position of the head, a small folded towel should be placed under the occiput, to leave the cervical spine free (see figure 6.7). An inflatable biofeedback pressure cuff is placed under the cervical spine to provide support. The inflatable cushion should not push the cervical spine forward, as this takes it out of the neutral position. Once the ideal position is established, the cushion is inflated to 20 mmHg. The pressure cuff dial can be turned toward the patient, so that he can see that the dial is set to 20 mmHg. The patient is then instructed to gently nod the head to a target of 22 mmHg on the cuff and to hold the dial steady for 10 s while breathing normally. If successful, the patient is instructed to relax to 20 mmHg and, after resting, to perform the chin nod movement to a target of 24 mmHg and hold for 10 s. This procedure is repeated to target pressures of 26, 28, and 30 mmHg; each time the patient should maintain the target pressure for 10 s. Ideal performance is when the patient holds the pressure steady for 10 s at 28 or 30 mmHg. Failure occurs if the patient is unable to reach the target pressure or hold the target pressure for 10 s. Another sign of failure is overactivation of the superficial SCM muscles. Both patients with insidious-onset cervical pain and patients with whiplash demonstrate significantly increased SCM EMG activity when compared with control subjects at each test level, regardless of whether the pain is acute or chronic (Jull, Kristjansson, and Dall'Alba 2004). Falla, Jull, and Hodges (2004) have shown the association between poor performance of this test and dysfunction of the deep cervical flexors. The CCF test may provide a more specific method to assess and retrain the deep cervical flexors when compared with the conventional cervical flexion exercises in which superficial muscle activity may mask impaired performance of the deep cervical flexors (O'Leary et al. 2007).

Transversus Abdominis Test

A latent or absent recruitment of the TrA and activation of the multifidi have been demonstrated in both acute and chronic low back pain cases (Richardson, Jull, Hodges, and Hides 1999; Hodges and Richardson 1996, 1998). The Queensland group has observed that a drawing in, or hollowing, of the abdominal wall recruits the TrA and so has developed an assessment and treatment tool to target the motor reeducation of this muscle. Independent activation of the TrA is a skill and requires practice, even in people without a history of low back pain. The clinician must carefully observe the contraction of the superficial abdominal muscles to flatten the abdominal wall.

The abdominal hollowing test can be performed in any body position, but it is useful to have the patient perform the test in the prone position to increase the awareness of the abdominal movements (figure 6.8a). The clinician monitors the active contraction of the TrA by palpation medial to the anterior superior iliac spines. The patient is instructed to gently draw her lower abdomen and navel inward toward the spine without moving the spine or pelvis. Once the patient has practiced several times, the formal testing can be performed.

A pressure cuff is positioned under the abdomen so that the navel lies in the center of the cuff and the distal edge of the cuff is at the level of the ASISs (figure 6.8b). The cuff is inflated to 70 mmHg and the patient is instructed to draw in the lower abdomen gradually, as performed in the practice sessions. Ideally, the patient is able to reduce the pressure by 4 to 6 mmHg by contracting the TrA and then maintain this reduced pressure for 10 s. This maneuver is repeated 10 times. Inadequate TrA contraction results in a pressure reduction of less than 4 mmHg, whereas excessive contraction of the superficial abdominal muscles results in a pressure reduction of greater than 10 mmHg. The clinician must also watch for thoracolumbar hypertonus, lumbar extension, posterior pelvic tilt, and breath holding.

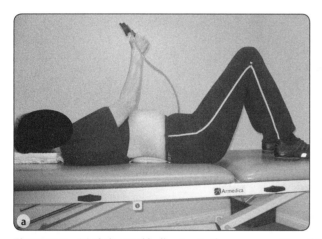 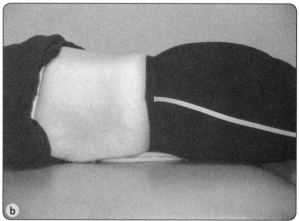

Figure 6.8 *(a)* Abdominal hollowing in the prone position. *(b)* Pressure cuff placement for the prone position.

Abdominal Bracing

Recruitment of the TrA has been shown to be impaired following injury (Richardson et al. 1999) and abdominal hollowing has been advocated by the Queensland group as a means to increase TrA recruitment. While hollowing may be used for motor reeducation, McGill and colleagues have argued that hollowing does not ensure or enhance spinal stability (McGill 2002; Grenier and McGill 2007).

Sufficient spinal stability can be ensured by abdominal bracing. Abdominal bracing does not entail a hollowing or pushing out of the abdominal wall. Rather, it requires maintaining a mild isometric contraction in the abdominal wall, or stiffening up the entire abdominal wall without changing it geometrically (Juker et al. 1998; McGill 2002). The coactivation of the TrA and external and internal obliques has been demonstrated to ensure spinal stability in various possible positions of instability (Lehman and McGill 2001; McGill 2002; Grenier and McGill 2007). High levels of co-contraction are rarely required: McGill (2002) proposes that 10% or less maximal voluntary co-contraction of the abdominal wall is sufficient for ADL. However, if a joint has lost stiffness because of damage, more co-contraction may be required.

The clinician introduces the concept of abdominal bracing by asking the patient to stiffen up one joint, perhaps an elbow, by simultaneously contracting the flexors and extensors. The patient is then asked to palpate her muscles and joints and to compare the co-contraction and relaxation of the muscles in various positions of the joint. Once the patient can successfully stiffen up various peripheral joints, she is asked to replicate the technique on her torso. It is important to observe how the patient performs an abdominal brace. An ideal technique does not involve a geometric change in the shape of the belly. The clinician should not see excessive sucking in or a pushing out of the abdominal wall as in a Valsalva maneuver. The patient is then instructed to add some level of abdominal bracing to independent arm or leg movements and eventually incorporate bracing into her exercise program or ADL.

Breathing Patterns

Breathing is regulated and coordinated by the autonomic nervous system. The rate and volume of breath is influenced by physical, chemical, and emotional factors. Under normal functioning circumstances, the rate and volume of breathing return to the relaxed baseline state once a demand or threat has been removed. Faulty respiration develops subcortically to compensate for injury or pain or to maintain the blood pH in response to stress, altitude, infection, or pathology. A faulty breathing pattern may perpetuate on a subcortical level and lead to an ingrained motor program, even when the initial trigger no longer exists. This is often seen in chronic hyperventilation (Gardener 1996), in which the faulty pattern often becomes self-perpetuating.

Correcting a faulty respiratory pattern is integral to the success of any rehabilitation program addressing the movement system. Treatment must be directed at restoring normal subcortical motor programs through motor training. For respiratory training to be effective, the new motor program must be practiced repeatedly under various conditions until it becomes the program of choice. When voluntary motor training is unsuccessful, reflex therapy as described by Vojta and Peters (2007) and Kolář (2007) is necessary to activate postural reactions including physiological respiration. Lewit (1980) contends that no other movement can be normalized if the breathing pattern is not. Thus, a routine examination of the neuromuscular system must include an evaluation of the respiration pattern, especially for patients with chronic musculoskeletal pain symptoms and limited response to previous therapies.

The primary muscles responsible for respiration are the diaphragm, intercostals, scalenes, TrA, pelvic floor muscles, and deep intrinsic spinal muscles (Hruska 1997). Each of these muscles plays a role in both respiration and spinal stabilization. According to Kendall, McCreary, and Provance (1993), of the 20 primary and accessory muscles associated with respiration, almost all of them have a postural function.

Some patients may show relatively normal respiratory patterns when relaxed in a supine position but may change into accessory-muscle or chest breathers when challenged in a functional position such as sitting at a computer or standing erect. Thus respiration patterns should be assessed with the patient in various positions, especially any painful positions used in ADL. A simple test is for the clinician to gently rest her hands on the patient's shoulders during quiet breathing to note any upward movement of the shoulders that would indicate accessory respiration (figure 6.9). There are several things to observe in assessing respiration:

- Initiation of breath—the initiation of breathing should be at the abdominal region and not the chest.
- Lateral excursion of the lower rib cage during inspiration—movement of the rib cage is best assessed with the patient in the seated or standing position.

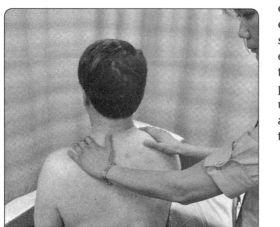

Figure 6.9 Assessment of accessory respiration with the patient in sitting position.

- Upper-chest expansion during the final phase of inspiration—the most common faulty pattern is the superior or cranial excursion, or lifting of the upper ribs by the scalenes and upper trapezius to substitute for inefficient or inhibited diaphragm activity.

There are several primary respiratory faults:

- Superior excursion, or lifting of the entire rib cage during inspiration
- Chest movements that predominate over abdominal movements
- Minimal or absent lateral excursion of the lower ribs
- Paradoxical breathing, or hollowing of the abdomen during inhalation and bulging of the abdomen during expiration
- Inability to maintain an abdominal brace during normal breathing

The following secondary respiratory faults may also be present:

- Shallow breathing with minimal or absent movement in the abdomen or rib cage
- Asymmetrical rib cage or abdomen movements
- Alterations in the sequencing of motion from lower abdomen to middle chest to upper chest
- Observable or palpable excessive tension in face, neck, or jaw
- Frequent sighs or yawns

Selected Manual Muscle Tests

MMT has been covered extensively in many texts. This section focuses on MMT of a few key muscles that are often tested weak with the movement pattern tests. Aside from quantifying the strength of the muscle, noting the quality and intensity of the muscle contraction is important; hence, the clinician should palpate the muscle that is being tested. The gluteus maximus and medius are involved in stabilizing the pelvis, particularly in stance and gait. These are the muscles that commonly are weakened or inhibited in the LCS. The middle and lower trapezius are weakened or inhibited in the UCS, often resulting in shoulder and cervical pain dysfunctions. Latency in recruitment in these muscles has been demonstrated in subjects with shoulder impingement syndromes (Cools et al. 2003).

Gluteus Maximus

Gluteus maximus strength is tested with the patient in the prone position with the knees flexed to 90° in order to place the hamstrings in a mechanically disadvantaged position for assisting in hip extension (see figure 6.10). The clinician moves the patient's thigh into hip extension, ensuring that the lumbar spine is neutral (neither flexed or extended). Once this position is established, the patient is instructed to hold the leg up actively as the clinician gradually removes the support under the thigh. At the same time, the clinician monitors the quality of the muscle contraction with her other hand over the gluteus muscle belly and observes for compensatory movements at the lumbar spine and pelvis. If the patient is able to hold the thigh against gravity, the clinician provides gradual downward resistance at the distal thigh. The muscle is graded according to how much resistance the patient is able to hold against.

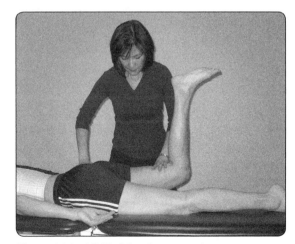

Figure 6.10 MMT of the gluteus maximus.

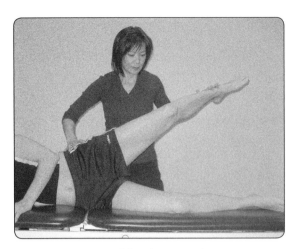

Figure 6.11 MMT of the gluteus medius.

Gluteus Medius

Gluteus medius strength is tested with the patient in the side-lying position (see figure 6.11). The patient's bottom leg is flexed at the hip and knee, and the pelvis of the top leg is rotated slightly forward to place the posterior fibers of the gluteus medius into an anti-gravity position (Kendall, McCreary, and Provance 1993). The clinician then abducts the leg. A slight external rotation of the hip is added to challenge the posterior fibers of the gluteus medius. The patient is then instructed to hold the leg in the test position. If the patient is able to hold the position, the clinician applies resistance near the ankle in the direction of adduction and slight flexion. Weakness of the gluteus medius may become apparent by the inability of the patient to hold the test position, by the tendency of the muscle to cramp, or by the posterior rotation of the pelvis in an attempt to substitute with the TFL and the gluteus minimus.

Middle and Lower Trapezius

The tests for the middle and lower trapezius are especially useful for patients with faulty shoulder positions or upper-back, cervical, and arm pain. These muscles are often weak or inhibited in the UCS. The middle and lower trapezius are tested with the patient in a prone position. The patient's arm is abducted at 90° or 130°, respectively, and slightly externally rotated (see figure 6.12, *a-b*). Care is taken to place the shoulder in external rotation to ensure the upward or lateral rotation of the scapula. The patient should be able to hold the test position of adduction and upward rotation without shoulder girdle elevation. Resistance is applied in a downward direction (toward the table) at the distal forearm. Weakness in the middle and lower trapezius is apparent when the patient is unable to hold the test position. Weakness may also result

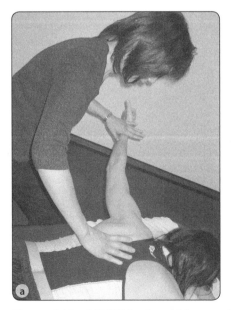
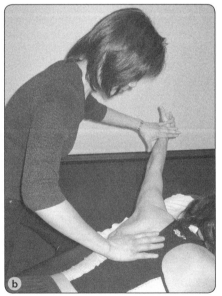

Figures 6.12 *(a)* MMT for the middle trapezius. *(b)* MMT for the lower trapezius.

in scapular abduction and a forward position of the scapula due to the dominance of the pectoral muscles or scapular elevation due to the dominance of the upper trapezius. Another common faulty pattern is increased medial rotation of the shoulder and downward or lateral rotation of the scapula through increased rhomboid muscle activity. The muscles of the middle and lower trapezius reinforce the thoracic spine extensors, and when they are weak they increase the tendency toward kyphosis at the midthoracic spine.

Janda suggested another way to test the lower trapezius (figure 6.12c). The patient lies down in a prone position with the test arm overhead, in line with the line of pull of the lower trapezius. The clinician places her hand on the lower trapezius at the medial edge of the scapula. The patient is then instructed to adduct and depress his scapula against the clinician's resistance. The clinician grades the quality and quantity of lower-trapezius activation while noting any compensatory movements of the cervical spine and lumbar spine into extension or any overactivation of the thoracolumbar paraspinals and latissimus dorsi.

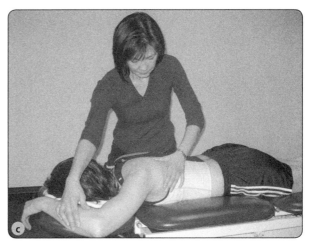

Figure 6.12c Janda's test for the lower trapezius.

Summary

In functional pathology, the quality of movement is more important than the test for muscle strength. The clinician focuses on the quality, sequencing, and degree of activation of the muscles involved in the movement pattern in order to evaluate the coordination of the synergists. The quality and control of the movement pattern are imperative, as the movement pattern may contribute to or perpetuate adverse stresses on the spine and other joint structures.

MUSCLE LENGTH TESTING

As described in chapter 4, Janda identified a group of muscles prone to tightness (see table 4.2 on page 48). Muscle tightness decreases ROM, facilitates (often unwanted) activation, or causes inhibition of a reciprocal muscle. Clinicians must be able to quantify muscle tightness and determine its possible causes in order to provide the most effective treatment. Generally, assessment of muscle length is performed after the movement pattern assessment and is used to confirm the clinical observations made during the posture and movement pattern evaluations.

According to Mense and Simons, "Muscle tone or muscle tension depends physiologically on two factors: the basic viscoelastic properties of the soft tissues associated with the muscle, and/or the degree of activation of the contractile apparatus of the muscle" (Mense and Simons 2001, p. 99; see figure 7.1). The basic viscoelastic properties of the muscle involve muscle tightness, stiffness, and loss of extensibility (length), whereas the contractile apparatus involves increased contractile activity as seen in trismus spasms of TMJ muscles or spasmodic torticollis. With respect to the viscoelastic changes, the muscle may shorten or stiffen (decrease in extensibility) secondary to the shortening of the contractile muscle fibers or the retraction of the intramuscular connective tissue or adjacent fascia. On the other hand, contractile muscle tone may involve the majority of muscle fibers in the muscle or a selected number of muscle fibers as seen in taut bands in TrPs (see chapter 8).

Clinically, resting muscle tone is a combination of both contractile and viscoelastic properties. Tight muscles have a higher resting muscle tone and a lower irritability threshold, meaning that these muscles are more readily recruited in movements. The presence of a higher muscle tone and its presence and its lower irritability threshold contribute to the inhibition of the reciprocal muscle. The perpetuation of this pattern contributes to the perpetuation of muscle imbalance, often leading to pain and dysfunction. Stretching a tight muscle or inhibiting the resting muscle tone of a tight muscle may spontaneously improve the strength of the inhibited reciprocal muscles; this improvement is probably mediated via Sherrington's law of reciprocal inhibition (Sherrington 1906).

Muscles that are moderately tight generally test stronger than normal. However, in the case of pronounced muscle tightness, some decrease of muscle strength occurs. Janda referred to this weakness as a *tightness weakness* indicating long-standing tightness (Janda 1986a). The treatment for this kind of tightness is not strengthening, as strengthening results in further shortening and thus further weakness. Instead,

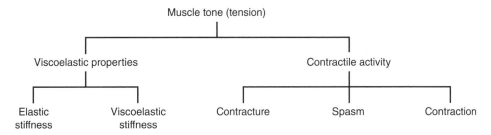

Figure 7.1 Factors influencing muscle tone.

Adapted, by permission, from S. Mense and D.G. Simons, 2001, *Muscle pain: Understanding its nature, diagnosis, and treatment. Pain associated with increased muscle tension* (Baltimore: Lippincott, Williams & Wilkins), 100.

treatment is directed toward stretching the viscoelastic property, or the noncontractile but retractile connective tissue, of the muscle.

Muscle length testing is most useful for patients with recurrent or chronic pain. Increased muscle tone or decreased muscle length may provide an explanation for limited success of a strengthening program of weak muscles. This chapter presents detailed techniques for testing key lower- and upper-quarter muscles and provides a commentary on joint hypermobility.

Muscle Length Assessment Technique

Muscle length testing involves elongating the muscle in the direction opposite of its action while assessing its resistance to passive lengthening. Precise testing requires that one of the bony attachments of the muscle (usually the origin) be in a fixed position while the other bony attachment is moved passively in the direction of lengthening the muscle. In other words, muscle length testing assesses the resistance to passive movement. This is in contrast to typical flexibility or ROM testing. The actual ROM can be measured for documentation purposes, but it gives limited clinical information in muscle imbalance syndromes. The most valuable clinical information is the muscular end feel and the location of the ROM end feel. The elongation of the muscle should be performed slowly to avoid eliciting a quick stretch of the muscle spindle and subsequently inducing a twitch response and muscle contraction. In addition, for the best accuracy and precision, muscle length testing should be performed when the patient is not in acute pain in order to avoid pain inhibition and muscle guarding. In summary, there are four steps to assessing muscle length:

1. Ensure maximal lengthening of the muscle from origin to insertion.
2. Firmly stabilize one end (usually the origin).
3. Slowly elongate the muscle.
4. Assess the end feel.

Following are the procedures for testing key muscles. Clinicians do not have to perform muscle length testing on every muscle listed; instead, they should assess the muscles that the postural and movement pattern analysis indicate as being possibly tight. Once tight muscles have been identified, the clinician can establish a muscle imbalance pattern (if present) and begin to look for causes of the tightness. Table 7.1 provides the normal results of muscle length for flexibility testing.

Table 7.1 Normal Results of Muscles Tested for Length

Muscle	Normal ranges or end feel
Iliopsoas	0° hip extension, 10° with overpressure
Rectus femoris	90° knee extension, 125° with overpressure
TFL-IT band	0° hip abduction (neutral), 15°-20° with overpressure
Adductors	0° hip abduction (neutral), 20°-25° with overpressure in the modified Thomas test position 45° hip abduction in supine position
Hamstrings	80° hip flexion with contralateral leg extended 90° hip flexion with contralateral leg flexed

Muscle	Normal ranges or end feel
Triceps surae	0° ankle dorsiflexion
Quadratus lumborum	Thoracolumbar curve should be smooth and gradual
Piriformis	Gradual soft end feel
Upper trapezius	Gradual soft end feel
Levator scapulae	Gradual soft end feel
SCM	Gradual soft end feel
Pectoralis major	*Sternal portion (lower fibers):* with shoulder abducted at 150°, arm should be horizontal to table and 15°-20° with overpressure *Sternal portion (midfibers):* with shoulder abducted to 90°, arm should be horizontal to table and 30° with overpressure *Clavicular portion:* with shoulder abducted to 60°, arm should hang freely over table
Paraspinals	Schober's test: excursion of >2.4 in. (6 cm)

Lower-Quarter Muscles

The muscles of the lower quarter include those of the leg, pelvis, and lower back. The muscles prone to tightness are those involved in maintaining a single-leg stance (Janda 1987). Tightness of the hip flexors and tightness of the thoracolumbar extensors are hallmark signs of Janda's LCS.

Modified Thomas Test for Hip Flexor

The modified Thomas test (figure 7.2, *a-e*) allows the clinician to assess four different muscles prone to tightness namely, the one-joint hip flexor, iliacus and psoas major, and the two-joint hip flexors, rectus femoris and TFL-ITB. Tightness of the hip flexors limits hip hyperextension in gait and may cause an anterior pelvic tilt. Weakness of the gluteus maximus often is due to facilitation of the hip flexors.

Patient Position

The patient is asked to sit on the edge of the table, with the coccyx and ischial tuberosities touching the table and one foot on the floor. Then, the patient is asked to flex the opposite hip and knee toward the chest and maintain the position with the hands (see figure 7.2*a*).

Clinician Position

The clinician stands beside the leg not being tested, facing the patient. While supporting the patient by placing one hand on the midthoracic spine and the other on the knee, the clinician passively rolls the patient down to the table to the supine position. The clinician needs to ensure that the patient's knees are flexed, lumbar spine is flexed, and pelvis is in posterior rotation to fix the origin of the hip flexors.

Test

The clinician passively lowers the tested leg until resistance is felt or movement at the pelvis is detected. With the patient's thigh in the final resting position, the clinician observes whether it is in neutral and parallel to the table or abducted. A normal length of the one-joint hip flexors with the lumbar spine and sacrum flat on the table is indicated by the posterior thigh touching the table (0° of hip extension). With slight overpressure, the thigh should reach 10° to 15° of hyperextension (figure 7.2, *b-c*). Prominence of a superior patellar groove (figure 7.2*d*) suggests a short rectus femoris, while prominence of a lateral IT groove suggests a short IT band (see figure 7.2*e*).

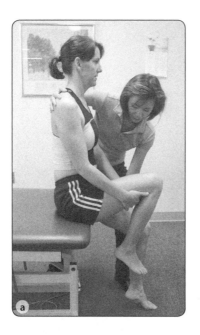

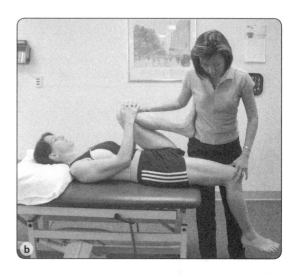

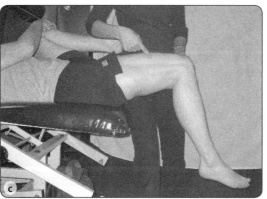

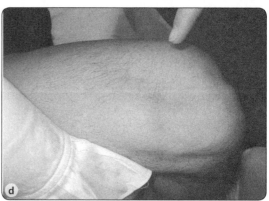

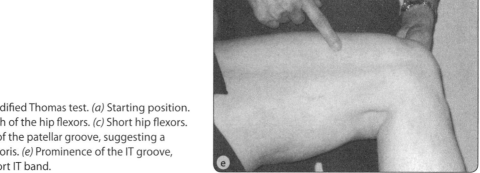

Figure 7.2 Modified Thomas test. *(a)* Starting position. *(b)* Normal length of the hip flexors. *(c)* Short hip flexors. *(d)* Prominence of the patellar groove, suggesting a short rectus femoris. *(e)* Prominence of the IT groove, suggesting a short IT band.

The position of the thigh should be examined for the following:

- **Flexed position of the hip.** To differentiate between the one- and two-joint hip flexors when the thigh does not reach or touch the table, the clinician should extend the knee to place the two-joint hip flexors on slack. If the range of hip flexion decreases and moves closer to the table, the two-joint hip flexors are predominately short. If the hip flexion range remains unchanged, the one-joint hip flexors are predominantly short.

- **Abducted position of the thigh.** The clinician should be able to move the patient's hip into 15° to 25° of passive abduction and 15° to 20° of passive adduction. The clinician brings the patient's thigh to neutral; if hip flexion increases, a TFL-IT band shortness is confirmed. A lateral deviation of the patella may also be observed when the TFL is tight.

- **Knee flexion less than 80°.** Ideally, the rectus femoris lengthens to provide about 80° of knee flexion with the hip at 0° of extension. A short rectus femoris is suggested by knee flexion less than 80°. Prominence of a superior patellar groove may also be observed when the rectus femoris is short.

Hamstring Muscle Length Test

The gluteus maximus and hamstrings are synergists for hip extension. However, when the gluteus maximus is weak, the hamstrings often act as the primary hip extensor in order to compensate for the gluteus maximus, and this altered muscle imbalance eventually leads to faulty movement and recruitment patterns. Hamstring length should be assessed in patients who display altered hip extension or increased muscle bulk in the distal two thirds of the hamstrings on postural assessment.

Patient Position

The standard position is supine with the opposite leg extended. Alternatively, the opposite leg can be flexed to allow the back extensors to relax or to accommodate a patient with short hip flexors.

Clinician Position

The clinician stands beside the leg being tested, facing the patient. In order to control for leg rotation, the clinician cradles the patient's heel in the crook of her elbow and places slight pressure on the tibia in order to maintain knee extension during the straight-leg raise. The clinician places her other hand on the ASIS of the leg being tested; this is done in order to detect pelvic movement (see figure 7.3).

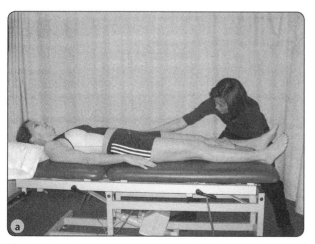 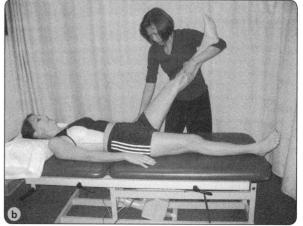

Figure 7.3 Hamstring length test. *(a)* Starting position. *(b)* Ending position.

Test

The clinician passively raises the leg being tested until the pelvis moves upward, which indicates the end of the hamstring length. The normal length of the hamstrings, as indicated by Kendall, McCreary, and Provance (1993), is 80° of hip flexion with the contralateral leg extended and 90° with the contralateral leg flexed. Hip flexion of 70° or less reveals a significant loss of hamstring extensibility that may lead to reflexive inhibition of the quadriceps or gluteus maximus.

Adductor Muscle Length Test

The adductors stabilize the hip in conjunction with all the other pelvic girdle and trunk muscles. When the adductors are tight or hypertonic, their antagonists (the gluteus medius and deep hip external rotator intrinsic muscles) may experience reciprocal inhibition. Adductor muscle length should be tested when an adductor notch is noted during the postural assessment or when a patient stands with excessive hip adduction with or without excessive medial femoral rotation. Single-leg balance and gait analysis may reveal inadequate lateral pelvic stability.

Patient Position

The patient lies supine with the legs extended. The leg not being tested is placed into 15° of abduction in order to assist with stabilization of the pelvis.

Clinician Position

The clinician stands beside the leg being tested, facing the patient. In order to control for leg rotation, the clinician cradles the patient's heel in the crook of her elbow and places slight pressure on the tibia in order to maintain knee extension during the straight-leg raise. The clinician places her other hand on the ASIS of the leg being tested; this is done in order to detect pelvic movement.

Test

The clinician passively slides the patient's leg into abduction until lateral movement of the pelvis is detected. The normal length of the adductors, as stated by Kendall, McCreary, and Provance (1993), is hip abduction to 45° without lateral movement of the pelvis (figure 7.4a). If the adductors are found to be short, the one- and two-joint hip adductors can be differentiated by passively flexing the knee to 15°. Doing so places the two-joint hip adductors (adductor longus, gracilis, and medial hamstrings) on slack. An increase in the range of hip abduction when the knee is flexed indicates that the shortness is in the two-joint hip adductors. If the hip abduction remains unchanged, the one-joint hip adductors are likely short (figure 7.4b).

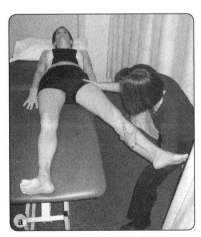 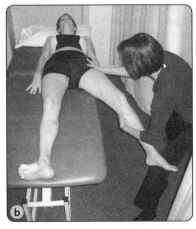

Figure 7.4 (a) Ending position of the adductor muscle length test. (b) Differentiating the one- and two-joint adductors.

Triceps Surae Muscle Length Test

Triceps surae tightness is often the hidden cause of low back pain (Janda 1987; Janda, Frank, and Liebenson 2007). When the triceps surae are tight, the body's center of mass shifts anteriorly, often causing compensatory overactivation of the thoracolumbar paraspinals to maintain erect posture during quiet stance and gait. This overactivation places abnormal compressive stresses on the lumbar segments and helps perpetuate the chronic low back pain cycle.

Patient Position

The patient lies supine with the leg not undergoing testing flexed and the corresponding foot resting on the table. The leg being tested is extended with the foot hanging over the edge of the table.

Clinician Position

The clinician sits or stands at the edge of the table, facing the patient. The clinician's hand should be in a hook position, with the third, fourth, and fifth metacarpophalangeal joints flexed (see figure 7.5a). Starting at the patient's calf muscle, the clinician slides her hand along the leg, coming to a stop at the calcaneus. At this point, the clinician holds the calcaneus between the hook and the fleshy part of the thenar eminence.

Test

The clinician distracts the calcaneus caudally until all the slack is taken up by the triceps surae or no further movement is detected. Then the clinician rests the thumb of her other hand on the lateral border of the patient's forefoot; the thumb rests on the fifth metatarsal head (see figure 7.5b). While maintaining the calcaneal distraction, the clinician passively applies pressure to the forefoot in the direction of dorsiflexion, keeping the subtalar joint neutral as much as possible (figure 7.5c).

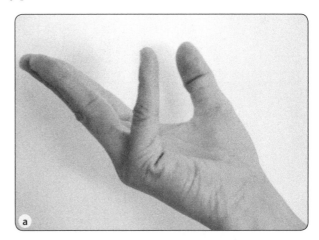

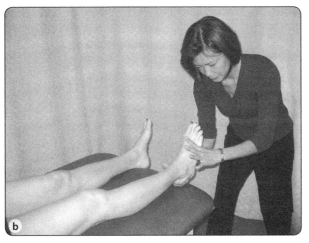

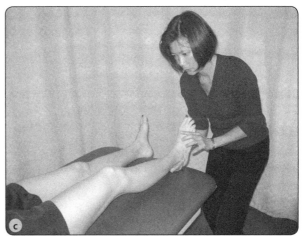

Figure 7.5 *(a)* Hook position. *(b)* and *(c)* Triceps surae length test.

The normal length of the triceps surae allows for the foot to be in 0° of dorsiflexion. If muscle shortness is noted, the clinician can differentiate whether the two-joint gastrocnemius or the one-joint soleus is the primary muscle contributing to the shortness. To do this, the clinician flexes the patient's knee joint while maintaining the calcaneal distraction and forefoot pressure. If the range of ankle dorsiflexion increases, the shortness is caused by the gastrocnemius by virtue of relaxing the muscle at the knee joint. The soleus is the tight muscle if the ankle range is unchanged when the knee is flexed.

Quadratus Lumborum Muscle Length Test

Hip abduction is performed primarily by the hip abductors (namely the gluteus medius and minimus) and the TFL, with synergistic activity and stabilization provided by the quadratus lumborum, abdominal muscles, and deep intrinsic back extensors. When the gluteus medius and minimus are weak or inhibited, the TFL or quadratus lumborum compensates by becoming the primary mover. The hip abduction movement test provides the clinician with a picture of the participation of these muscles. As described in chapter 6, the most impaired movement pattern of hip abduction is when the quadratus lumborum initiates the movement, which results in hip hiking. Hip hiking places excessive side-bending compressive stresses on the lumbar segments. Thus, a tight quadratus lumborum may be another hidden cause of low back pain (Janda 1987 ; Janda, Frank, and Liebenson 2007).

The quadratus lumborum is a difficult muscle to test because of the multiple spinal segments that it spans. The true length test should be performed passively with the patient in a prone position, but this test may be impractical in the clinic because it requires two clinicians. The side-lying and standing tests may be more practical.

Quadratus Lumborum Muscle Length Test in Prone Position

Two clinicians are required to administer the quadratus lumborum muscle length test when the patient is in a prone position to ensure a true passive muscle length test. The patient's pelvis is stabilized by one clinician, while the other clinician passively side bends the patient's torso.

Patient Position

The patient is prone with the torso supported on a rolling stool. The lumbar spine is in a relatively neutral position (figure 7.6a).

Clinician Position

The patient's pelvis is fixed by the one of the clinicians. The other clinician stands at the head of the patient, facing the patient.

Test

While the patient's pelvis is fixed by one of the clinicians, the other clinician passively bends the patient's torso toward one side until pelvic movement is detected (figure 7.6, b-c). The smoothness or straightening of the thoracolumbar spinal curve is then observed.

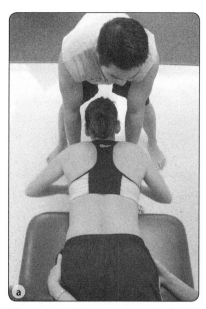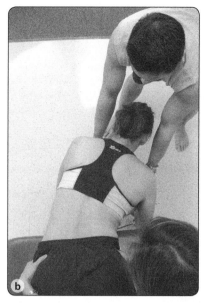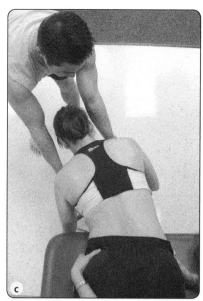

Figure 7.6 *(a)* Starting position for testing the quadratus lumborum. *(b)* Ending position. *(c)* Ending position on other side. Note the decreased smoothness of the spinal curve with Left lateral trunk side bending.

Quadratus Lumborum Muscle Length Test in Side-Lying Position

The side-lying test was advocated by Janda to provide a fixed stable base at the pelvis while the trunk is bent to the side by virtue of extending the lower arm. This test is possible only if the patient has a relatively pain-free shoulder and adequate strength and stability in the shoulder girdle musculature to lift the torso.

Patient Position

With the patient in standing, the clinician makes a mark on the inferior angle of the scapula. Then, the patient lies on the side that is being tested, with the bottom arm flexed under the head and the top arm on the table for stability (see figure 7.7). The clinician ensures that the patient's spine is in a neutral position with respect to flexion and rotation.

Clinician Position

The clinician stands behind the patient and places one hand just below the iliac crest of the patient. This allows the clinician to monitor movement of the pelvis during the test.

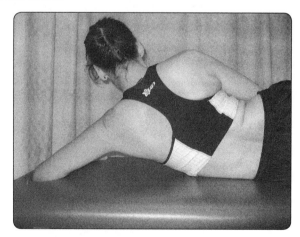

Figure 7.7 Testing the quadratus lumborum with the patient in a side-lying position.

Test

The patient extends the bottom arm to raise the upper trunk laterally. The movement is stopped when the clinician detects pelvic motion. The distance between the table and the mark on the inferior angle of the scapula is measured. The inferior angle of the scapula should be raised 2 in. (or 3-5 cm) off the table. The quality and smoothness of the spinal curve are also noted. If the quadratus lumborum is shortened, the lumbar spine remains straight.

Standing Lateral Trunk Flexion Test for the Quadratus Lumborum

The simplest clinical screening test for the quadratus lumborum is to observe the spinal curve during active lateral trunk flexion. The curve of the thoracolumbar spine should be relatively smooth with most of the curve occurring above the lumbar segments (see figure 7.8a), owing to the fact that there is more segmental joint play in the thoracic versus lumbar segments. The curve is also observed for any sharp fulcrum areas where the primary side bending is occurring from.

Patient Position

The patient stands erect with the arms relaxed at the sides.

Clinician Position

The clinician stands behind the patient.

Test

The patient bends to each side while the clinician observes the smoothness of the spinal curve. If the quadratus lumborum is shortened, the lumbar spine appears straight when the patient bends to the opposite side, and a fulcrum is seen above L4-L5 (see figure 7.8b).

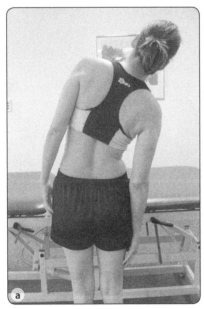 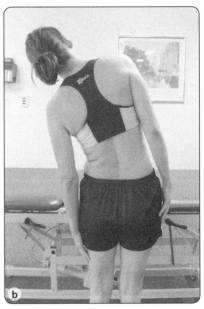

Figure 7.8 Testing of the quadratus lumborum. *(a)* Smooth spinal curve. *(b)* Curve fulcrums above L4-L5; note the fulcrum from which side bending occurs.

Paraspinals Muscle Length Test

The paraspinals are often overactivated in response to insufficient deep spinal stabilization by the abdominal, pelvic floor, and gluteal muscles. Overactivation also is found when the hip flexors are tight, as in Janda's LCS. A clue to overactive and dominant paraspinals is the observation of excessive paraspinal muscle bulk when the patient is standing quietly or in prone position. Another clue is an inability to flatten the lumbar spine when in the supine position. A confirmatory test is prone hip extension in which an increased lumbar extension or anterior pelvic tilt is observed.

Like the quadratus lumborum, the paraspinals are difficult to assess because of the multiple segments they span. A screening test for the paraspinals is the modified Schober's test, which is described later.

Patient Position

The patient sits with the hips and knees bent at 90° and with a slight posterior pelvic tilt. The clinician makes a mark on the sacrum at the level of the posterior superior iliac spine (PSIS) and another mark on the spine 4 in. (10 cm) from the mark made on the sacrum.

Clinician Position

The clinician stands or squats behind the patient and places the hands on the patient's iliac crest to monitor pelvic movement when the patient flexes forward.

Test

The patient flexes forward until movement at the pelvis is detected. At this time, the clinician measures the distance between the two marks at the end of the movement (figure 7.9). An excursion of 2.4 in. (6 cm) or more suggests a normal length of the lumbar paraspinals. A more reliable test, however, is to use an inclinometer to make objective measurements of lumbar flexion mobility.

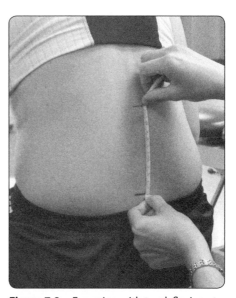

Figure 7.9 Excursion with trunk flexion at the end of the movement.

Piriformis Muscle Length Test

The piriformis is prone to hypertonicity because of its attachments from the sacrum and greater trochanter. Positional changes straying from the ideal alignment of the pelvic girdle and hip often cause tonal changes in the piriformis secondary to its low irritability threshold. The piriformis, along with its synergists, namely the gluteus maximus, quadratus femoris, obturators, and gemelli, is an external rotator of the hip. In addition, the piriformis may assist in hip abduction and extension. Its role becomes more pronounced when the gluteal muscles are weak or inhibited and hence movement patterns deviate from the ideal.

Patient Position

The patient lies supine with the legs extended.

Clinician Position

The clinician stands beside the leg being tested and places that leg into hip flexion less than 60°.

Test

The clinician stabilizes the pelvis by applying compression toward the hip joint via the long axis of the femur. While maintaining the compressive force into the hip joint, the clinician adducts and medially rotates the hip (see figure 7.10*a*). The normal end feel is a gradual soft resistance toward the end of the ROM. If the muscle is tight, the end feel may be hard or abrupt and the patient may perceive a deep ache in the buttock region.

Janda noted that the piriformis acts as a hip internal rotator when the hip is flexed past 60° due to its orientation in that position. Therefore, he suggested testing the piriformis in hip flexion at 90°. This is done by following the procedure just described but flexing the hips to 90° and then externally rotating the hip (figure 7.10*b*).

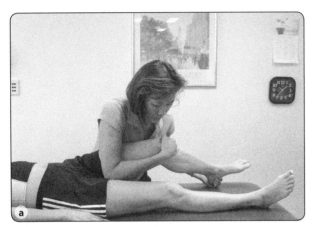 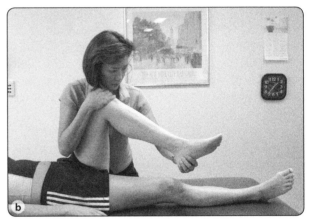

Figure 7.10 *(a)* Piriformis test at 60° of hip flexion. *(b)* Piriformis test at 90° of hip flexion.

Palpation of the Piriformis Muscle

Palpation of the piriformis is performed in addition to testing its length in order to provide further information on the degree of muscle tension and irritability.

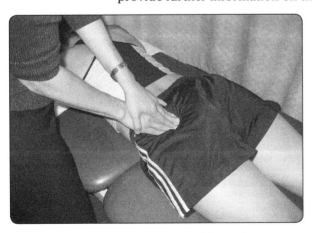

Figure 7.11 Location and palpation of the piriformis.

Patient Position

The patient lies prone with her head comfortably turned to one side and her feet hanging over the table to ensure neutral rotation of the hips.

Clinician Position

The clinician stands on the side of the leg being tested. Four landmarks are used to determine the location and palpation of the piriformis: the ischial tuberosity, the ASIS, the greater trochanter, and the PSIS (see figure 7.11). The muscle is found at the intersection of the lines drawn between the ASIS and the ischial tuberosity and between the PSIS and the greater trochanter.

Test

Using a flattened hand position, the clinician gently sinks her hand into the gluteus muscle and pushes it caudally. The clinician then places her other hand on top of the flattened hand to palpate the piriformis. A patient with a nonirritable piriformis perceives a pressure on the muscle. On the other hand, a tight piriformis is extremely sensitive and tender to palpation. In the case of an irritable piriformis with an entrapped sciatic nerve, the patient might perceive a reproduction of sciatic symptoms.

Upper-Quarter Muscles

The muscles of the upper quarter include those of the cervical spine, shoulder, and arm. The muscles prone to tightness are those involved in a protective flexor response. Tightness of the upper trapezius, pectoral muscles, and suboccipitals in particular is a hallmark sign of Janda's UCS.

Pectoralis Minor Muscle Length Test

Because of its attachments onto the coracoid process and the superior margins of the third, fourth, and fifth ribs, the pectoralis minor muscle tilts the scapula anteriorly and assists in forced inspiration respectively (Kendall, McCreary, and Provance 1993). Pectoralis minor tightness contributes to a faulty position of the scapula that in turn changes the force couples and muscular balance in the shoulder girdle. Pectoralis minor shortness is observed during postural analysis as an excessively anteriorly translated or protracted humeral position.

Patient Position

The patient lies supine with the knees flexed and the arms resting by the sides. The clinician makes a mark on the posterior border of the acromion. The distance between this mark and the table is measured.

Clinician Position

The clinician views the mark on the patient from a superior view.

Test

The normal distance between the acromion and the table is 1 in. (or 2 cm; Sahrmann 2002). The horizontal levels of the anterior aspects of the acromions can be compared with each other (see figure 7.12). The two acromions should be on the same level; a higher acromion indicates possible pectoralis minor tightness.

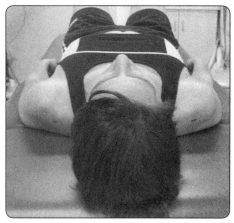

Figure 7.12 The pectoralis minor muscle length test.

Pectoralis Major Muscle Length Test

A short pectoralis muscle holds the humerus in medial rotation and adduction that in turn abducts the scapula away from the spine. This may be observed during postural analysis as excessive medial rotation of the shoulder and protraction of the scapula. In addition to changing the biomechanical alignment of the shoulder complex, a short or hypertonic pectoralis major inhibits its antagonists, namely the shoulder external rotators and scapular adductors, through reciprocal inhibition.

Patient Position

The patient lies supine with the glenohumeral joint that is being tested at the edge of the table. The corresponding scapula should be supported on the table.

Clinician Position

The clinician stands on the side of the shoulder being tested, facing the patient. The clinician places his forearm on the patient's sternum to stabilize the thorax during the test.

Test

The different portions of the pectoralis major are tested separately. The clinician is able to target the specific portions by changing the amount of shoulder abduction.

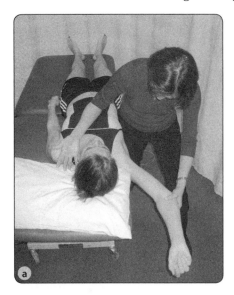

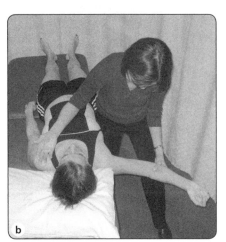

- **Lower sternal fibers.** The clinician abducts the patient's arm to 150° with slight external rotation. The normal length of these pectoral fibers allows the patient's arm to rest in a horizontal position; slight overpressure produces end-feel resistance (figure 7.13*a*). The clinician should also palpate the sternal fibers medial to the axilla for tenderness. Shortness or hypertonicity of the muscle is indicated by an inability of the arm to reach horizontal or a palpable tenderness in the muscle.

- **Midsternal fibers.** The clinician abducts the patient's arm to 90° and palpates the muscle fibers at the second rib interspace. The normal length of these fibers allows the patient's arm to rest below the horizontal (figure 7.13*b*). There is gradual end-feel resistance when the clinician applies slight overpressure. Palpation does not produce tenderness.

- **Clavicular fibers.** The clinician places the patient's arm in an extended position close to the body and allows the arm to come to a rest. The normal length of these fibers allows the patient's arm to rest below the horizontal (figure 7.13*c*). The clinician applies a gentle anteroposterior and caudal pressure through the glenohumeral joint as well as palpates the fibers just inferior to the clavicle. Resistance to this pressure should be gradual and fibers should not be tender to palpation.

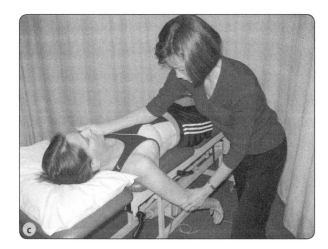

Figure 7.13 Pectoralis major muscle length test for *(a)* lower sternal fibers, *(b)* midsternal fibers, and *(c)* clavicular fibers.

Latissimus Dorsi Muscle Length Test

The latissimus dorsi is a large, flat muscle spanning the last six thoracic vertebrae, the last four ribs, the thoracolumbar fascia from the sacral and lumbar vertebrae, and the external lip of the iliac crest to its insertion onto the intertubercular sulcus of the humerus. Because of its many attachments, the latissimus dorsi can medially rotate, adduct, and extend the humerus as well as extend the lumbar spine and anteriorly tilt the pelvis. A short latissimus dorsi is observed as excessively medially rotated shoulders and contributes to a decreased ROM for shoulder flexion.

Patient Position

The patient lies supine with the hips and knees bent to relax the paraspinals.

Clinician Position

The clinician stands beside the arm being tested.

Test

The clinician passively elevates the patient's arm toward the head of the table. The normal length of the latissimus dorsi allows the arm to rest horizontally to the table with the lumbar spine flat on the table. Tightness of this muscle is indicated by the arm resting above horizontal or by the lumbar spine going into extension (see figure 7.14).

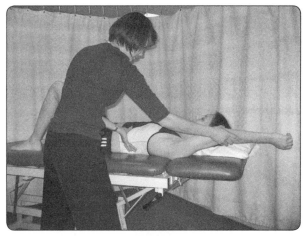

Figure 7.14 Tightness of the latissimus dorsi.

Upper-Trapezius Muscle Length Test

The force couples among the upper, middle, and lower muscles of the trapezius provide dynamic stabilization to the scapula, contributing to the upward rotation of the scapula necessary for shoulder elevation. Excessive scapular elevation and inadequate upward rotation often result from a tight upper trapezius and a weak middle trapezius or lower trapezius. This force-couple imbalance affects not only the shoulder girdle complex but also the cervical spine because of the attachments of the upper trapezius onto the superior nuchal line, ligamentum nuchae, and spinous processes.

Upper-trapezius tightness or hypertonicity is often associated with the gothic shoulder seen in postural analysis. Another indicator of upper-trapezius tightness is excessive shoulder elevation before 60° of shoulder abduction.

Patient Position

The patient lies supine with the hips and knees bent to relax the paraspinals.

Clinician Position

The clinician stands or sits at the head of the table, facing the patient. The clinician then fully flexes the patient's head, laterally flexes the head away from the tested side, and finally rotates the head toward the tested side. The position of the patient's head is supported on the side not being tested by the clinician's hand and forearm or gently supported by the clinician's abdomen.

Test

While maintaining the patient's head in a stabilized position as just described, the clinician depresses the shoulder girdle on the tested side by applying a caudal pressure on the acromion and clavicle (figure 7.15). The length of the upper trapezius is assessed qualitatively by noting the end-feel resistance. The normal end feel is gradual rather than abrupt. The upper trapezius can be palpated on the belly of the muscle at the midclavicular area. The right and left sides should be compared. The clinician can selectively increase the tension in the upper fibers of the upper trapezius by adding ipsilateral neck rotation.

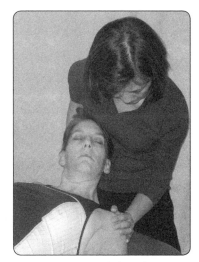

Figure 7.15 Muscle length testing of the upper trapezius.

Levator Scapulae Muscle Length Test

The levator scapulae and its synergist the upper trapezius are strong elevators of the shoulder girdle. Additionally, the levator scapulae is a downward rotator of the scapula; this may impair the ideal movement of the shoulder into full elevation. Tightness of the levator scapulae is associated with the presence of a levator notch during postural analysis and excessive shoulder elevation before 60° of shoulder abduction.

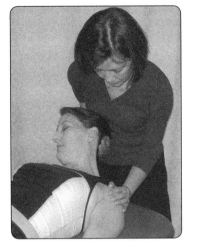

Patient Position

The patient lies supine with the hips and knees bent to relax the paraspinals.

Clinician Position

The clinician stands or sits at the head of the table, facing the patient. The clinician positions the patient's head the same way it is positioned for the upper-trapezius muscle length test. However, for this test the head is rotated to the side being tested (figure 7.16).

Test

The clinician notes the quality of the resistance and compares resistance from side to side. To look for tender points, the clinician palpates the levator scapulae at the area of the superior angle of the scapula.

Figure 7.16 The levator scapulae muscle length test.

Sternocleidomastoid Muscle Length Test

Head flexion is performed primarily by the longus colli, longus capitis, and rectus capitis. These muscles are assisted by the secondary muscles, which are the SCM and anterior scalenes. When the primary deep cervical flexors are weak, the secondary muscles often perform the movement, resulting in hyperextension of the cervical spine during the head flexion movement test as described by Janda. Tight SCM muscles are often associated with a forward head posture as well as prominence of the muscle in the midbelly to distal attachment.

Patient Position

The patient lies supine with the head off the table. The clinician supports the patient's head.

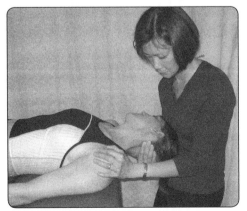

Clinician Position

The clinician stands at the head of the table, supporting the patient's head. Because of the vulnerability of the vertebral artery and the stress this position places on this artery, the vertebrobasilar artery insufficiency (VBI) test must be performed first.

Test

Once the VBI test has been ruled negative, the clinician first rotates the patient's head away from the tested side and then gradually extends the head, supporting it all the while (figure 7.17). The end feel is assessed.

Figure 7.17 The SCM muscle length test.

Hypermobility

Constitutional hypermobility is a vague nonprogressive clinical syndrome that is characterized by a general laxity of connective tissues, muscles, and ligaments in particular. It involves the entire body, although not all areas are affected to the same extent. It is found more frequently in women than in men and typically involves the upper part of the body. The classic sign of hypermobility is excessive ROM in various joints throughout the body. Other signs include lower muscle tone upon palpation and decreased evident muscle hypertrophy even with vigorous strengthening exercises. Patients with constitutional hypermobility may develop muscle tightness with increased tone as a compensatory mechanism to stabilize the unstable joints, particularly the weight-bearing joints. When a muscle is tight, gentle stretches, if necessary, should be conducted. Muscles in constitutional hypermobility tend to have a lower muscle tone and in general are weaker. Hence, they are more prone to overuse and more likely to develop TrPs. Inhibition and release of these TrPs are imperative.

Assessment of hypermobility is the estimation of muscle tone via palpation and ROM. However, in the clinic, ROM tests usually are sufficient to provide information about the status of hypermobility in a patient. The most useful upper-body tests include the high arm cross (figure 7.18*a*), touching the hands behind the back (figure 7.18*b*), elbow extension (figure 7.18*c*), and hyperextension of the thumb (figure 7.18*d*). In the lower part of the body, the most useful tests are bending forward (figure 7.18*e*),

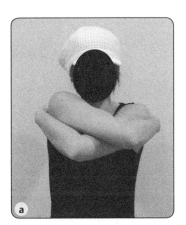
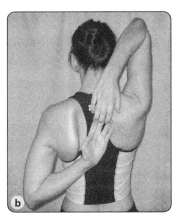
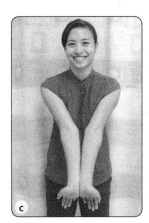
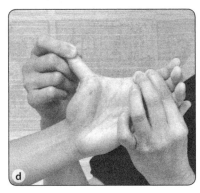
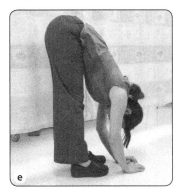

Figure 7.18 Hypermobility tests. *(a)* High arm cross. *(b)* Touching the hands behind the back. *(c)* Elbow extension. *(d)* Hyperextension of the thumb. *(e)* Forward bending.

(continued)

the straight-leg raise test for determining hamstring length (figure 7.18*f*), and ankle dorsiflexion (figure 7.18*g*).

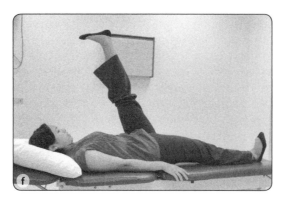
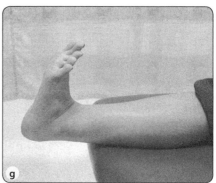

Figure 7.18 *(continued)* Hypermobility tests. *(f)* Straight-leg raise. *(g)* Ankle dorsiflexion.

Summary

Muscle imbalance is the altered relationship between the muscles that are prone to inhibition or weakness and the muscles that are prone to tightness or shortness. Imbalance is not an isolated response of an individual muscle but rather a systemic reaction of a whole series of striated muscles. Janda proposed that the development of tightness or weakness does not occur randomly but occurs in typical patterns. Muscle length tests, end-feel assessment, and muscle palpation are integral to the functional evaluation of musculoskeletal pain syndromes.

SOFT-TISSUE ASSESSMENT

The final step in the functional evaluation is soft-tissue assessment through palpation. Before the soft-tissue assessment, information gathered through visual inspection of posture, balance, and movement patterns is combined with specific testing of muscle length and strength. Soft-tissue assessment is performed near the end of the evaluation since it can be both facilitatory and painful, thus giving inaccurate information about a functional pathology. The soft-tissue assessment includes the examination of tender points and TrPs as well as an examination of soft tissue.

As noted in previous chapters, muscle dysfunction manifests itself as abnormal muscle tone, which is either increased (hypertonic) or decreased (hypotonic). The term *global muscle dysfunction* or *global muscle tone* is used to describe the clinical scenario in which one or several entire muscles undergo abnormal changes in tone. Unlike global muscle dysfunction, the TrP is a focal or localized type of dysfunction. TrPs are focal areas of hypertonicity that are not painful during movement but are painful upon palpation. They are localized, hyperirritable taut bands within the muscle (Travell and Simons 1992; Simons, Travell, and Simons 1999; Mense and Simons 2001). The overall tone and length of the muscle harboring these TrPs are not necessarily abnormal: Only one or more subsections of the muscle may be affected. These hypertonic taut bands have a decreased threshold to stimulation and tend to contract first but inefficiently in voluntary movement. This type of focal muscle dysfunction typically is associated with myofascial pain syndrome (MPS).

The brain controls all movements of the body through muscles. Hence, it should follow that alterations in muscle tone are typical neurological reflex responses to the irritation of spinal nerves, joints, discs, muscles, or ligaments (Mense and Simons 2001; Simons 1996). These responses lead to a reflex arc of reciprocal inhibition for protection and subsequently cause impaired function of the motor system (Janda 1986, 1991). These reflex responses typically are seen in acute disc herniations in which there is inhibition of the deep multifidus and concurrent excitation and muscle guarding in the more superficial erector spinae. Another typical example of these protective reflex responses is seen in ACL tears, when inhibition of the quadriceps occurs concurrently with excitation or hypertonicity of the hamstrings. A muscle can also be inhibited reflexively when its antagonist is activated, as described by Sherrington's law of reciprocal inhibition (see chapter 2). TrPs found in globally hypotonic muscles such as the gluteus medius have been described by Janda as *areas of muscle incoordination* (Janda 1986; Jull and Janda 1987). This type of muscle incoordination likely is due to alterations in the neural control of muscle tone.

The two-volume textbook by Travell and Simons (Travell and Simons 1992; Simons, Travell, and Simons 1999) provides a complete and comprehensive understanding of focal muscle dysfunction, TrPs, and myofascial pain patterns commonly found in the various regional pain syndromes. TrPs found in focal muscle dysfunction are associated with MPS. These myofascial TrPs occur in a characteristic pattern for each skeletal muscle in the human body (Travell and Simons 1992; Simons, Travell, and Simons 1999). Like the dermatomal patterns seen in inflamed nerve roots, the myofascial referred pain patterns can serve as important diagnostic criteria.

Chapter 3 of this text described the TrP chains (Hong and Simons 1992; see table 3.3) and Lewit's nociceptive chain (in Lewit 2007) of tender points and TrPs. A key TrP in a particular muscle can induce a satellite TrP in other muscles that are functionally related to the muscle harboring the key TrP. Inactivation of the key TrP often spontaneously inactivates the satellite TrP.

Clinicians should sometimes consider TrPs and tender points as indicators or symptoms rather than pathologies. For example, tender points and TrPs associated with fibromyalgia (FM) may in fact be a symptom of an underlying neuromuscular pathology. Often clinicians can determine the effectiveness of a treatment by evaluating the tenderness of these points before and after treatment. If the points decrease in pain after treatment, the treatment may have had a positive global effect. Direct treatment of TrPs includes spray and stretch, heat, electrical stimulation (TENS [transcutaneous electrical nerve stimulation therapy] and interferential therapy), and active ROM. Combinations of these treatments, as well as ischemic compression, are effective at reducing TrP pain (Hou et al. 2002).

This chapter begins with a description of TrPs commonly found in MPS and distinguishes these TrPs from tender points commonly found in FM. The etiology and pathophysiology of both TrPs and tender points are summarized based on current available evidence. In addition, the concept of developmental kinesiology is presented to provide further understanding of the correlation and interplay of the components of the motor system and how a disturbance of this motor system equilibrium or a muscle imbalance often manifests as TrP chains. The latter part of this chapter describes the palpatory assessment of soft tissue for key tonic muscles that tend to become tight or hypertonic as described in Janda's UCS and LCS.

Characteristics of Trigger Points

Active TrPs often manifest as pain that the patient describes as his primary complaint. Latent TrPs exhibit the same characteristics that active TrPs exhibit, although to a lesser extent. In addition, latent TrPs do not reproduce the patient's primary comlaint or symptoms. However, both can cause significant motor dysfunction. A TrP is often activated by mechanical abuse of the muscle in the form of muscle overload, be it acute, sustained, or repetitive trauma. Active TrPs are often found in patients with a current complaint of pain. Deep manual palpation of an active TrP reproduces the patient's pain. On the other hand, latent TrPs may reside in muscles not actively causing any symptoms. Patients often do not perceive any spontaneous symptoms from a latent TrP at rest or during ADL. However, pain from a latent TrP may become familiar or apparent when provoked by deep palpation. An acute TrP may revert spontaneously to a latent state when perpetuating factors cease to irritate the tissue (Travell and Simons 1992; Simons, Travell, and Simons 1999; Simons 1996; Mense and Simons 2001). Pain symptoms may disappear, but the latent TrPs can be reactivated when the muscle stress is induced. This may explain the recurrence of similar pain episodes over several years. The symptoms associated with myofascial TrPs include pain, weakness, paresthesias, loss of coordination, and decreased work tolerance. Active TrPs are common in postural muscles in the neck, shoulder, and pelvic girdle and in the masticatory muscles. Also commonly involved are the upper trapezius, levator scapulae, SCM, scalene, and quadratus lumborum. Incidentally, these are the same muscles described as the tonic muscles that Janda recognized as being prone to tightness or hypertonicity.

The type of pain described by a patient often provides a clue as to the source of the pain. Patients with active myofascial TrPs often describe their pain as aching pain, and typically their pain is poorly localized. However, localized pain can be induced by deep palpation over the TrP nodule, or knot. Patients with myofascial pain may also describe a referred pain, or a perception of pain in a body region that is anatomically distant from the pain generator. The severity, constancy, and extent of the referred pain depends on the irritability or sensitivity of the TrP. Myofascial pain frequently, but not always, occurs within the same dermatome, myotome, or sclerotome a TrP occurs in (Travell and Simons 1992, Simons, Travell, and Simons 1999). Active myofascial TrPs can disturb motor coordination, as is seen in patients who complain of giving way of the knee; this giving way is caused by a TrP in the vastus medialis that produces a profound inhibition of the quadriceps. Due to referral, TrPs can influence muscles at a considerable distance. In addition, TrPs cause stiffness and weakness of the involved muscles. Myofascial stiffness of the muscle is often reported after inactivity or resting in a sustained position.

Trigger Points Versus Tender Points

Tender points need to be distinguished from TrPs for effective treatment. Tender points associated with FM are widespread and nonspecific. The etiology of tender points is still unknown, and it is uncertain which specific soft tissues are tender in these patients. Hence, local treatment applied to tender points is ineffective. On the other hand, specific treatment of TrPs associated with myofascial pain often is dramatically effective owing to the fact that myofascial pain arises from muscle dysfunction (Schneider 1995). Tender points are often found in FM, a condition characterized by widespread, nonspecific soft-tissue pain and a lowered threshold to any type of firm palpation of the muscles and soft tissues. Biopsy studies of tender points have shown no significant abnormalities or tissue changes of the myofascial tissues in the area of complaint, a finding that has led to a current theory that patients with FM have a dysfunction in pain processing by the CNS and not a dysfunction in the peripheral soft tissues. FM is a systemic disease and is hypothesized to be caused by a dysfunction in the limbic system or neuroendocrine system. It often requires a multidisciplinary treatment approach that includes psychotherapy, antidepressant medications, and a moderate exercise regime (Salter 2002; Hendriksson 2002; Schneider 1995; Simons 1996; Simons, Travell, and Simons 1999).

On the other hand, the MPS is a condition with regional and typical referred pain patterns characterized by TrPs. Myofascial TrPs are found within a taut band of skeletal muscle and have a characteristic nodular texture upon palpation. TrPs are thought to develop after trauma, overuse, or prolonged spasm of muscles. They show specific biochemical and histological abnormalities in biopsy studies, and they display spikes of spontaneous electrical activity while the adjacent tissue remains electrically silent (Mense and Simons 2001; Hong and Simons 1992, 1998; Simons 1996, Simons, Travell, and Simons 1999). Janda's description of myofascial TrPs as muscle incoordination (Janda 1991) appears to be quite appropriate, in that the affected muscle features hypertonic areas surrounded by adjacent normotonic muscle fibers. Thus, myofascial TrPs often respond to manual treatment methods such as TrP pressure release (formerly known as *ischemic compression),* specific stretching, and postisometric relaxation (Simons, Travell, and Simons 1999; Janda 1987; Janda, Frank, and Liebenson 2007). Table 8.1 summarizes the differences between TrPs and tender points.

Table 8.1 Characteristics of Tender Points and Trigger Points

	Tender points	**TrPs**
EMG	No abnormalities in myofascial tissues in the area of complaint	Spikes of spontaneous electrical activity while the adjacent tissue remains silent
Tissue texture	No tissue texture change; tissue merely exhibits tenderness or hyperalgesia upon light palpation	Distinct palpable small nodules found within a taut band of muscle tissue
Location	Pervasive tenderness and global hyperalgesia	Any skeletal muscle but especially muscles that are prone to repetitive overuse (microtrauma) or frank injury (macrotrauma)

Myofascial TrPs and tender points are equally tender at the cutaneous, subcutaneous, and intramuscular levels. However, myofascial TrPs are abnormally tender only at circumscribed TrP sites, which are invariably found in the midbelly of skeletal muscles (Hong 1999; Simons, Travell, and Simons 1999), and at specific sites of referred tenderness. On the other hand, abnormal tenderness in patients with FM is widespread, without any specific pattern. Muscles harboring TrPs often feel tense because of the palpable small nodules or taut bands within the muscle itself, whereas muscles of a patient with widespread tenderness often feel softer and more doughy (Travell and Simons 1992; Simons, Travell, and Simons 1999).

Developmental Kinesiology Approach to Trigger Points

As described in chapter 3, developmental kinesiology provides a better understanding of the correlation and interplay of all components of the motor system. Humans are immature at birth, both in function and morphology. After birth, development continues in both function and morphology and is completed at the age of 4, when gross motor function reaches full maturity. The shape of the hip joint, plantar arch, and spinal curve in a newborn changes during the course of normal development. Motor development in infancy is automatic and depends on the optical orientation and emotional needs of the child. Motor development is genetically determined, and motor functions develop on an automatic, subconscious level. The morphological development of the skeleton as well as joint positions and posture greatly depends on the stabilizing function of the muscles necessary for resultant movement. Each joint has a well-determined movement as part of a motor pattern. The anatomical structure determines the biomechanical ideal joint movement. Each position that a joint adopts is dynamically controlled by specific parts of muscles that stabilize the joint at any given time. The position and stabilization of joints through coordinated muscular activity between the phylogenetically older tonic muscles (flexors) and the phylogenetically younger phasic muscles (extensors) result from CNS control. The muscle function that is encoded by motor programs develops as the CNS matures. Disturbance of the equilibrium between the tonic and phasic muscles by CNS lesions, immaturity, pain, trauma, habitual patterns, or repetitive overuse often results in dominance by the tonic system, or the muscles that tend to tightness or hypertonicity.

When the tonic system dominates, there is always a corresponding inhibition of the phasic muscles as well as inhibition of the postural function of the diaphragm and pelvic floor muscles (Jull and Janda 1987; Lewit 1999, 2007; Kolář 2001, 2007). Disturbance of the tonic–phasic system equilibrium or muscle imbalance often manifests as painful lesions in the form of TrPs. While typically more prevalent in tonic muscles, TrPs can exist in either tonic or phasic muscles because of their functional anatomical interconnections. The spread of these TrP or nociceptive chains depends primarily on the chronicity of the dysfunction.

Lewit (1999, 2007) described a nociceptive chain related to TrPs throughout the body. Nociceptive chains develop with the progression of time and the chronicity of a painful dysfunction. Lewit observed that patients with chronic pain often exhibit TrPs on one side of the body. He postulated that the spread of muscular dysfunction throughout one side is related to postural balance. For example, dynamic right shoulder girdle and right pelvic girdle stabilization is required to push an object with the right arm while in the standing position. The head is also stabilized by the right shoulder girdle musculature. This chain is mainly unilateral and characteristic of chronic painful conditions. The contralateral side often demonstrates a marked reduction in response and activity. Upon palpation, TrPs are found mainly on one side, as is shown in table 8.2.

Table 8.2 The Trigger Point or Nociceptive Chain

Trigger point location	Associated TrP chains
Cervical area	SCM, scalene, deep extensors of the craniocervical junction, splenius, upper trapezius, levator scapulae
Thoracic area	Pectoralis major, pectoralis minor, diaphragm, subscapularis, serratus anterior, iliocostalis
Lumbar (abdominal) area	Abdominal muscles (rectus abdominis, obliques), longissimus, quadratus lumborum, psoas major
Pelvic girdle	Pelvic floor, diaphragm, short adductors, hamstrings, glutei (maximus, medius), piriformis, rectus femoris, iliacus, TFL
Lower extremity	Long toe extensors, tibialis anterior, soleus, short toe flexors and extensors
Shoulder girdle	Subscapularis, infraspinatus, supraspinatus, deltoids, teres major, triceps long head
Forearm and hand	Pronators, supinators (biceps brachii), long and short finger extensors and flexors

Adapted, by permission, from K. Lewit, 2007, Managing common syndromes and finding the key link. In *Rehabilitation of the spine*, edited by C. Liebenson (Philadelphia, PA: Lippincott, Williams, and Wilkins), 784.

Kolář (2001, 2007) proposed that the functioning of any muscle is determined not only by its specific function or action but also, and more importantly, by its stabilization. Insufficient stabilization is often the cause of muscular dysfunction. It is well accepted that proximal stability is necessary for distal movements. For instance, the quality of wrist flexion depends on shoulder stability, which in turn depends on abdominal stabilization of the trunk. Thus the condition of the abdominal muscles can affect the quality of wrist flexion.

Localized changes in muscle tension affect joint function via force-couple imbalances and vice versa. The chain reaction of local tonal differences in muscles, especially those harboring TrPs, is not haphazard or random. A TrP is never an isolated phenomenon; it always has an interconnected chain of TrPs, as described in chapter 3. When a key TrP is released, the interconnected chain of TrPs is also released. A TrP freezes, or immobilizes, a joint in a certain position and also changes its articular pattern. A TrP found in an area of muscle that stabilizes a particular joint position affects the corresponding sections of the muscle as well as the muscles functionally connected to it. For example, in order to maintain a given position of the arm (see figure 8.1), specific fibers of the pectoralis major contract. Meanwhile, the pectoralis major attachment point is stabilized by

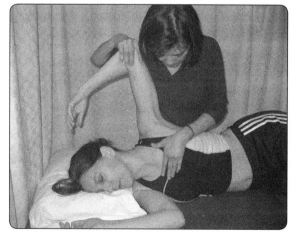

Figure 8.1 The pectoralis major when a patient is in a side-lying position.

the activation of other functionally related muscles, such as the abdominal muscles, scapular adductors, serratus anterior, and even muscles at the hip. Hence, when the pectoralis major harbors a TrP, it is not uncommon to locate associated satellite TrPs in the muscles that are related functionally to the pectoralis major.

Additionally, the close interplay between joint restrictions and muscular TrPs can enhance or perpetuate dysfunction. For example, in the forward head posture, movement restrictions at the cervicocranial junction often relate to hypertonic or tight and short cervicocranial extensor and SCM muscles. The head is stabilized by muscles in the shoulder girdle, which in turn is balanced over the trunk and lower extremities. Thus dysfunction in any part of the neuromusculoarticular system is never localized; it affects the function and movement of all or part of the whole kinetic chain. Table 8.3 provides an example of the effect that forward head posture has on TrPs throughout the body.

Table 8.3   Trigger Points and Joint Dysfunction in the Forward Head Posture

Area	TrPs and joint dysfunction
Cervical area	Hypertonic or short SCM muscles and deep craniocervical extensors produce reclination at the craniocervical junction and movement restrictions. TrPs occur in the upper trapezius and levator scapula and produce associated movement restrictions at the cervicothoracic junction.
Thoracic area	TrPs occur in the pectoralis major, diaphragm, and dorsal erector spinae and restrict movement of the thoracic spine and rib cage. An inspiratory position of the rib cage is often observed in rib cage and thoracic spine stiffness due to the dominance of the accessory inspiratory respiratory muscles over the diaphragm.
Lumbar area	Most prominent TrPs in the rectus abdominis are particularly painful and are found at the attachments at the lower arch of the ribs, xiphoid, pubic symphysis, erector spinae, and gluteus maximus. TrPs are often found in the pelvic floor, psoas, quadratus lumborum, and adductors. Movement restrictions are often found at the lumbar and hip joints.
Lower extremity	TrPs occur in the biceps femoris with movement restrictions at the fibular head and occur in the short plantar flexors (soleus) with movement restrictions at the tarsometatarsal joints.

Adapted, by permission, from K. Lewit, 2007, Managing common syndromes and finding the key link. In *Rehabilitation of the spine*, edited by C. Liebenson (Philadelphia, PA: Lippincott, Williams, and Wilkins), 784.

Assessment of Trigger Point or Tender Point Chains

The first rule of palpation is that the muscle should be relaxed as much as possible. Knowledge of the anatomy and mechanical actions of muscles is important for locating the muscles. If active contraction is performed initially by the patient in order to help the clinician locate the muscles of interest, the clinician needs to ensure that the patient is completely rested before beginning palpation.

Palpation Techniques

Travell and Simons (1992) and Simons, Travell, and Simons (1999) have advocated three key palpation techniques for the morphological assessment of TrPs: flat, snapping, and pincer palpation. Although these methods are differentiated for teaching purposes, clinicians often overlap them once expertise is established. All require the muscle to be as relaxed as possible before being palpated.

Flat Palpation

In flat palpation, the clinician uses the pads of the fingers to move across the fiber orientation of the muscle while compressing over a firm or bony underlying structure (see figure 8.2). This movement allows detection of changes in the underlying structures. In this way, a TrP can be trapped and the nodule assessed. Further direct compression over the nodule often provokes a pain response from a patient and concomitantly elicits a stereotypical referral pattern. Flat palpation works well on broad, flat muscles as well as muscles that are not easily accessible, such as the diaphragm or psoas major.

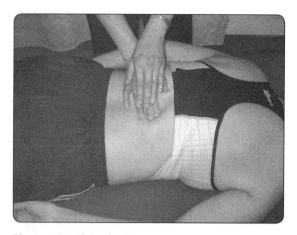

Figure 8.2   Flat palpation.

Snapping Palpation

When a taut band is detected by flat palpation, the clinician uses a rigid finger to perform a brisk transverse snapping of the taut band (see figure 8.3). The snapping motion is likened to the motion used to pluck a guitar string, except that in snapping palpation, contact with the surface is maintained. A local twitch response is elicited when a TrP is provoked. Snapping palpation is quite effective on superficial long muscles such as the erector spinae and rectus abdominis.

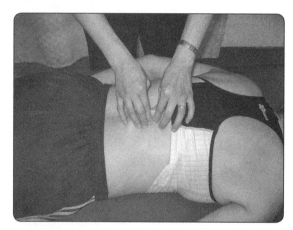

Figure 8.3   Snapping palpation.

Pincer Palpation

To form the pinch position, the thumb and a rigid finger assume a C shape (see figure 8.4). The target tissue is pinched to locate TrPs between the thumb and finger while allowing the tissue to roll between the fingers. The clinician assesses for local taut bands and a local twitch response.

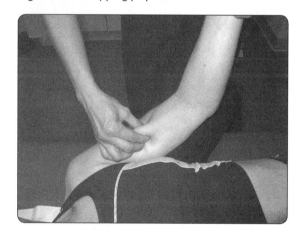

Figure 8.4   Pincer palpation.

Palpation Procedures

The clinician first instructs the patient about what to expect from deep palpation of the muscles. The patient is then asked to assess the pressure: whether it feels like pressure or pain and how it compares from side to side. The patient can also be instructed to rate the pressure sensation on a scale of 0 to 10. Using the pads of the fingers as in the flat palpation technique, the clinician applies a firm and gradual pressure to the muscle, while assessing the tone and texture of the soft tissue. The clinician repeats the procedure on the other side while having the patient compare the pressures from side to side. The clinician must take care to use equal pressure on both sides when palpating TrP chains. The clinician then proceeds to test other muscles in the chain, as shown in figure 8.5, taking note of how the TrPs are linked. A diagram is helpful for charting TrP chains; the clinician looks for consistent patterns and areas where chains cross over to the opposite side of the body.

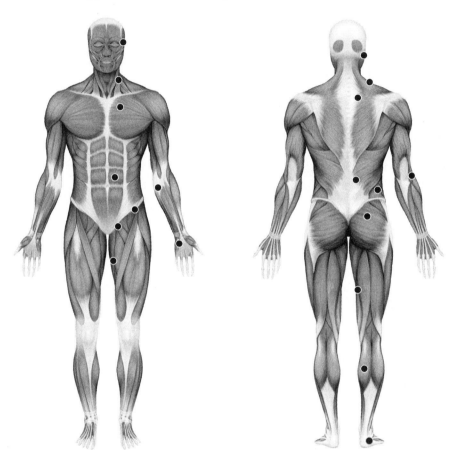

Figure 8.5 TrP and tender point palpation diagram.

Adapted from NSCA, 2008, Biomechanics of resistance exercise, by E. Harman. In *Essentials of strength training and conditioning*, 3rd ed., edited by T.R. Baechle and R.W. Earle (Champaign, IL: Human Kinetics), 68.

A pain algometer can be useful in quantifying TrP or tender point pain (see figure 8.6). Using the algometer to gradually increase the pressure on a painful point provides an objective measure of pain. The resulting number can be documented and used to track progress.

Palpation of key muscles that tend to become tight or hypertonic in Janda's UCS and LCS is presented in the sidebar that follows. Key muscles include quadratus lumborum, thoracolumbar fascia, psoas major, piriformis, adductor magnus, hamstrings, medial gastrocnemius, medial soleus, sole of the foot, subocciptials, sternocleidomastoid, upper trapezius, levator scapulae, pectoralis major, and lateral wrist extensors.

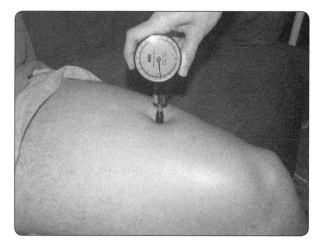

Figure 8.6 Using a pain algometer to quantify TrP or tender point pain.

Palpation of Key Tonic Muscles

This section describes the procedures for palpating trigger points in key tonic muscles.

Quadratus Lumborum

Locate the posterior aspect of the 12th rib and follow the rib with your fingers until you reach the lateral edge of the erector spinae. The quadratus lumborum is a deep muscle located laterally to the erector spinae between the lower arch of the posterior ribs and the posterior iliac crest. Sink your fingers slowly into the quadratus lumborum and assess the quality of the soft tissue. Note the patient's response.

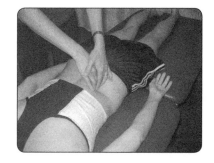

Palpation of the quadratus lumborum.

Posterior Crest of the Ilium (Thoracolumbar Fascia)

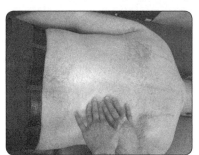

Locate the posterior crest of the ilium where the thoracolumbar fascia attaches itself. The thoracolumbar fascia serves as an attachment of multiple muscles such as the latissimus dorsi and abdominal muscles. Palpate for tenderness along the posterior crest of the ilium.

Palpation of the thoracolumbar fascia.

Psoas Major

Ask the patient to lie supine with the hips and knees slightly bent. Locate the ASIS and the umbilicus and draw an imaginary line between these two points. The psoas major is located midway between these two points, lateral to the rectus abdominis. Slight active hip flexion will help you locate this muscle. Once the psoas muscle is located, gradually sink your fingers into the muscle and assess its quality. Note the patient's response.

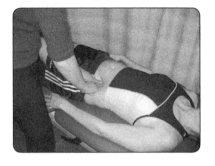

Palpation of the psoas major.

Piriformis

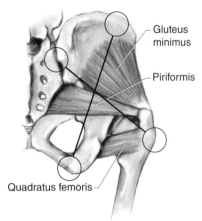

Gluteus minimus

Piriformis

Quadratus femoris

The location of the piriformis.

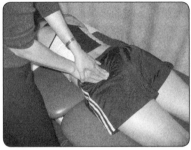

Palpation of the piriformis.

Ask the patient to lie prone. Locate the greater trochanter, ischial tuberosity, ASIS, and PSIS. Draw a pair of imaginary lines: one between the ASIS and ischial tuberosity and one between the PSIS and greater trochanter. The piriformis muscle is located at the intersection of these two lines. Using a flat hand position, gently sink into the gluteus muscle and push it caudally. Place your other hand on top of the flattened hand to palpate the piriformis muscle. A patient with a nonirritable piriformis will perceive a pressure on the muscle. In contrast, a patient with a tight piriformis or a TrP will be extremely sensitive and tender to palpation. A patient with an irritable piriformis associated with an entrapped sciatic nerve may perceive a reproduction of the sciatic symptoms.

Adductor Magnus

The adductor magnus is located between the adductor longus and the gracilis. You may direct your palpation of this muscle at the proximal or middle portion of the medial thigh.

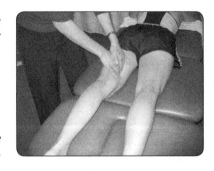

Palpation of the adductor magnus.

Hamstrings

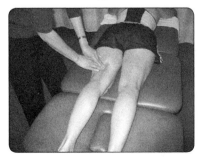

The hamstring muscles are located on the posterior portion of the thigh. The medial hamstrings, namely the semimembranosus and semitendinosus, attach distally to the medial condyle of the tibia. The lateral hamstrings, namely the long and short head of the biceps femoris, join together to form the biceps femoris tendon at the lateral aspect of the knee, just proximal to its insertion into the head of the fibula. Direct your palpation of the hamstrings at the middle portion of the muscle belly.

Palpation of the hamstrings.

Medial Gastrocnemius and Soleus

Direct your palpation of the gastrocnemius at the proximal aspect of the muscle belly on the medial leg. Direct your palpation of the soleus at the distal aspect of the leg.

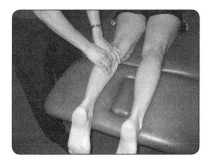

Palpation of the medial gastrocnemius.

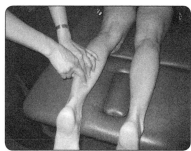

Palpation of the medial soleus.

Sole of the Foot

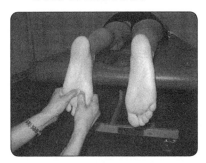

Palpate the sole of the foot first on the plantar surface at the first metatarsal interspace. Examine the entire plantar fascia from the metatarsals to the calcaneus for tender points.

Palpation of the first metatarsal interspace.

Suboccipital and C2 Region

The most prominent bony structure below the occiput is the spinous process of C2. Locate the suboccipitals by asking the patient to slightly extend the head. Palpate each side of C2.

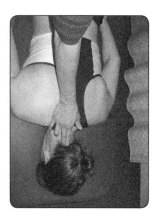

Palpation of the suboccipitals.

Sternocleidomastoid

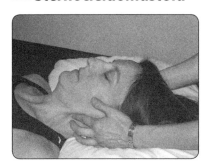

Locate the SCM by having the patient bend to the ipsilateral side and contralaterally rotate the head. Once this muscle is located, palpate for tenderness.

Palpation of the SCM.

Upper Trapezius

The upper trapezius spans the area between the spinous process of the cervical spine and the lateral third of the inferior border of the clavicle. To locate this muscle, have the patient bend to the ipsilateral side and contralaterally rotate the head and elevate the shoulder. Once this muscle is located, the patient is asked to relax the head completely and the clinician palpates it at its midpoint on the shoulder and neckline. Palpation of the upper trapezius can be performed in an erect or recumbent position.

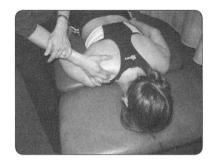

Palpation of the upper trapezius.

Levator Scapulae

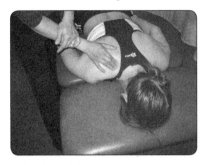

The levator scapulae spans the area between the transverse processes of the cervical spine and the superior angle of the scapula. To locate this muscle, have the patient slightly extend, bend to the side and rotate ipsilaterally, and elevate the shoulder until the superior angle of the scapula reaches its highest point. Once this muscle is located, the patient is asked to relax completely and the clinician palpates the muscle towards the superior angle of the scapula. Palpation of the levator can be performed in an erect or recumbent position.

Palpation of the levator scapulae.

Pectoralis Major

Muscle length tests of the pectoralis major are described in chapter 7. You may palpate the three portions of the muscle simultaneously with the muscle length tests or perform palpation and testing separately. Palpate the lower fibers of the pectoralis major at the anterior axillary wall. Palpate the middle fibers of the sternal portion at the second sternocostal interspace. Palpate the clavicular portion of the pectoralis major inferiorly to the clavicle.

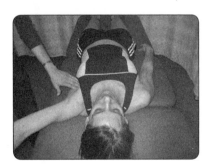

Palpation of the pectoralis major: sterna portion, lower fibers.

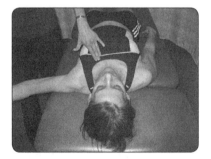

Palpation of the pectoralis major: sternal portion, middle fibers.

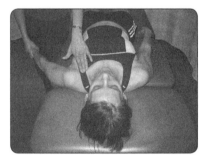

Palpation of the pectoralis major: clavicular fibers.

Lateral Wrist Extensors

First locate the lateral epicondyle of the humerus. Direct your palpation of the wrist extensors to the musculature just inferior to it.

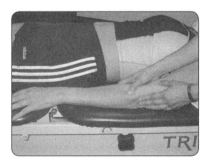

Palpation of the lateral wrist extensors.

Scars

Soft-tissue assessment should always include the evaluation of scars. A scar penetrates all layers of soft tissue from the skin to the fascia overlying the bone. Under normal healing circumstances following an injury, scar tissue should adapt fully to the surrounding layers of soft tissue and should function normally. However, if inadequate or abnormal healing occurs, the soft tissue around the scar becomes restricted and its ideal function is affected. This finding is termed an *active scar.* Active scars and their associated dysfunctional fascia are often chained up with TrPs and joint dysfunction at a location away from the site of the scar. Patients do not normally seek help for scars; instead, they may report symptoms of low back or cervical pain, headaches, difficulty breathing, and so on. Thus, the clinician must determine the relevance of a scar (if present) to the patient's symptoms. If palpation of an active scar reproduces a patient's symptoms, there is a key link between the scar and the patient's complaint or dysfunction.

When assessing scars, the clinician should note the appearance and temperature as well as note if the scar appears highly vascularized or if erythema is present or remains after light palpation. Warmth at the site of the scar may signify ongoing inflammation. An active scar often exhibits an increased skin drag. In other words, the skin at the site of the scar does not stretch or move easily. In many instances, there may be a thicker skin fold. The resistance to movement of the scar is assessed in all directions until a barrier is reached. The barrier is described by Lewit as the first palpable sign of resistance of the tissue, where the spring quality of the tissue is altered. The pliability or loss of springing in the tissue assists the clinician in identifying areas for treatment and reassessment. The scar is also evaluated for its sensitivity to palpation, stretching, or compression. Pain points are frequently found at the end of scars (Lewit 2007).

Myofascia

Janda noted the importance of fascia linking the entire musculoskeletal system into one unit. Fascia is made of collagen protein, which is very strong and has little elasticity. Collagen is produced by fibroblasts, and it orients itself along the lines of tension. This connective tissue not only links muscles and other body organs but also creates compartments or layers of muscle groups.

Fascia has been viewed clinically as a potential source of dysfunction, particularly in chronic MPS (Travell and Simons 1992; Simons, Travell, and Simons 1999). MPS and FM are characterized by TrPs or tender points, respectively. Specific treatment techniques such as soft-tissue mobilization, myofascial release, spray and stretch, and instrument-assisted soft-tissue mobilization such as the Graston technique may be helpful in these conditions. Chapter 9 provides more details on soft-tissue treatments. While it is possible for myofascial structures to be the primary cause of pain, clinicians should look for the source of dysfunction elsewhere in the sensorimotor system.

Summary

Muscle dysfunction manifests as either increased (hypertonic) or decreased (hypotonic) muscle tone. TrPs and tender points are often found in muscles that undergo tonal changes. TrP and tender point chains can be found in both tonic and phasic muscles and play an important role in perpetuating chronic musculoskeletal pain syndromes. Clinicians must remember that TrPs are often not the cause of dysfunction; rather, they are a symptom. Clinicians are encouraged to look for the functional cause of the soft-tissue dysfunction, which may be related to joint pathology, sensorimotor dysfunction, or other soft-tissue dysfunctions such as scars and hypomobile fascia.

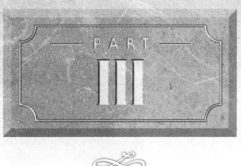

TREATMENT OF MUSCLE IMBALANCE SYNDROMES

The rehabilitation of the musculoskeletal system is based on the strong relationship between the CNS and the motor system; the logical assumption is that improving the quality of information improves the quality of CNS decision making in motor execution. The motor system acts as a window into the function of the CNS and frames the quality of its performance and its limits. Within the rehabilitation process, the diagnosed pathology may be clinically irrelevant. It is often the ensuing functional pathology that is the obstacle and that requires treatment. As a rule, the clinical picture correlates better with functional change than with structural pathology (Lewit 1997).

Improving CNS function is the ultimate goal of rehabilitation. This is accomplished by achieving efficient brain function through full processing and integration of afferent information from the senses and full expression of the motor system within its biomechanical capabilities, thus achieving physical, emotional, and chemical homeostasis and flexibility.

The three subsystems described by Panjabi (1994) are the control, passive, and active subsystems. They form a didactic triad and are linked and altered by their proprioceptive relationship. Change in any one system, or wheel, alters the position of the other wheels. Janda strongly felt that the evaluation of any patient must recognize the functional indivisibility of the subsystems. Muscles, ligaments, tendons, and fasciae form a single functional unit rather than separate entities, and the division between joint and muscle afferents is artificial (Gillquist 1996). Along with the viscera and skeleton, they make up the framework for collecting and expressing data processed by the CNS in response to the internal and external environment. Janda firmly believed that the CNS and motor system function as one unit, the sensorimotor system. He suggested treatment be organized into three stages:

1. **Normalization of the peripheral structures.** All peripheral structures outside the CNS must be treated in order to improve the quality of afferent information being received by the CNS.

2. **Restoration of muscle balance.** The balance between the phasic and tonic muscle systems must be improved as a prerequisite for improving coordination.

3. **Facilitation of afferent system and sensory motor training.** This training improves movement coordination and therefore promotes ideal mechanical loading of biological structures and efficient motor execution.

An optional but important addition to sensory motor training has always been the activation of primitive locomotor reflexes. Coordination and joint stability are improved by evoking complex reflex synergies that are stored at the midbrain level and that form the basis for gross motor system maturity. These synergies can be considered key factors in improving the quality of motor execution. However, this is a relatively complex approach to master, and proficiency and supervised training in learning and performing this approach are necessary. This Vojta approach is therefore beyond the scope of this text.

Part III details the different components of muscle imbalance intervention. Chapter 9 describes the procedures for normalization of the peripheral structures. Chapter 10 describes different techniques for restoring muscle imbalance through facilitation and inhibition techniques. Finally, chapter 11 reviews Janda's facilitation of the afferent system and his sensorimotor training program.

NORMALIZATION OF PERIPHERAL STRUCTURES

This chapter briefly discusses why peripheral structures are treated and then looks at techniques directed at the CNS to bring about profound peripheral changes as well as techniques directly aimed at the peripheral structures. The reason for looking at both types of techniques is that the strong link between the CNS and the periphery has shown certain global techniques to be vital in rapidly improving the status of the peripheral structures. These global techniques can reduce the amount and time spent on localized techniques.

Treatment approaches to the periphery can be divided according to the tissue type, the nature of the dysfunction, and the degree to which the dysfunction has a systemic effect. Janda defined peripheral structures as all tissues and organs lying outside the CNS and its meninges. Janda considered normalizing and treating the peripheral structures as the first step in the rehabilitation process, as a prerequisite for improving the quality of afferent input to the CNS. Accurate information from the proprioceptors is necessary to coordinate movement and protect joints (Freeman, Dean, and Hanham 1965; Freeman and Wyke 1967a). Therefore, improving the quality of the afferent input is a priority. Restoring this input augments the potential ability to improve motor control. However, the influence of proprioceptors on the nervous system is relatively subordinate in comparison with the driving influence of higher centers. This way, the integrated processes of the CNS avoid being overwhelmed constantly by prioritized but unnecessary external stimuli. However, this situation may be altered if the incoming information serves a protective function (Lederman 1997).

There are claims based on the current accepted knowledge of the properties of mechanoreceptors and reflex activity that manual reflexive techniques are ineffective in controlling the motor system (Lederman 1997). However, we see evidence to the contrary daily in the clinical setting. The means by which these motor changes effected by manual reflexive techniques occur may be unexplained as of yet, and our current knowledge may fall short in utilizing the correct parameters for measuring and researching these reproducible clinical phenomena. Nevertheless, they do exist and in the appropriate situation can be utilized with good effect as a useful adjunct to the more active phase of rehabilitation.

Techniques that normalize the peripheral tissue can be divided into two types. Central techniques indirectly affect peripheral structures, while local techniques directly affect the structures. A clinician cannot strictly treat the periphery without treating the CNS and vice versa. So it is up to the practitioner to utilize this relationship effectively both in treatment and in reassessment.

Central Indirect Techniques

Techniques that are not necessarily directed at manipulating the pathological tissues but have a powerful systemic or general peripheral effect on these tissues are considered to be central indirect techniques. A few examples of such approaches are the Vojta approach, primal reflex release technique (PRRT), and Feldenkrais. A detailed explanation of these techniques is beyond the scope of this text, but they are mentioned here to demonstrate their complementary role in Janda's approach.

Vojta Approach

The Vojta (pronounced *voy-tah*) approach is based on the genetically encoded motor function that is linked to development and maturation of the CNS. Specific positions and reflex points are used to summate afferent input to the CNS. This input can elicit partial patterns of movement that are related to the development of gross motor function and can enhance the quality of motor activation and joint stabilization by improving the body's ability to create the fixed points necessary for efficient muscle activity. Initially used by Václav Vojta, a Czech pediatric neurologist, to treat children with cerebral palsy and other motor developmental delays, the Vojta approach has been adapted for use with an adult population. One of its foremost pioneers is physiotherapist Pavel Kolář, of the Czech Republic, who developed his own techniques called *dynamic neuromuscular stabilization* (Kolář 2001; 2007). Patients are placed in certain neurodevelopmental postures to stimulate reflexive movement patterns. Certain pressure points are used to evoke motor patterns that are related to the gross motor patterns of creeping and turning (see figure 9.1, *a-b*). These postures

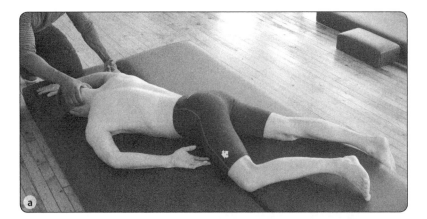

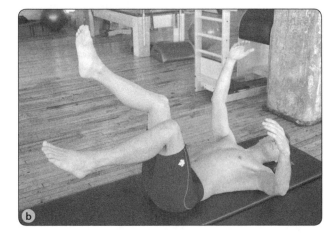

Figure 9.1   *(a)* Crawling neurodevelopmental posture. *(b)* Turning neurodevelopmental posture.

and patterns help to reset the motor system in cases of long-standing dysfunction. Clinically it is difficult for the patient to voluntarily replicate ideal gross motor synergies, especially after injury or in patients with long-standing compensatory motor strategies. It is therefore necessary to try to elicit a more effective and pure motor pattern—without the patient's compensatory voluntary input—by accessing the basic subcortical motor programs that are stored in the CNS. After summated reflex stimulation, voluntary exercises can be performed with increased quality and awareness of movement. Janda viewed the Vojta approach as a unique and integral part of rehabilitating patients who had poor motor control strategies that could not be easily influenced by more localized techniques and sensory motor training.

Primal Reflex Release Technique

The PRRT approach blends several simple manual procedures in an attempt to decrease the undesirable effects of startle, withdrawal, and joint protective reflexes that often accompany nociception and pain (Iams 2005). While these reflexes play an important role in the survival and coping strategies of humans, they can be overactivated and remain overactive in the form of undesirable physiological changes such as altered muscle tone or limited ROM. TrP and tender point chains exaggerate autonomic responses to mild stimuli, emotional overreaction, and so on; if the residual effects are left untreated they can plague the patient, resulting in continued symptoms that hamper expected recovery. Developed by the American physical therapist John Iams, PRRT is gaining popularity and is part of a paradigm shift within the rehabilitation process. The rapid physiological changes that can be achieved by PRRT make it a very useful clinical tool. Used as a stand-alone or adjunctive treatment, it can simplify the symptom presentation by eradicating unwanted tender points and subsidiary symptoms that often confuse the practitioner. For example, a patient who experienced recent trauma may present with significant pain and limited motion in his shoulder. If these findings are due to a protective response, then within one PRRT treatment session he may experience an 80% to 90% lasting improvement! Such results are not common in the traditional approach to treatment, since the traditional approach does not appreciate or totally ignores the vital role of the CNS in rapidly altering the patient's physiological and symptomatic presentation. In the traditional approach, local techniques are evaluated for their local effect, and no or little attempt is made at a centrally mediated intervention. The indivisibility of neurology and orthopedics is missed or not strongly utilized.

Feldenkrais

The Feldenkrais method, developed by Moshé Feldenkrais in the 1940s, changes movement strategies through verbal instruction for exercise performance (awareness through movement) and sensory integration, which involves manual movement manipulation of the patient by the practitioner. This manipulation improves the unconscious and conscious perception of movement, which in turn allows the patient to understand inefficient movement and explore acceptable alternatives. These alternatives are rapidly incorporated into the motor program, thereby eliminating undesirable motor strategies. Feldenkrais published the theoretical basis and basic exercises in his 1967 book, *Improving the Ability to Perform.* In 1972 the English version, *Awareness Through Movement,* was published. In it he describes awareness as taking place in the delay between thought and action and how awareness then relates to movement change (Feldenkrais 1972).

Local Direct Techniques

Techniques that are directed at the pathological or pathogenic tissues have a powerful local effect that may have a more general effect as well. The choice of techniques will depend on the patient evaluation, the practitioner's knowledge, the technique's suitability to the patient, and the desired goal. Local direct techniques include soft-tissue, neural tension, joint mobilization, Bowen, lymphatic, and orthotic techniques, just to name a few. There are a few indirect local techniques such as strain and counterstrain (Jones 1964) that do not engage the local pathological barrier of restriction but instead move away from it for treatment.

Soft-Tissue Techniques

Soft-tissue techniques are useful in managing scars, adhesions, and contractures. Any restriction in soft tissue (including skin, fascia, and muscle) affects movement and function both locally and globally. Scars may have a range of conditions that result in limited joint movement, pain, and postural changes. Cross-linking (chemical bonding), cellular matrix damage, adhesions, and contractions caused by myofibroblastic activity may all alter scar mobility, as is evidenced by postsurgical scars. Adhesions are abnormal deposits of connective tissue that occur between surfaces that should be able to glide by each other. Adhesions often result from some previous insult, infection, or inflammation between muscle layers or between tendons and their sheaths. Contractures are the shortening of connective tissue, which may be due to cross-linkages and adhesions that occur in muscles and ligaments and directly affect ROM. If the different fascial layers cannot move freely, they bias the movement of the underlying joint and can affect muscle function.

TrPs can be considered to be precursors to adhesions within muscle tissue. They can become hard, painful, palpable lesions that can be observed in muscles experiencing chronic overuse or injury. These hardened structures have been observed in cadavers (Schade 1919), a finding indicating that they are not due to muscle tonal changes alone but are structural alterations or contractures that affect the consistency of the tissue. Throughout several years, the observation of referred pain associated with these nodular phenomena and their identical qualities with TrPs became obvious (Reynolds 1983). The works of Simons and Travel (1999) and Mense and Simons (2001), among others, deal extensively with TrPs and acute and chronic pain generation within the motor system. Their effects can be multifactorial in affecting sensory motor function.

Since scars can involve adhesions and contractures and cause TrP formation in muscles, they can be used as a primary example for explaining soft-tissue assessment and treatment. Dormant scars are generally older, more mobile, and nonpainful. Active scars should be treated because they have an extensive effect on the sensory afferents to the CNS and can cause adverse motor function both locally and generally. Lewit (1997) and Janda have always given the treatment of scars a high priority in normalizing peripheral afferent information. The evaluation of soft-tissue restrictions includes several aspects:

- **Appearance.** If the scar appears highly vascularized or if erythema is present or is easily evoked by light palpation (and remains thereafter), then the scar is active and needs to be treated manually.

- **Temperature.** Warmth at the site of a scar may signify ongoing physiological activity that is either normal (a scar that is still healing) or abnormal (a scar with chronic inflammation).

- **Sensitivity.** All layers of the scar should be examined. If a part of the scar or the entire scar is painful to palpation, including stretching or compression, it may be active. Scars that are well healed should not be painful.

- **Hyperhydrosis.** Increased sweat production along the scar path can be tested by estimating the degree of skin drag and comparing sides or involved and uninvolved areas of skin. Skin drag is the feeling of increased resistance that is noted where there is increased moisture. The practitioner lightly strokes the skin of the scar by lightly running the fingers at a constant but moderate speed along the area of interest. Either simultaneously or in sequence, the practitioner strokes an area of unscarred skin and compares the amount of resistance felt to that felt on the scar. Hyperalgesic (skin) zones (Lewit 1999) often display increased skin drag due to autonomic activity. These zones are sensitive regions of skin related segmentally to other superficial or deep lesions, displaying decreased springing and elasticity.

- **Elastic quality.** The springing technique of assessing give and elasticity or pliability of the palpated tissue is applied and comparisons are made side to side. This helps identify areas for treatment or reassessment.

- **Soft-tissue texture.** The texture of the tissue is palpated for variations in consistency. The clinician assesses the tissue for uniformity, unevenness, or edema and compares the tissue with normal skin.

- **Mobility restriction.** The clinician first assesses the mobility at the barrier of the different layers of fascia and tissue that the scar traverses and of the scar itself. The physiological barrier is described by Lewit (1991) as the point where the first resistance at passive motion is met. It is also where the presence or absence of springing can be estimated. The loss of springing or the natural giving way of the elastic properties of tissues is of significant clinical value in determining if the tissue under inspection is normal or pathological.

- **Inhibition.** The muscles near or underneath the scar will often be inhibited. The muscles can be manually tested for strength loss and reassessed after treating the scar.

Specific techniques such as soft-tissue mobilization, instrument-assisted soft-tissue mobilization, cross-friction massage, and myofascial release (MFR) are useful in restoring normal soft-tissue movement. The primary goal is to eliminate abnormal nociception responses and movement restrictions. Many different myofascial techniques are available. These can be applied in increasing degree of force, from low-grade sustained gentle barrier release holds such as postisometric relaxation (PIR), which is the voluntary relaxation of hypertonic muscles achieved by the patient after a short mild isometric contraction of the same muscles (Lewit 1999), to grade 5 fascial thrusts (Iams 2005), until the elastic recoil properties of the tissue and mobility are normalized (see figure 9.2, *a-e*). In addition, respiratory or ocular synkinesis can enhance the effect of PIR. For example, relaxation of the masseters can be enhanced by oral inhalation during the relaxation phase (see figure 9.3). Likewise, gazing caudally during the contraction while supine and then looking cranially during the relaxation phase of a hip flexor stretch can speed up tone normalization and TrP resolution.

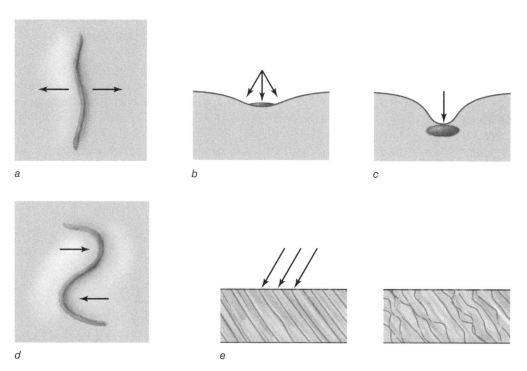

a   b   c

d   e

Figure 9.2 *(a)* Scar distraction. *(b)* Multivector dynamic release of a deeper scar. *(c)* Sustained static release of deeper scar tissue. *(d)* S-form mobilization of a scar. *(e)* The fascial barrier at which connective tissue thrust mobilization can occur.

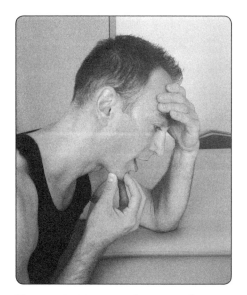

Figure 9.3 Masseter relaxation with respiratory synkinesis.

In addition to hands-on techniques, other modalities such as laser or ultrasound may be effective at breaking up active scar tissue. Whatever the technique, the tissue is restored to normalcy by making side-to-side comparisons. Often the autonomic reactions dissipate as the treatment progresses; this may take several sessions depending on the degree of dysfunction. The influence of scars can be far reaching because they can affect different tissues that in turn can affect other functions.

Neural Tension Techniques and Neurodynamics

The role of adverse neural tension (ANT) as a physiological and physical factor in limiting ROM and compromising sensory and motor function has been demonstrated by Butler (1991), Elvey (1986), and Shacklock (2005). ANT or altered neurodynamics can cause or aggravate existing symptoms and can hinder objective and subjective improvement of the patient.

The CNS is a dynamic continuum that is sheathed within the musculoskeletal system and must follow its every move. Therefore, the CNS is evaluated for ANT by loading the soft tissues through a base test system with sequential and variable joint movements. These include, among others, passive neck flexion, the straight-leg raise, the slump test, and four variations of upper-limb neurodynamic tests (ULNT; see figures 9.4 through 9.7). If symptoms are reproduced, increased, or decreased by these tests, then there is good reason to pursue a more thorough evaluation and treatment of ANT.

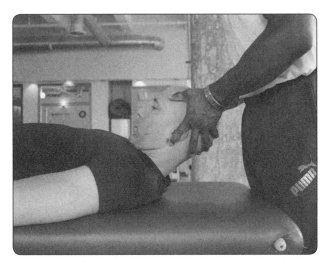

Figure 9.4 The passive neck flexion test.

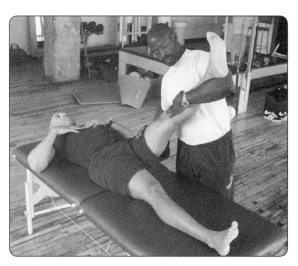

Figure 9.5 The straight-leg raise.

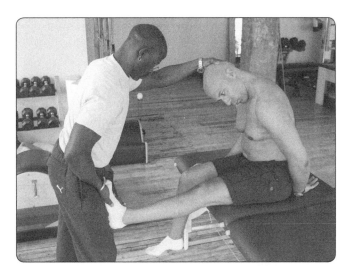

Figure 9.6 The slump test.

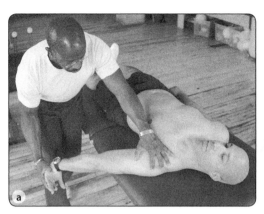
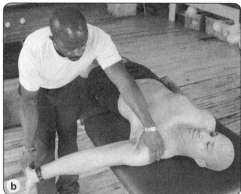
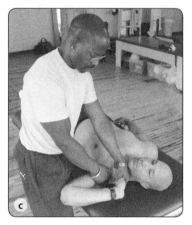

Figure 9.7 Upper-limb neurodynamic tests. *(a)* Radial nerve; *(b)* median nerve, and *(c)* ulnar nerve.

The cause of nociception or pain can be traced to either the nervous system (content) or the surrounding tissue (container) that protects the nervous system and to which the nervous system must adapt. The treatment of neurodynamic tension is a clinically significant intervention and one the clinician must address competently by utilizing the recommended techniques for resolving the issue of container versus content. The details of treatment techniques such as sliding and flossing or tensioning are beyond the scope of this chapter and are best reviewed in the texts by Butler (1991) and Shacklock (2005).

Joint Mobility Techniques

Joint mobility techniques such as joint mobilization and manipulation are valuable therapeutic techniques. The increase of physiological ROM, the reduction in nociceptive input to the dorsal horn, and the evoking of analgesia through manipulation have been supported in the literature (Herzog et al. 1999; Herzog 2000; Conway et al. 1993; Zusman 1986; Wright 1995). It can be inferred that graded mobilizations may have a similar but possibly milder effect compared to joint manipulation. Since mobilizations tend to be repeated many more times in one session than the manipulative thrust is repeated, it may be assumed that the mobilizations can create a cumulative effect.

The need for these techniques, which may be graded 1 through 5 in degree of intensity, should be carefully considered and evaluated. They are barrier techniques, involving the identification of a barrier restriction to normal mobility and then the application of force to overcome that barrier. The clinician must ensure that the choice of applying force to the barrier restriction is the best choice in light of the given evaluative information. Contraindications for the use of manipulation are well detailed (Barker et al. 2000; Grieve 1991; Gifford and Tehan 2003). Overcoming a barrier with force is not always the correct or ideal treatment because these restrictions may be protective. The cause for their protective strategy may not be localized to the restricted area, and the patient may not be well served by a local application of this type of barrier technique.

Lewit (1986, 1987) described the strong relationship between myofascial TrPs and articular dysfunction. He stressed throughout his teachings that both should be evaluated and, in light of the overall exam, prioritized and treated. The subsequent reexamination would then guide the therapist along the most effective path of dealing with the arthromyofascial dysfunction. For example, a patient's low back pain and altered pelvic mobility may have a relationship to limited fibula head mobility and the presence of a TrP in the hamstring belly of the biceps femoris. After a thorough exam and history—maybe a trip or stumble on that leg or a higher concentration of dysfunction in that limb—the release of the fibula head may be prioritized and the results seen in the abolishment of the hamstring TrP, the decrease in low back pain, and the improvement of pelvic mobility.

Remember, however, that restoring ROM through these techniques without ensuring that there are concomitant stability and strength through the new range is not good therapy. The active and control subsystems must be assessed for their ability to stabilize the motion made available.

Lymphatic Techniques

The flow of lymph has been considered to be an important factor in restoring normal physiological function. The human body is more than 60% water; one-third of its fluid is extracellular and two-thirds are intracellular (Lederman 1997). Localized pitting edema can often accompany injury following ankle sprains and surgery. (Pitting occurs when temporary deformation of the tissue—the pit—can be seen after applying point pressure to the edematous tissue.) Nonpitting edema is often related to more systemic pathology and often requires a more complicated treatment that may involve oral medication.

Muscles play an important role in moving lymph (figure 9.8). Manual techniques such as active muscle pump or rhythmic compression and decompression with external machines assist the hydrokinetic movement of extracellular fluid between the interstitial and lymphatic system and the blood plasma (Ganong 1981). Intermittent compression and decompression must be performed with sufficient pressure to affect the deeper vascular structures.

Fluid transport in and out of the joints depends on joint movement. Moderate amounts of active motion that do not aggravate pain in the involved joint are useful for decreasing joint edema given that the aggravating inflammatory cause has been addressed. Localized interstitial edema can be observed (along with muscle dysfunction) over the involved muscle belly or between the tendons and also at the tendino-osseous junction. It often resolves rapidly once the muscle chain has been treated and normal afference and function are restored.

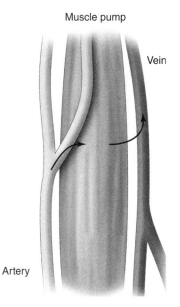

Figure 9.8 The role of the muscles in transferring lymph from artery to vein.

It has been suggested in the literature that modalities such as electrical stimulation (stimulation on the subsensory, sensory, and motor levels), iontophoresis, and ultrasound can be used to affect localized lymph movement and drainage in both acute and chronic situations by either inhibiting edema formation (sensory-level electrical stimulation) or aiding in its dispersal (Starkey 1999). However, it seems that significant results are obtained with some form of muscle activity (Walloe and Wesche 1988; Mann, Morrissey, and Cywinski 2007).

Orthotic Techniques

There is some evidence that orthotics can alter neural input and therefore affect posture and muscle function. Guskiewicz and Perrin (1996) reported that patients with acute

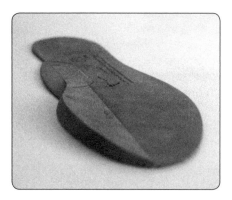

ankle sprains demonstrated significant decreases in postural sway after wearing custom-fit orthotics. Orthotics may enhance joint proprioception, increasing the patient's ability to detect perturbations and control postural sway. Similarly, Rothbart (2005) has cited changes in postural statics and the improvement of chronic musculoskeletal pain as a result of applying dynamic control insoles to the feet of patients (see figure 9.9). The global effects of microwedges on posture can be appreciated in the treatment approach of the posturology schools in Canada, France, and Italy.

Orthotics can be a useful adjunct to treatment; however, their introduction and use must be monitored by skilled practitioners. The effects of such devices must be weighed against the constraints they place upon the foot joints. Limiting the motion of the foot can have serious neurological consequences even if

Figure 9.9 Dynamic control insoles.

the biomechanical reasoning for the orthotic device appears sound and logical. Many practitioners have found themselves in the situation where the patient experiences a worsening of symptoms or develops new, unwanted symptoms from using orthotics despite all the positive indicators and carefully measured casting of the orthotic devices.

Pathogenic foot types can be observed in both planus (low longitudinal arched) and cavus (high longitudinal arched) feet. The structure of the feet may indicate the potential for pathology but may not necessarily determine or cause any pathology. The goal is to improve the stability of the foot and restore integrity during function, which involves ideal coordination, balance, strength, and power development to assist in locomotion and other general transfers associated with ADL. If these conditions are met irrespective of foot type, then the foot is biomechanically efficient and stable. There is evidence suggesting that stabilizing intrinsic muscle activity and function differ in shod versus unshod feet, in that the shod feet experience decreased intrinsic muscle development and depend more on passive structures for stabilization (Robbins and Hanna 1987).

Summary

After a comprehensive examination of the patient, peripheral structures are normalized by applying techniques appropriately targeting the different types of pathological tissue conditions. The goal is to normalize them as much as possible and enhance the quality of beneficial afferent input to the CNS as well as provide an environment that promotes healing and reactivation. The more powerful techniques target the CNS directly and achieve strong global responses from the sensory motor system. These techniques rapidly affect physiological processes and improve the symptoms and functional status of the patient. The more localized techniques address focused local deficits and complement each other. The unity of CNS and peripheral structures must be utilized and continually assessed by their response to treatment strategies. This helps clinicians zero in on the important deficits and create a more effective rehabilitation for their patients.

RESTORATION OF MUSCLE BALANCE

This chapter reviews different factors leading to muscle weakness and inhibition or tightness and shortening and the immediate treatment recommended by Janda. In addition, other therapies, some of which may be as effective or important procedures in light of new ideas and interventions, are also discussed. The goals of therapy are then summarized at the end.

Muscle imbalance must be viewed as both a local and a global response to afferent input. If treatment only targets imbalance as a local agonist and antagonist dysfunction, it will probably not have a lasting effect. The local and global imbalances are both expressions of CNS dysfunction between two complementary systems, the tonic and phasic systems. Muscle imbalances are discussed in detail in chapter 4.

The changes in muscle tone that result from aberrant afference lead to a cascade of events. The vicious cycle can continue and propagate, eventually leading to an acute breakdown of function at the weakest link; namely, that segment or part of a kinetic chain that is unable to adapt any further to the altered conditions. As a result, the weak link experiences an acute injury or inflammatory response and ultimately undergoes compensation or adaptation. Adaptation may progress vertically, in which case changes affect the CNS. Changes may also occur horizontally, affecting adjacent or contralateral joints and tissues.

Janda et al. (2007) recognized that different factors can alter muscle tone. Initially there is a neuromuscular response and then later more structural changes may occur within the contractile and noncontractile tissues. Changes in muscle tone that are not related to actual lesions of the nervous system (including upper and motor lower neurons) involve both the contractile and the noncontractile elements of the muscle: neuroreflexive and viscoelastic components, respectively.

- **Neuroreflexive factors.** There are many factors that alter muscle tone neuroreflexively. Many tissues can be involved in the reflexive responses of the CNS to positive or negative stimuli. These reflexes may be related to withdrawal, flight, fight, or freeze responses to stressors both mental and physical. Autonomous changes (e.g., changes in peristalsis, blood pressure, hydrosis, heart rate, or sphincter tone) and somatic changes (e.g., changes in muscle tone, nociception, resting posture, and skin sensitivity) have been demonstrated during these responses, and therefore global normalization of these observed symptoms can be an important indicator of the degree of homeostasis achieved postincident and posttreatment.

- **Viscoelastic and connective tissue changes.** The shortening of muscle and connective tissue over time can be seen as a long-term response to continued or intermittent stimuli. For example, shortened pectoralis muscles or hip flexors are a common clinical finding accompanied by limited ROM or movement substitution.

Lewit (1999) described the loss of springing and altered elasticity of the soft tissues in the presence of pathology. One example is the loss of springing in the interdigital connective tissues of the toes within the segmental dermatome of an active discogenic lumbar lesion.

In analyzing musculoskeletal dysfunction, limitation of motion itself is not necessarily a painful phenomenon. Joint blockage or limitation in joint play is also not painful unless accompanied by a change in muscle tone. Janda believed that muscle fatigue was often a predominating factor in dysfunction. The muscle, fascia, and nervous system span several segments, and this often leads to referred pain and the propagation of dysfunction. The initial treatment is to normalize muscle tone and results in the decrease of palpatory tone in the hypertonic muscles. Janda et al. (2007) described several causative factors that induce tonal changes leading to either inhibition and weakness or hypertonicity and tightness.

Factors Contributing to Muscle Weakness

Muscle weakness in chronic musculoskeletal pain must be differentiated from true weakness and from pseudoparesis, in which a muscle tests weak but is only temporarily inhibited (Janda 1986a). Several factors causing weakness may contribute concomitantly or separately in any given pathology, and careful analysis is needed to apply the appropriate treatment. Specific treatment techniques addressing the various causes of weakness are described shortly.

Tightness Weakness

With overuse or trauma, muscle becomes tight. There is a shift of the muscle length–strength curve, and the muscle may appear stronger. However, continued overuse increases the amount of noncontractile tissue, decreases elasticity, and then causes ischemia leading to degeneration of muscle fibers and eventual weakness. Tightness weakness is considered to be the most severe form of muscle shortening.

• **Treatment:** The involved muscle is stretched with the necessary techniques for contractile or noncontractile elements. Usually, stretching must be performed daily for 2 to 3 wk. The muscle must be checked to ensure that it is not inhibited by the stretching procedures, and then it can be strengthened through gradual progression.

Arthrogenous Weakness

Arthrogenous weakness is inhibition of muscle activity via the anterior horn cells secondary to joint dysfunction or swelling. For example, a meniscal derangement in the knee may lead to joint dysfunction and edema with resulting tendency for inhibition of the vasti muscles.

• **Treatment:** The normalization of joint function can be aided by direct mobilization or manipulation. Facilitation and activation of exteroceptors can be achieved with techniques such as brushing, which is lightly stroking the limb or the segments adjacent to the involved joints. The involved muscles can then be strengthened through gradual progression.

Trigger Point Weakness

TrPs can develop in response to a variety of stressors or stimuli (Mense and Simons 2001). Hyperirritable fiber bands decrease the stimulation threshold of the muscles unevenly, leading to inefficient activation, overuse, and early fatigue and weakness.

• **Treatment:** TrPs can be selectively deactivated using any of many different techniques such as PIR, spray and stretch, and strain and counterstrain. The involved muscles can then be strengthened through gradual progression.

Stretch Weakness

Prolonged and repeated elongation of muscle inhibits muscle spindle activation and can contribute to the addition of sarcomere units. In addition, habitual positions can place a muscle on stretch for significant durations. Also referred to as *positional weakness,* the resulting weakness is due to inhibition by antagonist tightness.

• **Treatment:** Relaxation and stretching of the short, overactive antagonist or synergist is performed initially. Then facilitation of the muscle spindle and strengthening of the lengthened muscle are initiated gradually, by often training the muscle within a shortened arc.

Reciprocal Inhibition

Reciprocal inhibition occurs when an antagonist for a specific movement has increased in tone and as a result inhibits force production by the agonist during that movement. This imbalance of forces can alter joint motion, cause pain, and reduce overall ideal function. A classic example is lateral epicondylitis, which can be driven by the increased tone of the pronator and flexor groups of the forearm and the inability of the extensors to maintain their strength and provide balanced movement.

• **Treatment:** Muscle tone and strength are normalized via direct relaxation or other inhibitory techniques for the antagonistic muscles. If strength is not completely restored to the inhibited agonist, then facilitatory techniques are also applied. These include brushing, drop and catch, origin–insertion facilitation, and dry needling.

Additional Treatment Techniques for Muscle Weakness

Because the muscle spindle plays an important role in regulating muscle tone and the reactivity of the muscle to a stimulus, treatment of muscle weakness aims at stimulating and increasing the response of the muscle spindle of the pseudoparetic muscle. The initial effect that an exercise activity has on strength may be caused by different factors. Strength changes are specific not only to task, speed, and angle but also to technique and learning (Jones et al. 1989) and the CNS response to the stimuli (Manion et al. 1999). Facilitation techniques are not strengthening exercises but should stimulate and prepare the muscle's contractile ability and coordinated response to loading. These preparations should precede the strengthening intervention. Resistance training of pseudoparetic muscles is contraindicated, as it decreases the muscle's efficiency in responding to loading. This inhibition of motor units may be due to direct overload or to substitution of movement by synergistic muscles (Janda 1986a in Grieve; Janda 1987).

Facilitation techniques address four basic proprioceptors: muscle spindles, GTOs, mechanoreceptors, and exteroceptors. Table 10.1 summarizes these techniques.

Table 10.1 Common Treatment Techniques for Weak Muscle

Procedure	Tightness weakness	Arthrogenous weakness	TrP weakness	Stretch weakness	Reciprocal inhibition
Stretching + exercise	■				
Skin brushing, stroking + exercise		■			
TrP deactivation + exercise			■		
Muscle spindle facilitation	■	■	■	■	■
Vibration	■	■	■	■	■
Oscillation		■	■	■	■
Brushing, tapping	■	■	■	■	■
Drop and catch		■		■	■
Origin–insertion stimulation	■	■	■	■	■
Kinesio taping, taping	■	■	■	■	■
Isometrics	■	■	■	■	■

The Brügger exercises, acupuncture, and PNF affect both facilitation and inhibition and therefore have not been placed in the table.

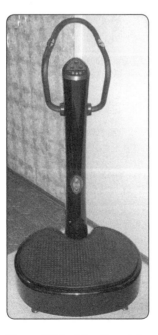

Figure 10.1 Vibration plate.

Vibration

Research has demonstrated that applying vibration either locally or generally has a positive effect on the force of muscle contraction (Bosco et al. 1999; Luo, McNamara, and Moran 2005). The muscle spindle is sensitive to small-amplitude vibrations of 50 to 200 Hz and will increase force output during a voluntary contraction. Placing the targeted muscle group in a lengthened position can enhance the effect.

Isometric and limited dynamic exercises can be performed on a vibration plate (see figure 10.1). Doing so improves muscle performance parameters such as strength and power afterward (Bosco et al. 1999). Frequencies that are used clinically range from 30 to 200 Hz with amplitude ranges in millimeters. The tonic vibration reflex (TVR) described by Hagbarth and Eklund (1966) is a reflex contraction induced by vibration that can be demonstrated in all skeletal muscles. Local application of vibration to the inhibited antagonist can normalize the tone of the agonist muscle groups. The effect can last up to 30 min, during which time functional movement can be trained with an altered muscle input that facilitates more normal physiology.

Oscillation

Oscillation involves rapidly alternating directions of motion over very short amplitudes. Amplitude, intensity, frequency, and method of application can be modulated to deliver an engaging series of exercises for facilitating muscle activation and coordination of movement. Several oscillating tools can be used to facilitate muscle activation. For example, oscillation with a Flexbar can activate muscles in the entire upper quarter (see figure 10.2; Page et al. 2004).

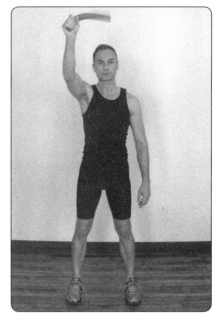

Figure 10.2 Flexbar oscillation in the upper extremity.

Brushing and Tapping

Brushing has been advocated by Rood to facilitate the spindle via the anterior horn cell and gamma loop (Carr and Shepherd 1980). Local or generalized brushing may be performed manually or electrically and may improve muscle activity as well as the patient's perception and experience of the muscle group or segment. Brushing the bottom of the foot may stimulate proprioceptors in the sole to increase the amount of afferent information (figure 10.3). Tapping over the muscle belly can be facilitatory, as it promotes localized quick stretching of the muscle fibers that enhances the myotatic reflex and therefore the contractility of the muscle.

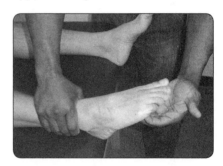

Figure 10.3 Brushing the bottom of the foot for proprioceptive stimulation.

Drop and Catch

Drop and catch is basically a quick stretch technique to facilitate the muscle spindle and muscle contraction via the myotatic reflex. It must be used with good control of all involved segments by the therapist and a short amplitude of application to minimize injury risk. It may be useful for an aberrant movement pattern of a segment or an inhibited muscle or muscle group. The inhibited muscle group is shortened passively and then placed in a supported static position. The clinician explains to the patient that at a randomly selected moment the support will be removed. The patient must initiate a rapid active contraction to prevent the segment from dropping uncontrollably out of the assumed position. This sequence is repeated 5 or 6 times. The drop and catch technique is often preceded just before by rubbing, tapping, or vibrating the involved muscle and its overlying skin for several seconds. It is best suited to large muscle groups and more robust joints such as the hip, knee, or elbow (see figure 10.4).

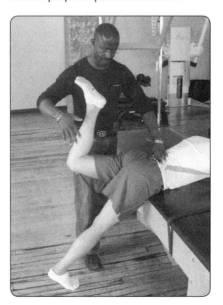

Figure 10.4 The drop and catch technique.

Acupuncture and Dry Needling

Given the high correlation between acupuncture points and TrPs (Melzack, Stillwell, and Fox 1977), using acupuncture needles to dry needle into the motor points and TrPs of muscles is very effective in eliminating TrPs or tender points that affect muscle contraction and performance (Hong 1994; Jaeger and Skootsky 1987). In addition to providing central analgesic effects (Hsieh et al. 2001), the stimulation of acupuncture points affects the limbic system and subcortical gray structures of the brain (Hui and Lui 2000), thereby influencing muscle tone throughout the motor system. This influence can aid in the normalization of ROM and muscle function.

In their book *Biomedical Acupuncture for Pain Management: An Integrative Approach*, Ma, Ma, and Cho (2005) provide a logical and structured approach to the dry needling of palpable tender points (that may include TrPs). Dry needling can improve motor function and modulate pain locally and centrally, among other things. The evaluative process and treatment differs significantly from those of traditional Chinese medicine in that the choice of points is determined by palpable tenderness in specific anatomical locations and is not related to meridians or the attributes traditionally assigned to them. Also, no herbs are recommended or administered as part of the treatment. Dry needling can be performed three times a week or more in conjunction with other therapies. Reassessment after each session determines the need for subsequent treatments. Unfortunately dry needling is not an option for many physical therapists, although it should be.

Proprioceptive Neuromuscular Facilitation

Proprioceptive neuromuscular facilitation (PNF), developed by Kabat (1950) and Knott and Vossin the 1950s, has provided a useful basis for facilitating and guiding movement synergies that reflect natural components of gross motor function and development while at the same time inhibit unwanted hypertonicity and hypotonicity. With the use of maximum available resistance, quick stretches, spiral and diagonal patterns, and rhythmic and combined motions, PNF restores and improves motor control and movement perception in patients. Exposing the CNS to familiar synergistic movement components can guide the therapist in choosing appropriate movements and emphasis. In chronic pain situations in which altered movement and degraded quality of movement may be a limiting factor, PNF can serve as an entry portal for change.

Origin–Insertion Facilitation

Origin–insertion facilitation, introduced by G. Goodheart in 1964 (Goodheart Jr. 1964; Walther 1988), led to the development of applied kinesiology and eventually clinical kinesiology. It focuses on the indirect facilitation of a neurologically inhibited muscle via the anterior horn. Facilitation is achieved by manually stimulating receptors and nerve endings as well as cutaneous receptors located at the origin and insertion of muscles. The suspected muscle is isolated as much as possible via positioning and is tested with a patient-initiated MMT. The practitioner observes the muscle's ability to contract isometrically on command; any sign of lag or give during the initial 2 to 3 s of the test is interpreted as neural incoordination and a sign of inhibition—in other words, hyperpolarization of the motor neuron. The origin and insertion of the muscle are then massaged for several seconds, and the muscle is reevaluated for an improvement in its ability to contract swiftly and effectively and to stabilize the assumed position isometrically without lag or give. This technique is suitable for many muscles, large or small, and can be very effective in improving muscle contractility and strength output (Walther 2000).

Muscle testing, origin–insertion manual therapy, and isometrics are also important aspects of the muscle activation techniques (MAT) developed by Greg Roskopf. However, the evaluative premise and thought process for MAT differ significantly from those of applied kinesiology. MAT is a system of biomechanical evaluation and treatment designed to address muscle imbalances and to restore agonist–antagonist balance. It includes a joint-specific ROM exam and the assessment of weakness and inhibition of correlated positional muscles. This approach to muscle activation is an important and basic aspect of the initial rehabilitation phase.

All muscles under voluntary control must be able to contract sufficiently and within sufficient time to maintain a direct relationship to the imposed load and speed of loading in order to satisfy the demands of any required task. If this basic criterion cannot be met, strengthening exercises will not be as effective. The Web site www.muscleactivation.com can furnish the reader with more information.

Brügger Concept

The Swiss neurologist Alois Brügger treated functional pathology by evaluating posture and movement to establish a neurophysiological basis for a patient's symptoms and a possible treatment strategy (Pavlu et al. 2007). Factors causing intermittent or constant disturbances give rise to physiological overload and nociception. The response is protective hypertonic or hypotonic arthro-tendo-myosis. Adaptation manifests as an altered posture, ROM, or movement pattern and symptoms of pain and discomfort. The exercise choices are based on deficits in the range of movement and signs of imbalance rather than pathology displayed by the patient. Treatment includes several components, which are described in the following sections.

Interstitial Edema Control

Edema control is performed before exercise by applying a hot compress massage to the edematous areas identified during the evaluation. Deep transverse friction massage is also performed on the heated tissue. The control of and decrease in edema can aid in limiting not only unwanted cross-linkage within damaged tissue, but also inflammation and resulting pain. These are important factors in improving overall function and achieving a satisfactory treatment outcome.

Postural Correction

Postural correction includes elongation of the spine with head centration. The spinal coupling of movement is conceptualized as a series of interlocking cogwheels (see figure 3.1 on page 28) that represent the cervical, thoracic, and lumbar segments and their synergistic relationship to each other during uprighting or collapsing movements with a concomitant increase or decrease in sternosymphyseal distance. An increase in palpable tenderness of the superficial musculature indicates a decrease in the sternosymphyseal distance associated with a slumped posture.

Local and Global Movement Exercises

These exercises restore muscle balance through functional synergism (i.e., cooperation among agonists, antagonists, and synergists). The goal is to eliminate the undesirable hyper- or hypotonicity within the region and throughout the motor system by increasing activity in hypoactive muscle chains and inhibiting overactive muscle chains. This is achieved through a series of isometrics, or smooth and rhythmic concentric and eccentric agistic movements that are resisted with elastic bands (see figure 10.5). Emphasis is placed on the eccentric phase of movement, which should be twice as slow as the concentric phase. Mild to moderate elastic resistance is used to enhance the effects of the exercises; however, the quality of the movement is definitely more important than the quantity or the loading of the movement. Several basic movement tests are performed for clinical evaluation, including active ROM tests, to tailor the intensity and volume of the exercise program to the patient. The procedures just described are combined with manual therapy, positioning, interstitial edema control, and modifications for posture and ADL. The principles incorporated into the Brügger approach are important, as they stress the respect for synergistic muscle systems whose balance governs the resting posture of patients and whose activation must be accounted for when prescribing therapeutic exercises. The Brügger exercises can be used in the initial phase of rehabilitation and also as prophylactic activities for situations involving ADL.

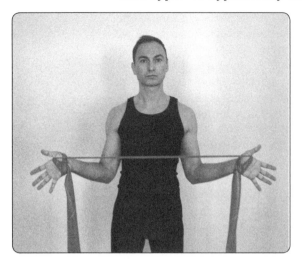

Figure 10.5 A Brügger upper-body exercise.

Kinesio Taping and Fascial Taping

Kinesio taping, which was invented by Kenzo Kase in the mid-1990s (Kase et al. 2003), has been popular due to the pain control and improvement in muscle function that it provides. Applying moderately contractile tape over affected muscle, joint, or soft tissue appears to cause gentle, passive, and constant contraction tension of the epidermis (see figure 10.6). There is no evidence as of yet to suggest that it improves joint position sense (Halseth et al. 2004; Murray 2000), but there is some

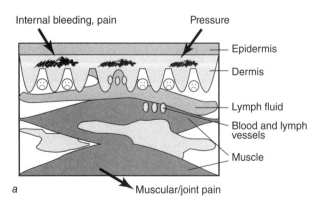

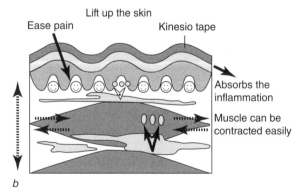

Figure 10.6 The physiological effects of kinesio taping.

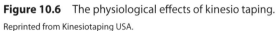

Reprinted from Kinesiotaping USA.

evidence that it can affect muscle strength (Murray 2000) and can change blood flow in the taped muscle of injured subjects but not in the muscle of healthy subjects (Kase and Hashimoto 1998). However, there are many clinical anecdotes on its usefulness in controlling pain. The mechanism by which pain control is achieved is unknown, but it is thought to involve proprioception and the sensorimotor system.

It is thought that kinesio taping can play either a facilitatory or an inhibitory role depending on the direction and amount of tension used during tape application, but this has not been verified. Inhibitory and facilitatory techniques can be used simultaneously to assist in muscle rebalancing. Figure 10.7 gives an example of combined facilitatory kinesio taping of the lower trapezius and inhibitive kinesio taping of the upper trapezius in UCS.

Good pain relief and improved function have also been reported by patients using functional fascial taping (FFT), a technique developed in 1994 by Ron Alexander (Alexander 2008). It is possible to conclude that any taping technique that modulates pain can normalize or improve muscle tone (whether it facilitates tone or inhibits unwanted tone), breaking the pain cycle and thereby improving patient comfort and function.

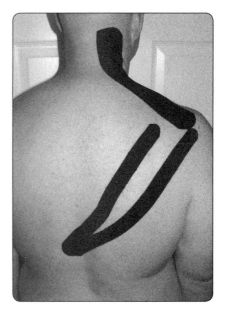

Figure 10.7 Facilitation of the lower trapezius and inhibition of the upper trapezius with kinesio taping.

Isometrics

In the 1950s, Charles Atlas popularized isometric exercises as a fitness activity. The dynamic tension exercises were the basis of his training program for very weak individuals. Dr. T. Hettinger and E. Muller, a pair of German scientists, gave isometrics a scientific popularity after publishing a paper showing that isometrics increase strength (Hettinger and Muller 1953).

The use of isometrics to facilitate tonic muscle fibers can be an important initial step in addressing submaximal muscle strength and restoring joint stability. Though the activation order of muscle fibers varies under different conditions, in general small, slow-twitch tonic fibers are activated first and may confer the joint stability and feedback needed for increased load and movement. While there are limitations to its use in task-specific dynamic movement, isometric movement is the basis of submaximal stabilization control, which is an integral part of many rehabilitation approaches.

The typical prescription of 1 or 2 sets of 5 to 10 repetitions of 5 s minimum contractions with moderate to high force is performed three times a week and can stimulate tonic muscle function and strength as well as prepare the patient for more dynamic exercises. However, specific dose recommendations cannot be made based on the available research. In PNF and Brügger techniques, isometrics are used extensively—though not exclusively—to stimulate agonist contraction and inhibit unwanted antagonist activation, thereby increasing active ROM. Umphred (2001) indicated that resistance is facilitatory to the muscle spindle afferents and tendon organs. She also noted that isometric and eccentric forms of resistance are more facilitatory to extensor muscle groups. Eccentric training of agonists results in concurrent strength gains in antagonists of 16% to 31% (Singh and Karpovich 1967). Gandevia, Herbert, and Leeper (1998) attributed the reflex facilitation of muscles to spindle afferents, which contribute up to 30% of the excitation of motor neurons in an isometric contraction. Multiangle isometrics are recommended, and contribution of the muscle spindles varies from one joint position to another.

Factors Contributing to Muscle Tightness

Several factors contribute to muscle tightness, which are described in the following sections. Specific treatment techniques are described later in this chapter.

Reflex Spasm

Tightness due to reflex spasm is nociceptive or pain generated. Examples are acute lumbar antalgia and abdominal spasm associated with appendicitis. In these cases, the patient cannot voluntarily relax the muscle.

- **Treatment:** Neutralization or elimination of the pain generator with a variety of suitable techniques such as cryotherapy, manipulation, traction, and so on can be performed to decrease the muscle spasm. Note that the spasm may not be the pain generator but can indicate the status of the pain-generating structure.

Interneuron Spasm

While joint dysfunction may cause inhibition in some muscles, in other muscle groups spasm may be observed. An example is torticollis with involuntary activities of muscles such as the SCM.

- **Treatment:** Joint manipulation or mobilization has been shown to not only improve ROM but also normalize abnormal muscle tone in muscles associated with the manipulated joint either directly or indirectly (Herzog et al. 1999). It also has been shown to reduce nociceptive input to the dorsal horn (Zusman 1986). There is evidence for inducing analgesia via facilitation of the descending inhibitory pain pathways (Wright 1995).

Trigger Point Spasm

In a muscle spasm caused by TrPs, the muscle fails to relax over time. This is commonly seen in the trapezius TrP due to prolonged repeated tension.

- **Treatment:** TrPs can be deactivated initially with an effective technique such as spray and stretch, active release, or strain and counterstrain (Jones 1964), among others. Thereafter, a more global approach that involves active CNS participation is necessary to avoid recidivism of symptoms. Failure to affect the central regulatory mechanisms via some type of neuromuscular reeducation that coordinates muscle function and tone will most likely allow the TrP spasm to return, especially in chronic conditions.

Limbic Spasm

Hypersensitivity of muscle spindles due to overactivity of the limbic system, which is caused by any number of stressors, leads to regional increased muscle tone with a uniform increase and change in tissue tone throughout. These changes usually occur in the cervical and shoulder girdle area or the low back, typically resulting in upper-quadrant pain or nonspecific low back pain. Janda noted that sensitivity of the scalp could be observed in such limbic-driven conditions (Janda, personal communication).

- **Treatment:** General relaxation techniques such as massage, self-hypnosis, stress reduction, and rest are recommended. These techniques are thought to lower the hyperaroused state of the limbic system, which then directly affects muscle tone, eliminating the nociceptive response.

Muscle Spasm Tightness

Muscle spasm is usually caused by overuse, secondary to injury, as in tennis elbow or trapezius syndrome. A muscle becomes gradually or acutely tight as it fails to relax and recuperate between activities. This tightness leads to spasm that may cause pain (Mense et al. 2001).

- **Treatment:** Facilitation of the muscle followed by stretching if necessary is the treatment of choice. If muscle stretching is introduced without previous facilitation, further inhibition of the muscle may occur. This leads to deafferentation and loss of joint protection.

Additional Treatment Techniques for Muscle Tightness

Muscle tightness and the eventual shortening of the noncontractile tissue can inhibit the antagonist muscle groups and alter the synergistic and stabilization functions of segments. Remember that muscles never act in isolation and thus the restoration of ideal coactivation for stability is key. Inhibitory techniques can be applied to the involved agonist in order to decrease muscle tightness and normalize tone. Restoring agonist tone improves the activity of the antagonist and abolishes its resulting inhibition and weakness. Table 10.2 summarizes various techniques used to address muscle tightness and the indications for their use.

Table 10.2 Common Treatment Techniques for Muscle Tightness

Procedure	TrP	Tight muscle	Short muscle	Pain relief
PIR	■	■		■
PNF: hold relax	■	■		■
PNF: contract relax		■	■	■
PFS			■	
Static stretch		■	■	■
Cryotherapy	■	■		■
Spray and stretch	■	■		■
Yoga	■	■	■	■
Massage	■	■		■
Strain and counterstrain	■	■		■
Meditation		■		■

Postisometric Relaxation

Postisometric relaxation (PIR) was first described by Mitchell et al. (1979) as an osteopathic technique called *isometrics*. It was later modified by Karel Lewit (Lewit 1991, 1986). PIR is a method of muscle relaxation aimed at neural modulation. It is guided by the therapist, but its success is totally dependent on the client. Primarily used to affect the contractile component of the muscle tissue, it helps eliminate abnormal muscle tone, abolish TrPs and tender points, and improve loss of motion due to altered muscle tone.

In PIR, the muscle is isolated biomechanically as much as possible. The patient is asked to imagine the contraction or to barely contract the affected muscle and to maintain this contraction for 20 to 30 s. This allows for the hypertonic foci of the TrPs to be activated and fatigued without much unnecessary activation of the surrounding muscle fibers. Then the patient is asked to relax the muscle as completely as possible. As the patient relaxes, the limb can be allowed to move to a new position, thereby gaining ROM through relaxation as opposed to stretching. This procedure can be repeated 3 or 4 times. At that point the tenderness or abnormal tone and ROM are reexamined for positive changes. The result is relaxation of the muscle and deactivation of hypertonic areas within the muscle.

There is no physical stretching of the muscle and therefore the effects of PIR are due to changes in neural function. These effects can be enhanced by respiratory or ocular synkinesis (Lewit 1986; Lewit et al. 1997). Figures 10.8 through 10.17 demonstrate PIR techniques for the muscles prone to tightness in Janda's syndromes. PIR techniques for other muscles are described thoroughly in Lewit's text (Lewit 1991).

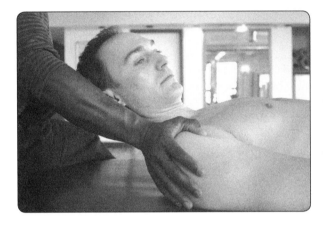

Figure 10.8   PIR for the upper trapezius.

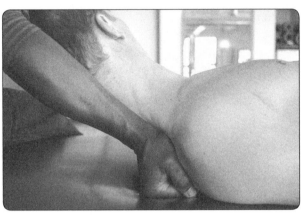

Figure 10.9   PIR for the levator scapulae.

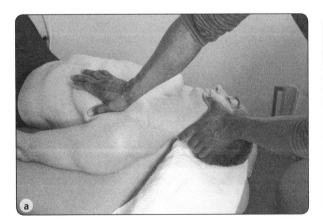

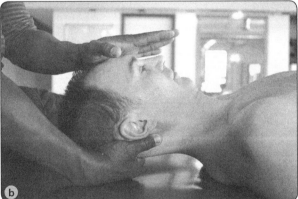

Figure 10.10   *(a)* PIR for the posterior scalenes and *(b)* PIR for the SCM and anterior and mdidle scalenes.

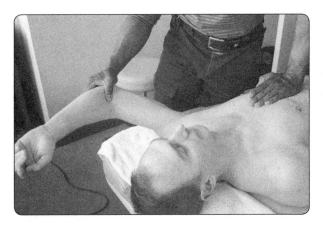

Figure 10.11 PIR for the suboccipitals.

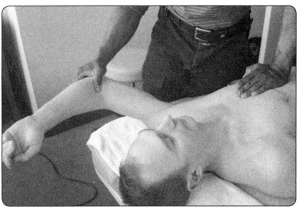

Figure10.12 PIR for the pectoralis major.

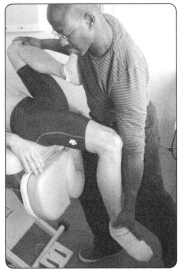

Figure 10.13 PIR for the hip flexors, including the iliopsoas and rectus femoris.

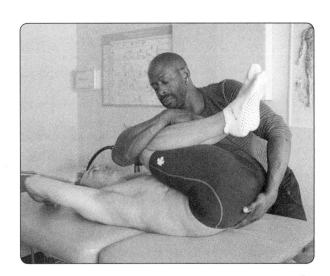

Figure 10.14 PIR for the thoracolumbar extensors.

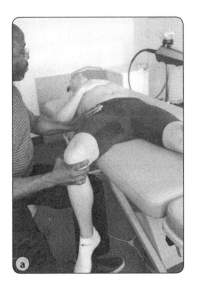

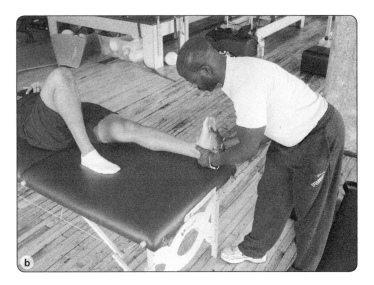

Figure 10.15 PIR for the *(a)* one-joint and *(b)* two-joint hip adductors.

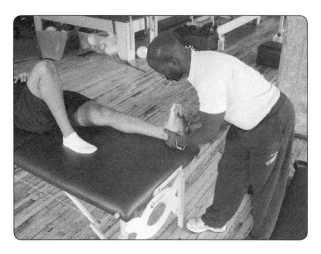

Figure 10.16 PIR for the triceps surae.

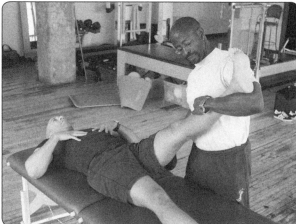

Figure 10.17 PIR for the hamstrings.

In all of the stretching techniques discussed in the following sections, some degree of mechanical stretch is applied to the tissue. The stretch causes viscoelastic and thixotropic (the quality of a solid or gel to become more liquidlike when agitated and to return to its former state at rest) effects, which do not change the stiffness of the muscle but improve its extensibility. There seems to be confusion regarding the terms *extensibility* and *stiffness* in the literature. In the case of true structural contractures, stretching can be judiciously applied in order to improve the tissue mobility.

PNF Techniques

Primarily used to affect the contractile component of the muscle tissue, stretches called *hold relax* and *contract relax* are adaptations of the original PNF techniques described by Kabat, Knott, and Voss in the 1950s and 1960s (Knott and Voss 1968). The muscle involved is lengthened to the barrier, which is the first sign of palpable resistance to further elongation.

• **Hold relax.** The patient performs an isometric contraction for up to 20 s and is then asked to relax and allow the therapist to guide the segment further in the direction of resistance. The therapist applies a mild stretch and holds the stretched position for another 10 to 20 s. From this new position the procedure is repeated and so on for 3 to 4 repetitions. This effectively increases the available ROM the muscle or muscle group can allow. In a study performed on rabbits, 80% of tissue elongation took place in the first four cycles of stretching, and thereafter very little elongation was observed (Taylor et al. 1990).

• **Contract relax.** Primarily used to elongate contractile tissue, this method is a slightly more aggressive form of hold relax in which the affected muscle is taken to the barrier, but instead of performing an isometric contraction, the patient performs an isotonic shortening contraction, allowing the segment to move away from the barrier to a midpoint where the isometric contraction is then maintained for 10 to 20 s. After the patient has been asked to relax, the segment is taken to a new but comfortable position past the original barrier that provides a moderate stretch, which is maintained for another 10 to 20 s. The procedure is repeated 3 to 4 times, each time from a new barrier further into the desired ROM.

• **Hold relax and contract relax with antagonist contraction.** This is essentially the same as the procedures just described, but in addition the antagonist is contracted either at the end of the passive stretch or during the stretch to enhance the inhibitory effect on the agonist being stretched.

Postfacilitation Stretching

The postfacilitation stretching (PFS) advocated by Janda et al. (2007) affects both contractile and noncontractile tissue elongation. The patient's ability to relax rapidly and as completely as possible is essential; otherwise this method is contraindicated as it can lead to injury of the muscle. Therefore the patient must demonstrate the ability to relax immediately on command. This can be done as a test run where the limb or segment is lifted and held by the patient and the therapist places his hands below the segment and asks the patient to relax and let the segment drop into the therapist's hands. The patient should respond as rapidly as possible without hesitation or apprehension. If the patient can demonstrate this correctly, then PFS can be utilized. This stretch is performed over the most stable joint available in the following steps:

1. The available ROM is estimated. The stretch range is also estimated by going further into the desired ROM and eliciting mild to moderate patient discomfort. This will be the barrier at which the stretch is maintained.

2. The segment is brought back to midrange, and maximal isometric resistance is applied for 8 to 10 s. The patient is positioned in such a way that it is relatively easy for the therapist to apply significant resistance during the isometric contraction phase.

3. At the end of the contraction the patient is ordered to relax. The stretch is applied by the clinician rapidly and firmly moving the segment to the estimated stretch position and holding it still for about 15 s.

4. The segment is then returned to a resting position with complete muscle relaxation for 20 s.

5. The contract and stretch procedure is performed again three more times, with an estimated final barrier going further into the desired ROM.

6. The patient can rest a few minutes until any sensation of weakness has passed before attempting any significant loading of the muscle.

7. Exercise as such should be avoided immediately after the stretching procedure.

This procedure is contraindicated for spasticity, primary muscle diseases, and patients with heart problems, pregnancy, acute pain, and bone lesions. It is useful for larger muscles such as the iliopsoas, rectus femoris, hamstrings, or latissimus dorsi (see figures 10.18-10.21). Moderate

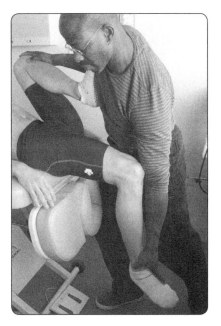

Figure 10.19 PFS for the rectus femoris.

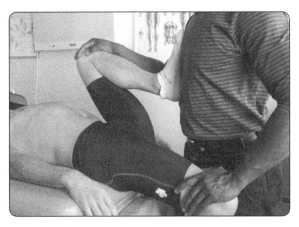

Figure 10.18 PFS for the iliopsoas.

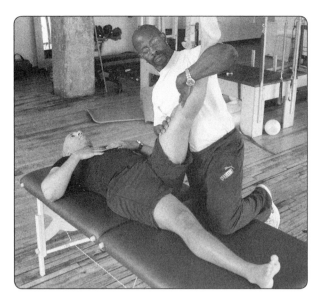

Figure 10.20 PFS for the hamstrings.

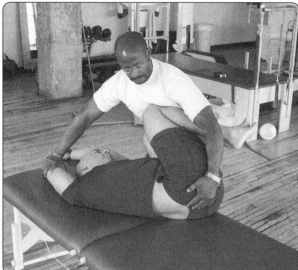

Figure 10.21 PFS for the latissimus dorsi.

discomfort is sometimes experienced. The muscle group may feel warm or weak after this stretch series. Due to transient inhibition, care should be taken that the muscle is not loaded too soon afterward in any particular function. Uncoupled spinal movements should be avoided.

Static Stretching

This technique affects both the contractile and the noncontractile tissue of the muscles involved. It is simply the placement of the segment at the barrier and allowing either gravity or an external force to stretch the muscle tissue over a significant length of time. No prestretch contraction is evoked, and the duration of the stretch can be significantly longer, such as 3 to 15 min, allowing creep deformation within the tissue. Creep deformation is the property of a material to deform over time due to applied external forces that do not exceed the integrity of the material; it can lead to temporary (elastic) or permanent (plastic) deformation. Stretching can be performed for up to 1 h with intermittent breaks of 30 to 60 s.

There are risks involved in stretching, as it can increase tissue plasticity, damage, and muscle inhibition. The greater the frequency, force, or velocity used, the greater the risk for negative side effects that may lead to chronic inflammation or to poor tissue repair (Lederman 1997).

Cryotherapy

Cryotherapy is the use of a cold medium to reduce the temperature of biological tissues in order to reduce the physiological and physical signs of inflammation, mitigate the tissue response to trauma, or provide analgesia for pain. It can be utilized with the involved muscle on a stretch (at the tissue barrier) or with the muscle on slack. Its analgesic effect can be utilized just before or after exercise to modulate pain and decrease the risk for unwanted inflammation. It works as an analgesic because cold reduces the firing rate of afferent nerves, thereby reducing pain perception. Muscle spasm and hypertonicity are reduced by the decreased firing rate of nerves and decreased muscle spindle activity and inhibition of the stretch reflex. Pain is also gated by the excitation and discharge of large-diameter neurons that in turn gate the smaller-diameter pain transmitting nerves. The usual application time of 15 to 20 min is often sufficient to achieve these effects. A plastic bag partially filled with crushed ice is most practical. Crushed ice remains colder for longer when compared with ice cubes. Unwanted air should be expelled and the bag sealed. Wrapping a damp towel around the bag provides better conduction. The bag should be secured to the desired area for 15 to 20 min. Directly applying ice to the skin should be avoided unless part of an ice massage. Ice application can be repeated every 1 to 2 h at most. Effective alternatives to ice are cooling topical analgesics such as Biofreeze. These topical agents can be applied as a gel, cream, or spray.

Spray and Stretch

A cooling agent such as Fluoro-Methane is sprayed as a stream several times over the skin of the muscle that contains the TrP or tender point. At the same time, the muscle is stretched through a comfortable ROM either passively or actively. To have good effect, the coolant must be sprayed across the whole length of the muscle during application. Spray and stretch has been demonstrated to relieve TrPs, normalize abnormal tone, and improve ROM. It creates strong centrally mediated and local effects, which are evidenced by the relaxation of the muscle through cutaneous cooling and the abolishment of referred pain of visceral origin. There is also a strong anti-inflammatory response with the application of the vapocoolant spray, a phenomenon possibly mediated by the autonomic nervous system (Travell and Simons 1983).

Yoga

Contractile and noncontractile tissue elongation can be achieved by combining relaxation with meditation and the assumption of end-of-range static or slow poses that either passively or actively elongate the muscles. This can affect the extensibility of muscles, which can help restore ROM and improve joint loading. For example, tight hip flexors that adversely affect lumbar lordosis in standing may lead to mechanical low back pain. Through yoga poses and stretching, the hip flexors may be relaxed and gain increased extensibility, allowing the lordosis to be less acute and thereby relieving back pain. There is also evidence that isometric contractions decrease passive tension in a muscle (Taylor et al. 1990). This response, elicited by the static holding postures of yoga, may also reduce undesired hypertonus and therefore provide pain relief. Yoga includes strengthening aspects and therefore cannot be considered to be a wholly inhibitory process.

Massage and Myofascial Release

Rhythmic stroking and soft-tissue mobilization are mentally relaxing, causing the limbic system and reticular formation to decrease their activity, which in turn lowers muscle tone (Sullivan et al. 1993). This effect can be beneficial, especially when stress factors are causing anxiety and the resulting increased muscle tone leads to incoordination or inefficient use of the muscular system, a possible cause for the development of muscle lesions and imbalance. More aggressive soft-tissue techniques may inhibit undesirable muscle tone, restore fascial mobility, and increase circulation and lymph flow. Factors that can signal local and regional tonal changes include improved and symmetrical ROM, decrease in tender points and pain, and improved strength and coordination.

Neurodynamic Treatment

Shacklock (2005) describes a continuum of nervous tissue being affected by compressive, tensional, longitudinal, and transverse sliding stressors that can compromise physiological and mechanical homeostasis. Due to the effect that stressed nervous tissue can have on surrounding tissues (both the interface and the innervated tissues), altered neurodynamic status should be evaluated and treated since muscular changes in tone, tenderness, and strength can sometimes be directly linked to this factor. For example, sciatic irritation often results in perceived tenderness and hypertonicity of the hamstrings, leading to decreased ROM in the straight-leg raise when compared with the unaffected side. Flossing or sliding techniques can restore mobility and physiological homeostasis of the nervous tissue. This in turn can have a profound effect on muscle tone, activity, and function.

Strain and Counterstrain

This technique, invented by Lawrence Jones (1964), has been an empiric procedure utilizing a working hypothesis based on the theory of the facilitated segment (Korr 1979) and its apparent effect on the excitability of the muscle spindle and indirect excitability of the extrafusal fibers of adjacent muscles or muscles served by the involved segment. The conclusions of Korr's work on the facilitated segment have been questioned by Lederman (1997). However, this does not disqualify strain and counterstrain as a useful adjunct in manual treatment. Prolonged central sensitization of the CNS can arise from brief, low-frequency stimulation of C fibers. This in turn can increase the size of the receptive field of dorsal horn neurons and increase their responsiveness to harmless stimuli. Any treatment that can break that cycle of sensitization can be a useful tool in combination with other interventions (Light 1992; Woolf 1987). The nociceptive model described by Van Buskirk (1990), among others, may also aid in understanding the process of strain and counterstrain. The procedure involves the temporary inhibition (up to 90 s) of aberrant spindle activity through passively positioning the body segments to allow muscle to shorten to the point where hypertonic or painful areas within the muscle are no longer palpably painful. This technique appears to allow the muscle spindle and CNS to reassert the ideal relationships between muscle length and reported muscle tension, joint position, and centrally regulated spindle sensitivity. If these factors are synchronized, the muscle often relaxes, and tone is normalized after the patient maintains this position for 1 1/2 min. Strain and counterstrain can help tremendously in alleviating muscular dysfunction, decreasing pain, and restoring motion.

Meditation

The relaxation response has been described in literature alluding to various autonomous reactions induced by relaxation techniques and rituals that may alter CNS states. These alterations are evidenced by changes in EMG and electroencephalogram (EEG) recordings and by positive subjective experiences of well-being. Benson (1984) has been instrumental in researching and describing several methods and results of meditation. Meditation can be useful when increased muscle tone and discomfort are supported by increased limbic and reticular formation activity in response to stressors that trigger physiological responses. These responses to stressors often manifest as regional hypertonicity of muscle groups in the shoulder, neck, or low back without any particular TrP representation. Stress-induced symptoms can be identified by their absence when the patient relaxes or is on vacation, for example.

Summary

The treatment of muscle imbalance is directed at correcting common syndromes observed in the patient, the most common of which Janda has classified as the UCS, LCS, and layer syndromes. These syndromes have been reviewed in earlier chapters and are the result of CNS disequilibrium. They may originate from postnatal developmental motor problems or from activities that force single or repetitive changes in motor planning. This in turn causes predictable systemic imbalances that may assert themselves over time or after injury, fatigue, or disease.

Muscle imbalance is a systemic phenomenon that develops gradually and does not involve all the muscles to the same extent. There are often two primary areas where it appears to originate. These areas are linked to the most demanding functions we have as upright beings: the pelvic girdle and the shoulder girdle.

To treat the UCS, the tight and shortened tonic muscles of the cervicopectoral region and posterior cervical region must be inhibited. Their antagonists, the scapular fixators and depressors along with the deep anterior cervical muscles, must be facilitated and their endurance improved before coactivation training.

In treating the LCS, the tight hip flexors and thoracolumbar erector spinae are relaxed and stretched using appropriate techniques. The abdominal and gluteal muscles are facilitated and strengthened, and coactivation exercises are utilized to coactivate and coordinate the activity initially of the weaker glutes and abdominal wall but finally all of the muscle groups involved in synergistic balanced activities for stabilization and improved muscle balance. Overall balance of the synergistic phasic and tonic muscle groups must be improved. The patient must therefore alter his habitual activities and exercise regimen if he is to achieve long-term beneficial changes. Reintegration of muscle activity under a variety of conditions and improved motor engrams is the goal.

SENSORIMOTOR TRAINING

Sensorimotor training (SMT) is the third and vital stage in the rehabilitation process outlined by Janda. Manual therapy techniques alone are insufficient to rehabilitate the motor system; stimulation and integration of improved movement and motor strategies are also needed. Cognition, memory, central motor, and sensory program adaptations are necessary to improve rehabilitation results. As nociception, pain, and inflammation are reduced and ROM and biomechanical loading can be tolerated, synergistic movements and integrated whole-body movements can be encouraged.

The concept of progressive stimulation of the subcortical centers for coordinated movement patterns and equilibrium reactions is based on the work of Kabat in the 1950s, Fay in the 1940s, and Freeman in the1960s. Janda emphasized the importance of stimulating the entire sensorimotor system through afferent and subsequent efferent mechanisms. He noted that peripheral information must be emphasized and corrected first (see chapter 9). The cerebellum and other subcortical areas provide templates of movement based on primitive movement patterns, while the cortical parietal and frontal lobes provide the motor programs that are sent via muscular efferents.

SMT involves the passive and active facilitation of afferents that have a strong influence on controlling equilibrium and posture. There is evidence proprioception plays a role in maintaining balance and proper function of the lower extremity and in limiting the risk for injury (Hrysomallis 2007; McGuine et al. 2000; Payne et al. 1997; Tropp, Ekstrand, and Gillquist 1984a, 1984b). In addition, stimulating the sole of the foot improves kinesthesia and postural sway (Maki et al. 1999; Watanabe and Okubo 1981; Waddington et al. 2003), demonstrating the effects of proprioception in maintaining proper posture.

When it comes to improving muscle reaction, neuromuscular exercise programs have been shown to be more effective than isolated strength training (Sherry and Best 2004; Risberg et al. 2007; Wojtys et al. 1996). This finding supports Janda's rationale for using functional training over strength training. In addition, SMT has been shown to be more effective than strength training in improving function and strength in ACL rehabilitation (Beard et al.1994; Pavlu et al. 2001). SMT has also been shown to improve muscle balance and strength significantly more than strengthening alone improves it (Heitkamp et al. 2001).

SMT affects the higher centers of subcortical structures through the spinocerebellar, spinothalamic, vestibulospinal, and vestibulocerebellar pathways that influence and provide key regulatory information to maintain coordinated posture and equilibrium (Janda et al. 2007). Janda noted that different layers of muscle with different functions must be stimulated differently. For example, the superficial layers of the lumbar spine are under direct voluntary control, whereas the deep spinal stabilizers are not. Therefore the deep muscles must be stimulated through reflexive stimulation via SMT, for example, rather than through voluntary exercise.

The goal is to transform motor execution from the first stage of motor learning (where new movements are learned and improved with strong cortical participation) to a situation where automatized reactions to unexpected perturbations and forces are sped up (the second stage of motor learning, with reduced cortical participation in motor decisions and execution). This is considered an important factor for avoiding damage to passive and active structures of the musculoskeletal system caused by erratic, uncoordinated, and delayed movement strategies that may be too late to avoid biomechanical overload and microinjury of the joints, ligaments, tendons, or muscles.

Evidence suggests that an intact motor system can function almost normally in the absence of proprioceptive feedback (Rothwell et al. 1982); this is observed in many daily activities such as running, jumping, and performing quick repetitive movements (such as when playing an instrument or table tennis) for which the preprogrammed execution of the movement pattern precedes sensory feedback (Cockerill 1972). However, in the absence of proprioception the motor system cannot control fine motor movements or recently learned movements—nor can it improve upon them.

SMT has been shown repeatedly to improve proprioception, postural stability, and strength (Wester et al. 1996; Ihara and Nakayama 1986; Pavlu et al. 2001; Cordova, Jutte, and Hopkins 1999). The initial strength gains and neuromuscular effects of training are thought to be due to factors involving neural plasticity, since strength is gained within the first 6 wk of training and there is no significant muscle hypertrophy (Moritani and deVries 1979; Sale 1988; Shima et al. 2002). CNS stimulation is the key to initial strength increases, especially when it comes to coordination and stability.

This chapter briefly examines the origins of SMT as developed by Janda. It then reviews the components of SMT and the progression suggestions for the three training phases: static, dynamic, and functional. Utilization of reflex creeping and turning as a fourth or adjunctive stage of motor retraining is not a commonly used option and is not discussed in this chapter.

Role of Sensorimotor Training in Janda's Treatment

Janda described three ways to facilitate afferent motor pathways:

1. Increase proprioceptive flow in three key areas: the sole of the foot, the cervical spine, and the SI joints.
2. Stimulate the vestibulocerebellar system through balance training.
3. Influence midbrain structures through primitive locomotor activities.

Several researchers (Ihara and Nakayama 1986; Bullock–Saxton et al. 1993; Balogun et al. 1992) have demonstrated that faster muscle contraction can be achieved by dynamic stabilization training and that order and degree of contraction synergy can also be improved; as a result, an improvement in strength is expected. Janda et al. (2007) believed that activation of the deep axial musculature during voluntary exercises was accidental at best and that this musculature could not be consistently or efficiently activated for training purposes (Arokoski et al. 1999).

Janda often stated that musculoskeletal injury usually results from one of two sources: (1) altered movement patterns due to muscle imbalance, which causes biomechanical inefficiency and overload of structures over time, and (2) sudden unexpected and uncontrolled end-range loading of tissues and joints that cannot be absorbed and deflected in a coordinated fashion due to poor reaction times and equilibrium strategies (e.g., poor COG control that has been acquired over time and has replaced the more efficient subcortical program strategies). Therefore Janda considered SMT an ideal intervention for retraining the reaction time and control of the motor system and thereby reducing the risk of reinjury (see table 11.1).

Table 11.1 Indications and Contraindications for Sensorimotor Training

Indications	Contraindications
Muscle imbalance syndromes	Acute rheumatologic conditions
Instability or hypermobility, either general or local	Severe bone weakening or degenerative disease
Idiopathic scoliosis, mild to moderate	Acute fractures or sprains
Postsurgical or posttraumatic rehabilitation	Severe knee or ankle instability
Chronic neck or back pain syndromes	Severe balance or vestibular disorders
Fall prevention	
Mild balance or vestibular disorders	

In SMT, the patient can progress through four levels, moving from simpler reflexive stabilization strategies to more involved automatized movement strategies:

1. The volume and intensity of proprioceptive input are increased. This can be done by stimulating the bottom of the foot, the deep cervical musculature, and the SI area with superficial brushing, tapping, or taping.

2. The subcortical pathways noted previously are stimulated by introducing a degree of challenge to postural stability stressing reflexive stabilization of the joints.

3. Rapid and active subconscious recovery strategies are provoked to excite and promote the use of complex and more efficient ingrained motor engrams. Engrams are motor patterns of familiar automatized movement stored within the CNS. In this case, unconscious reactions and speed of contraction are considered more protective than strength. Isolated segment and joint movements then build on each other to form more complex interactions and coordinated movements.

4. Through functional activities, these synergies and strategies are integrated automatically into skill building and ADL.

The criteria for successful SMT are that it elicits the following:

- Reflexive activation of the motor system
- Dynamic stabilization through the active control and limitation of undesired movement
- Postural control, with all movement based on maintaining economic and efficient posture
- Coordinated movement with smooth muscular chain interplay for the efficient execution of tasks

The patient must be monitored carefully during the training session to ensure that the highest possible quality of movement is provoked and obtained. Not just any movement will suffice!

Sensorimotor Training Components

SMT consists of several components that are progressed throughout the program (see table 11.2). These define the parameters of posture, BOS, and COG that the patient masters during different challenges administered by the therapist. Throughout the training, patients are challenged through the systems controlling postural stability, such as the visual, vestibular, and exteroceptive systems. The intensity, duration, rate of progression, and degree of difficulty depend on the patient's ability to maintain a high quality of motor response and overall endurance. A session may last up to 30 min, but the duration of any individual exercise is usually only 5 to 20 s and always less than 2 min (Pavlu et al. 2007). The number of repetitions can vary from 20 for easy exercises to 5 for more difficult exercises. The challenges are selected according to the deficits observed during the initial patient evaluation and the subsequent responses observed during the actual SMT. In this way the training becomes its own evaluation and guides the practitioner's choices for progression.

Table 11.2 Sensorimotor Training Components

Posture	BOS	COG	Systems challenge
Sitting	Two-leg and one-leg stances	Weight shift	External support
Standing		Perturbation	Visual system
Minisquatting	Stability trainer	Upper-extremity motion	Vestibular system
Half-stepping	Wobble board	Lower-extremity motion	Cognitive system
Walking	Rocker board	Oscillation	Exteroceptive system
Squatting	Posturomed	Spinal stability	Speed
Lunging	Trampoline		Volume, intensity, duration
Step jumping	Exercise ball		
Running	Balance sandals		

Preparatory Facilitation

Just before the exercise session commences, moderately vigorous stimulation is applied to the sole of the foot via stroking or tapping or walking on rough or knobbed surfaces for about 30 s. In addition, manual or mechanical vibratory oscillation is applied to the SI joints and the suboccipital extensors in an attempt to stimulate areas of high mechanoreceptor concentration and to increase patient awareness of these areas.

Posture

Different postures can be adopted depending on the stage of training. The initial and subsequent choice of postures depends on the patient's ability to control the various postures and the final goal of rehabilitation. Patients can be progressed along a continuum of developmental postures in a manner similar to neurodevelopmental progression. Supine and prone activities are progressed to quadruped, kneeling, and sitting activities. Standing is progressed to functional positions such as stepping or jumping.

Base of Support

Challenging the BOS begins with progressing from two-leg to one-leg activities. The BOS can be altered by changing its texture, firmness, or stability; alterations depend on the patient's ability to control movement. Using labile surfaces during exercises increases speed of contraction and motor output (Beard et al. 1994; Blackburn, Hirth, and Guskiewicz 2002, 2003; Bullock-Saxton et al. 1993; Ihara and Nakayama 1986). Progressive increases in instability elicit progressive increases in muscle activation (see figure 11.1; Rogers, Rogers, and Page 2006). The patient can be advanced from foam pads and stability trainers to air-filled disks. Janda (Janda and VáVrová 1996) described using rocker and wobble boards to introduce the patient to progressively unstable surfaces in order to elicit APRs (see figure 11.2). The Posturomed is a

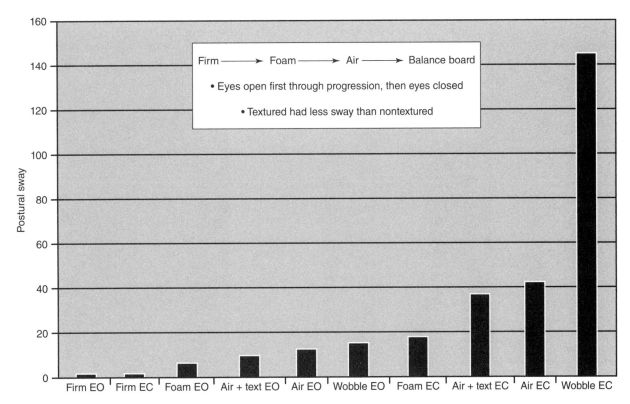

> Firm ——→ Foam ——→ Air ——→ Balance board
>
> • Eyes open first through progression, then eyes closed
>
> • Textured had less sway than nontextured

Figure 11.1 SMT progression used to measure degree postural sway. EO = eyes opened; EC = eyes closed; Air = air-filled disk; text = texture.

Data from N. Rogers et al., 2006, *Journal of Orthopeadic Sports Physical Therapy* 36(1): A53-54.

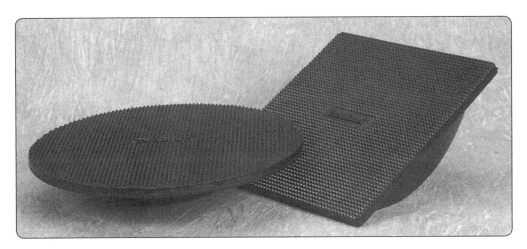

Figure 11.2 Rocker and wobble boards.

European balance device that provides a rigid platform with instability in the transverse plane (see figure 11.3). It has been used successfully in several SMT studies in Europe (Eils and Rosenbaum 2001; Heitkamp et al. 2001).

Exercise balls (see figure 11.4) can also be used as unstable surfaces for SMT. Recent research confirms that muscular activation is increased on exercise balls compared with firm surfaces (Behm et al. 2005. However, clinicians should avoid adding significant amounts of resistance or weight to the extremities while the patient is using unstable surfaces. The idea that an unstable base is an ideal platform for strength training and significantly loading the extremities and torso is misguided, dangerous, and unwise; it was never part of the original thought process of SMT. Research shows that muscle activation and force output in the extremities decrease significantly when the patient is using an unstable BOS (Anderson and Behm 2005; McBride et al. 2006).

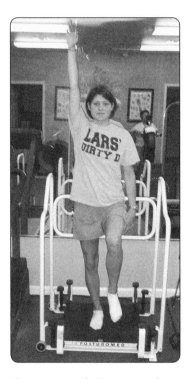

Figure 11.3 The Posturomed.

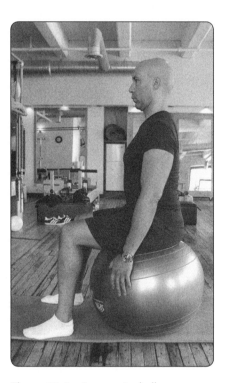

Figure 11.4 An exercise ball.

Center of Gravity

Once the goal for COG control is determined, the mode of challenge can be varied in order to provoke an array of recovery strategies throughout the training progression. Challenges to the COG include weight shifts, perturbations, movements of the upper and lower extremities, oscillations, and spinal stabilization.

Sensorimotor Training Progression

The three stages of SMT progression are the static, dynamic, and functional stages. Each is identified by increasingly difficult challenges to posture, COG, and BOS.

Static Phase

The goal of the static phase is to train control of the COG over the BOS while maintaining simple postural positions associated with sustaining uprighting and equilibrium functions. This stage improves the tonic or holding function of coactivation and stabilization of the axial skeleton. The static phase includes formation of the short foot, correction of posture, stimulation of proprioception, and progressive challenges to the BOS and COG.

Formation of the Short Foot

The short foot was described by Janda (Janda and VáVrová 1996) as a posture of the foot in which the medial and longitudinal arches are raised to improve the foot's biomechanical position. This posture relatively shortens the length of the foot (see figure 11.5). The short foot is taught by passive modeling by the therapist and then performed actively by the patient. The goal of the short foot is to activate the intrinsic muscles of the feet in a tonic manner; specifically, a sustained low-level activity is desired to increase afferent sensitivity and place the foot in a more neutral and less-pronated position in which the longitudinal and transverse arches are actively maintained. The short foot should be firm but not fixed or rigid.

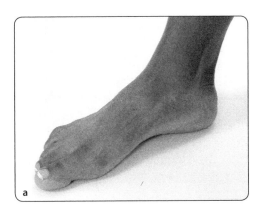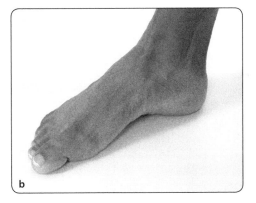

Figure 11.5 The short foot. *(a)* Beginning. *(b)* End.

Teaching of the short foot begins with the patient seated. The patient places the foot flat on the floor; the knee is flexed at about 80°. The clinician cups the heel in one hand and grasps across the dorsum of the foot so that the arch and foot can be controlled (see figure 11.6). The clinician slowly approximates the grasping hand toward the cupping hand that remains stationary, allowing the approximation of the metatarsal heads toward the heel. The clinician holds this position for a few seconds, making sure that the patient can perceive the change in foot form and is aware that the metatarsal heads all stay in contact with the floor. The clinician slowly returns the foot to the original position and then repeats the whole process 3

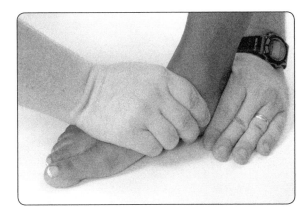

Figure 11.6 Manual short foot.

to 5 times, making sure that the tibialis anterior muscle is not overactive during training and that the tendon is not prominent during the formation of the short foot.

Next, the patient is asked to actively assist in the formation of the short foot for several repetitions and then finally to perform the action independently. The patient can then practice forming the short foot with the foot placed in different positions on the floor and with increasing loading through weight bearing until the patient can perform this exercise in the standing position. The goal is to train the patient's awareness of foot function and its role in maintaining stability while integrating this function into the initial postural correction and into the initial stages of weight transfer such as marching, half-stepping, or lunging.

The short foot was initially used on rigid unstable surfaces (such as rocker and wobble boards) to improve balance. Its use on softer unstable surfaces (such as foam or a minitrampoline) may not be as rewarding and may vary from one patient to another.

Visual imagery and guidance (both assistive and resistive) can play a very important role in the grooving in of new motor patterns (Kelsey 1961; Rawlings et al. 1972; Yue et al. 1992). The therapist and patient must focus on the qualitative goal of movement and make good use of the patient's cognitive skills.

Correction of Initial Static Posture

Postural correction for standing upright is introduced by correcting the patient's body segments. The correction progresses from the feet to the head: feet, knees, pelvis, shoulders, neck, and head. This helps the patient become aware of the alignment of segments in upright posture and of the muscle activity that can be used to control or move the COG.

The feet should be parallel and approximately shoulder-width apart. Active maintenance of the short foot is required. The COG should be slightly anterior, toward the metatarsals. The knees are slightly bent, but no more than 20°, to activate the co-contraction function of the lower-extremity muscles to stabilize the knee and hip. The hips are rotated externally by the hip external rotators and not by the supinators of the rear foot. The knees are aligned with the first and second metatarsals. The abdominal wall is activated, and the shoulders are kept as broad as possible with activation of the scapular fixators and external rotation of the arms. Centration of the head over the cervical column completes the postural correction. The perception should be one of spinal elongation cranially and of growing away from the support points of the arches of the feet and the fingertips. Common postural faults that can be seen during SMT include the following:

- Clawing and curling of the toes during short foot activation
- Exaggerated internal or external rotation of the knees
- Knee varus or valgus position
- Oblique pelvic position
- Lumbar hyperlordosis
- Thoracic hyperkyphosis
- Poor fixation of the shoulder blades
- Anterior head carriage

Stimulation of Proprioceptive Input

Localized areas with high mechanoreceptor densities, such as the sole of the foot, the sacral area, and the deep cervical muscles, are manually stimulated by percussive techniques. These techniques involve moderate, rapid tapping for 10 s or so over the area being stimulated and kneading or rubbing back and forth briskly over the same area just before training.

Challenge of Base of Support and Center of Gravity

The basic posture is maintained and reinforced by applying gentle static and then more rapid dynamic challenges to different body segments. This technique improves control and awareness of position and promotes reflex responses that should become automatic. The challenges should never exceed the patient's ability to stay in control or recover successfully, and they should be stopped when movement quality deteriorates so that the patient may recover and rest. Continued exercise should be based on the patient being able to maintain quality movement rather than be based on fatigue or a set timShort or sustained initial challenges are performed to test the patient's ability to maintain the COG within the BOS through stabilization. Gradually, challenges become more rapid and erratic so that they require the control of sway and displacement. The progression of BOS is from firm to increasingly labile. Rogers, Rogers, and Page (2006) established the following BOS progression, which the patient first performs with the eyes open and then repeats with the eyes closed:

Eyes Open	*Eyes Closed*
Two-leg balance, firm	Two-leg balance, firm
One-leg balance, firm	One-leg balance, firm
One-leg balance, foam	One-leg balance, foam
One-leg balance, rocker	One-leg balance, rocker
One-leg balance, wobble	One-leg balance, wobble

Exercise balls and minitrampolines can also be introduced as labile surfaces (see figure 11.7). Any time the patient works on an unstable surface, postural alignment and stabilization are critical in the static phase.

At all times during the training, the patient must show increasing control of her COG. Therefore, the clinician must observe the patient during the session to ensure quality of execution. The goal is to reflexively reestablish efficient strategies for COG control through subconscious regulation and facilitation. Progressive challenges to the COG in the static phase include weight shifts and perturbations. Weight shifts can be elicited by the clinician or an external force such as an elastic band (see figure 11.8).

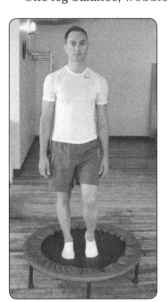

Figure 11.7 Minitrampoline.

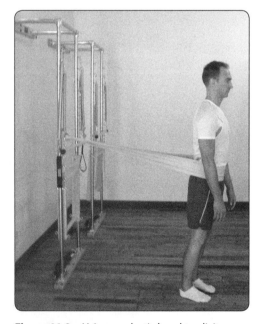

Figure 11.8 Using an elastic band to elicit weight shifts. The clinician provides elastic resistance of varying tensions to shift the COG within the BOS in varying vectors and at varying tempos.

Perturbations should be applied in different directions and at low intensities near the COG (figure 11.9) and then gradually increased in intensity and distance from the core.

The neural contribution to strength increases during the initial weeks of training is significant compared with the contribution made by structural changes such as muscle hypertrophy, which do not occur until several weeks later in the training. Therefore, efficiency of motor unit utilization and improved coordination interplay could account for the initial strength changes.

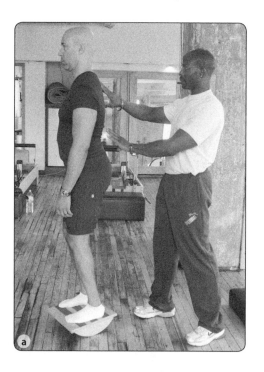
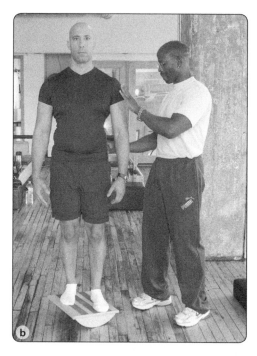
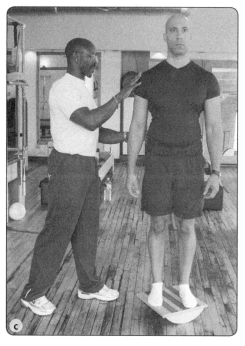
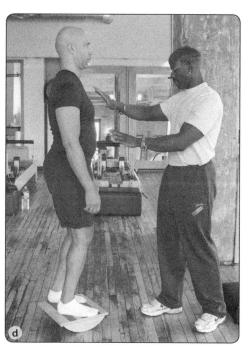

Figure 11.9 Applying perturbations: *(a)* anterior weight shift, *(b)* lateral right weight shift, *(c)* lateral left weight shift, and *(d)* posterior weight shift.

Dynamic Phase

Once the patient demonstrates adequate postural stabilization on various support bases and in response to various COG challenges, she can begin the dynamic phase of SMT. The dynamic phase builds on a stable core area by adding movement of the extremities, half-steps, oscillation, and spinal stabilization techniques.

Upper- and Lower-Extremity Movements

Active upper- and lower-extremity movements further challenge the postural system both biomechanically and reflexively. This exponentially increases the difficulty of COG control and increases demand on stabilization strategies. It also allows the BOS to change dramatically and to move in time and space. All the progressions follow logical increases in difficulty through judicious combination of the factors shown in table 11.2 on page 160. Again, the level of difficulty should not compromise the patient's motor quality. Movements in the cardinal planes are explored initially; these are followed by movements in more paracardinal and oblique plane vectors. The goal is to force the patient to reestablish axial equilibrium and simultaneously maintain good control of the extremities.

Reflexive stabilization of the stance leg has been demonstrated by EMG of elastic-resisted kicking (figure 11.10; Cordova et al. 1999; Schulthies 1998). The antagonistic supporting muscles of the stance leg are activated in the opposite direction of the kick: The hamstrings on the stance leg are activated during a front kick, while the quadriceps on the stance leg are activated during a back kick. The important factor in any case is not the activation of these muscles but the quality of the stabilization chain that includes these muscles in its function. There is also evidence of cross-training effects on the extensor muscle groups of the contralateral limb. These effects may have limited use in situations where the injury or patient endurance restricts the dosage of training that the impaired or immobilized leg can tolerate (Shima et al. 2002).

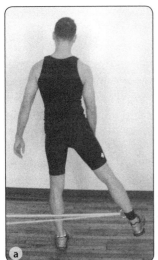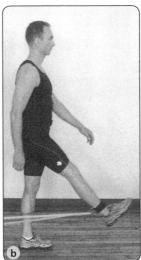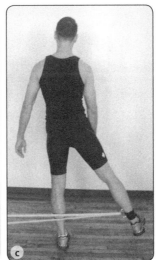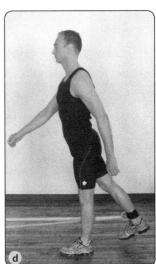

Figure 11.10 Thera-Band kicks: *(a)* medial, *(b)* anterior, *(c)* lateral, and *(d)* posterior.

Half-Step

The half-step is an important initial dynamic progression that challenges pelvic and lumbar control. The goal is to control weight transfer during load acceptance throughout the stance phase; from the heel strike, continuing along the lateral border of the foot and then across the metatarsal area to the big and second toes. Good cervicocranial alignment, thoraco-lumbo-pelvic alignment, and hip, knee, and foot alignment should be maintained during the activity so that the patient avoids unnecessary trunk flexion or lower-extremity deviation in the three cardinal planes (see figure 11.11). Once mastered, the half-step can be trained on different surfaces of increasing difficulty, such as foam stability trainers (figure 11.12). Backward stepping is also trained so the patient learns reverse weight transference from toe to heel.

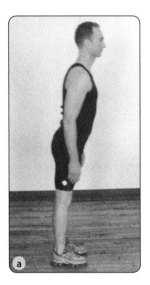 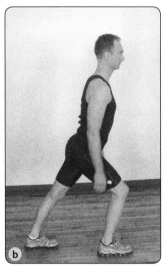

Figure 11.11   The half-step.

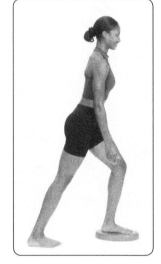

Figure 11.12   A half-step onto a stability trainer.

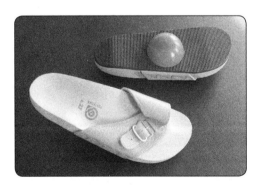

Figure 11.13   Janda's balance sandals.

Balance Sandals

Janda also described the use of balance sandals in SMT (see figure 11.13; Janda and VáVrová 1996). These balance tools are unique to Janda's SMT program and consist of relatively hard hemispheres attached to the soles of sandals. The sandals must be actively gripped by the formation of a short foot during use. The patient takes small steps in different directions and at different tempos to challenge distal–proximal stability via the lower extremities. Training during any given session should not exceed 2 min, though it can be repeated 5 to 6 times on the same day. Improved muscle activation speed and improved motor activation sequence were reported when the sandals were used to rehabilitate ankle sprains (Bullock-Saxton et al. 1994).

Oscillation

Oscillation is facilitatory to the muscle spindle (Umphred 2001). Several devices can be used during oscillation exercises to facilitate muscle activation. Page and colleagues (2004) quantified the EMG output of upper-extremity muscles during an oscillatory exercise with a Thera-Band Flexbar (figure 11.14). In addition to identifying key muscle activations (table 11.3), the researchers noted that the oscillatory exercise activated phasic muscles at higher levels than antagonistic tonic muscles. This technique may have potential for restoring normal muscle balance in patients with upper-extremity disturbances.

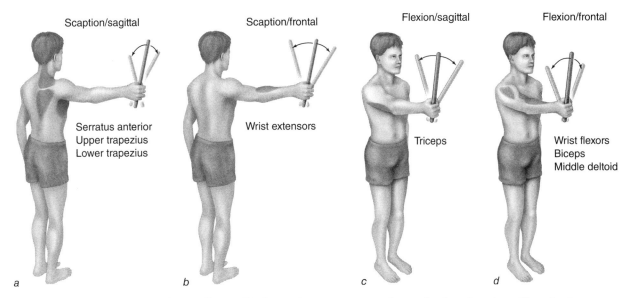

Figure 11.14 Thera-Band Flexbar oscillation. This figure demonstrates muscles predominately activated by using two shoulder positions. *(a)* Scaption position with sagittal oscillation, *(b)* scaption position with frontal oscillation, *(c)* flexion position with sagittal oscillation, and *(d)* flexion position with frontal oscillation.

Table 11.3 Muscle Activation with Flexbar Oscillation

Muscle	Position/plane	% Maximum contraction
Wrist extensors	Scaption/frontal	42.4
Serratus anterior	Scaption/sagittal	24.2
Wrist flexors	Flexion/frontal	22.3
Triceps	Flexion/sagittal	21.1
Biceps	Flexion/frontal	19.1
Middle deltoid	Flexion/frontal	18.9
Lower trapezius	Scaption/sagittal	17.9
Upper trapezius	Scaption/sagittal	9.5

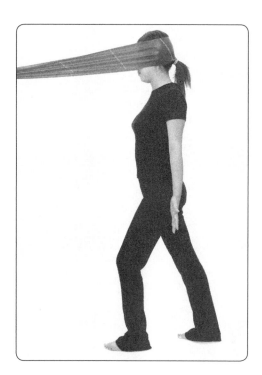

Spinal Stabilization

Challenges to spinal stabilization can be introduced in the dynamic phase. Generally, any exercise that challenges vertical stabilization is implemented at a level that allows the patient to maintain postural stability. Dynamic isometrics of the cervical spine are useful for facilitating dynamic stabilization during movement. For example, the patient may be asked to maintain correct cervical posture while stepping backward against an elastic band (figure 11.15). This exercise facilitates deep stabilizer muscles while imparting movement of the body. It allows the cervical flexors and extensors to stabilize the spine and head from their midthoracic origins.

Figure 11.15 Dynamic isometric resistance for the cervical spine.

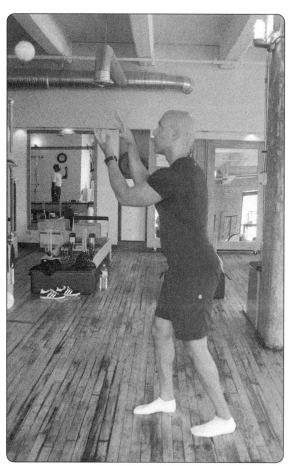

Figure 11.16 Tossing a soft weight.

Impulse training with a soft weight or plyometric ball (figure 11.16) can also be introduced at this stage. Patients throw a small medicine ball weighing from 1 to 11 lb (0.5-5 kg) at a rebounder or minitrampoline while maintaining postural stabilization on the catch and throw portions of the exercise. The weight of the ball and the surface the patient stands on can be progressed to add challenge.

Functional Phase

The final phase of SMT is the functional phase, which is characterized by the reintroduction and practice of complex synergies that are subsequently utilized in ADL. The goal of the functional phase is the automatization of more complex and purposeful synergies that require movement through space. This phase strengthens the quality and endurance of patient performance of ADL.

The complex movements of the functional phase include synergies that involve multiple joints, muscles, and planes of motion, such as a squat, press, or twist. Table 11.4 outlines these movements by body region. These movements are first introduced as generic movements that are subsequently built on and combined for more skilled and purposeful action.

Table 11.4 Functional Phase Synergies in Sensorimotor Training

Upper extremity	Trunk	Lower extremity
Push	Twist	Squat
Pull	Bridge	Leg press
Press up	Bend	Lunge
Reach	Stabilize	Step

Functional movements are made up of coordinated movement synergies. For example, bridging and reaching are components of moving from supine to standing. Lunging and pulling or pushing may be necessary when dragging heavy loads. Turning and thrusting may be utilized as defensive techniques within activities such as boxing, martial arts, or fencing. Turning or twisting the torso and reaching with the upper extremity is a daily requirement in so many activities. These movements in turn are incorporated into ADL, including occupational, leisure, and sport activities. External resistance can be added to make the activities more challenging as the patient progresses (see figure 11.17).

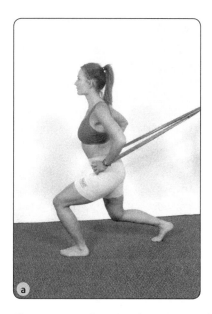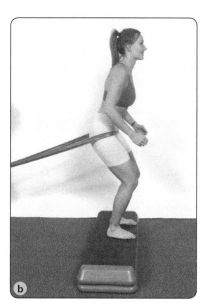

Figure 11.17 Functional activities performed against external resistance.

The functional phase reintegrates the patient into ADL with more specific exercises tailored to these needs. They may range from improving sedentary functions such as sitting time to ergonomic strategies to training for a particular sporting activity. The training approaches are too numerous to describe, but there are certain factors common to them all. Skill building within ADL is then fine-tuned when appropriate by increasing loading tolerance, accuracy, agility, plyometrics, cardiorespiratory capacity, power generation, and so on, which all may be necessary components that require practice.

The quality of functional movement and posture can be monitored through several key points:

- Breathing stereotype
- Stabilization strategies

- Lumbopelvic control and position relative to other body segments
- Shoulder girdle control and scapular position relative to other body segments
- Head placement and cervical control relative to other body segments
- Extremity placement and position relative to other body segments
- Fluidity of movement
- Speed of movement

Depending on the speed and type of movements or postures required, video observation and analysis may be necessary to give appropriate feedback for improving sensory motor skills.

Neuroreflexive Treatment (Vojta Approach)

As discussed in chapter 9, Janda considered reflex treatment of the motor system to be an important part of the rehabilitation process, especially when the patient had difficulty establishing improved motor patterns voluntarily and through sensory motor exercises. In its present form, neurodynamic stabilization, developed by Kolář for use within the adult as well as the pediatric population, is now considered an indispensable part of the treatment paradigm. It provides a logical and empirical basis for both the evaluation of biomechanically based pathology and faulty movement, and the subsequent treatment and choice of exercise and exercise progression. The details of neurodynamic stabilization are beyond the scope of this text. Further information can be obtained from the Web site www.rehabps.com.

Summary

Chronic musculoskeletal pain and overuse syndromes typically are associated with muscle imbalance syndromes. SMT is the critical intervention for muscle imbalance syndromes. Because these syndromes are centrally mediated, treatment must address the CNS rather than focus on the muscle imbalance itself. SMT integrates whole-body movement with automatic stabilization, progressing from static to dynamic to functional activities. As can be seen in table 11.5 the training aspect based on SMT is a more globally comprehensive attempt at training the musculoskeletal system by primarily improving CNS function through sensory awareness, coordination, motor control quality, and movement reprogramming. It is still undergoing development as we come to understand more about the brain.

Table 11.5   Comparison of Training Aspects

Training aspects	Janda approach	Traditional approach
Preparatory facilitation	Yes	No
Stage progressions	Yes	Random
Goal	Qualitative	Often quantitative
Intensity	Not to fatigue	Often to fatigue
Use of short foot	Yes	No
Cognitive challenge	Yes	Not usually
Used for initial strengthening	Yes	Not usually
Global approach	Yes	Not always

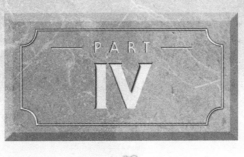

CLINICAL SYNDROMES

Clinicians treating patients with chronic musculoskeletal pain, particularly patients with Janda's muscle imbalance syndromes, must evaluate the body as a whole system because of the global influence of the sensorimotor system. The principles outlined in this text can also be applied to other clinical syndromes, particularly those involving localized muscle imbalances. It is beyond the scope of this text to review these clinical syndromes in depth; each has a variety of factors and considerations for the clinician. The following chapters provide an overview of the role of muscle imbalance and functional pathology of the sensorimotor system in common clinical syndromes.

Chapter 12 reviews common cervical pain syndromes related to muscle imbalance, including chronic neck pain and whiplash, headache, and fibromyalgia. Chapter 13 details common upper-extremity pain syndromes related to muscle imbalance, including shoulder impingement and instability and tennis elbow. Next, chapter 14 describes common syndromes of the lumbar spine related to muscle imbalance, including chronic low back pain and SI disorders. Finally, chapter 15 discusses common lower-extremity pain syndromes related to muscle imbalance, including anterior knee pain and chronic ankle sprains. Each chapter also presents a case study of the various syndromes.

.

CERVICAL PAIN SYNDROMES

T he cervical spine orients the head for visual alignment, positions the mouth for feeding, and positions or protects the sensory organs (eyes, ears, and nose). The cervical spine is one of the key areas of proprioception identified by Janda, and thus many cervical pathologies can create global problems in posture and balance.

This chapter begins by reviewing regional considerations of the cervical spine, including functional anatomy and chain reactions. It then discusses chronic neck pain and whiplash, describing cervical assessment and rehabilitation following Janda's approach. Next, several other pathologies of the cervical region are addressed, including cervicogenic headache, facial pain, TMJ disorders, and fibromyalgia and myofascial pain. Finally, a case study using Janda's approach to cervical rehabilitation is presented.

Regional Considerations

The cervical spine is a relatively mobile area of the body, with several unique articulations providing a variety of motions. Humans typically use 30% to 50% of their cervical ROM in ADL (Bennett, Schenk, and Simmons 2002). Generally, males have 40% more strength than females have in the neck (Garces et al. 2002). Although absolute strength of the neck muscles is not critical for function, quick and coordinated activation is essential for efficient movement and stabilization.

Functional Anatomy

The neck flexors and extensors coactivate to maintain alignment and smooth movement of the cervical spine and head in both extension (semispinalis capitis and cervicis and splenius capitis) and flexion (SCM). The normal flexion-to-extension strength ratio is 60% (Garces et al. 2002). The deep neck flexors (longus capitis, longus coli, and rectus capitis anterior) function more to retract the cervical spine than to flex it (figure 12.1). Deep neck flexors maintain posture (cervical lordosis) and equilibrium; they do not provide dynamic movement (Abrahams 1977). In particular, the longus colli is a postural muscle that counteracts the cervical lordosis produced by the weight of the head and cervical extension (Mayoux-Benhamou et al. 1994).

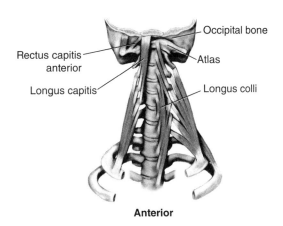

Anterior

Figure 12.1 The deep neck flexors.

Reprinted from R.S. Behnke, *Kinetic anatomy*, 2nd ed. (Champaign, IL: Human Kinetics), 130.

The finding of mechanoreceptors in the cervical facet capsules suggests that these capsules play an important role in the function and protection of the cervical spine (Chen et al. 2006; McLain 1994). Both mechanoreceptors and muscular afferents within the cervical spine provide important proprioceptive information for postural control (Gregoric et al. 1978; Lund 1980). The longus colli is particularly rich in muscle spindles, unlike the cervical extensors (Boyd-Clark, Briggs, and Galea 2002). Proprioceptive information is also critical for the newborn learning to align the eyes with the horizon for early mobility. Visual alignment is probably the most important function of the cervical spine (Zepa et al. 2003).

The feed-forward mechanism of the cervical muscles is important for stabilization preceding arm movement. Falla and colleagues (Falla, Jull, and Hodges 2004; Falla, Rainoldi,, et al. 2004) reported that the SCM, deep neck flexors, and cervical extensors are activated before arm movement in normal subjects. Fatigue of the neck muscles reduces balance (Gosselin, Rassoulian, and Brown 2004; Schieppati, Nardone, and Schmid 2003). Patients with chronic neck pain exhibit impaired proprioception (Heikkila and Astrom 1996; Loudon, Ruhl, and Field 1997; Revel et al. 1994) and postural sway (Karlberg et al. 1995; McPartland, Brodeur, and Hallgren 1997; Sjostrom et al. 2003; Treleaven, Jull, and Lowchoy 2005). These findings suggest that the sensorimotor system, including cervical proprioception and feed-forward mechanisms, may be disrupted in neck dysfunction.

Chain Reactions

It's important to remember the interplay between the cervical spine and the shoulder girdle. In particular, the upper trapezius and levator scapulae originate on the cervical spine. This relationship may have implications for assessment and exercise prescription addressing patients with cervical spine conditions and patients with shoulder conditions. For example, poor scapular stabilization increases activity of the upper trapezius for stabilization, which in turn increases scapular elevation and stress on the cervical origin of the trapezius.

Developmental reflexes such as the ATNR are an example of primitive reflexive chains in the cervical spine. Infants typically extend the upper extremity on the side to which the head is turned and flex the opposite upper extremity. While the ATNR usually is not seen past 1 y of life, this reaction demonstrates the effect that proprioceptive input of the cervical spine has on the rest of the body.

Common Pathologies

Patients with cervical spine dysfunctions often exhibit UCS (see chapter 4). In this syndrome, inhibited and weak muscles include the deep neck flexors, serratus anterior, rhomboids, and middle and lower trapezius. The upper trapezius, levator scapula, suboccipitals, SCM, and pectoralis major and minor are facilitated and tight.

Specific postural changes are also seen in UCS, including forward head posture, increased cervical lordosis and thoracic kyphosis, elevated and protracted shoulders, and rotation and abduction and winging of the scapulae (figure 4.26). This postural change also causes a decrease in glenohumeral stability as the glenoid fossa becomes more vertical due to serratus anterior weakness leading to abduction, rotation, and winging of the scapula. In response, the levator scapulae and upper trapezius increase activation to maintain glenohumeral centration (Janda 1988).

Chronic muscle imbalances of UCS often lead to C5-C6 pathology (Janda 2002). Radiographic findings often demonstrate osteophytes and narrowed foramen in the C5-C6 region. Remember that 20% of younger patients and up to 60% of older patients demonstrate radiographic abnormalities without symptoms. These abnormalities lead to many false positives (Boden et al. 1990) if the clinician relies on X ray or MRI alone for diagnosis.

Lund and colleagues (1991) described the pain adaptation model, reviewing the muscular changes in several chronic musculoskeletal pain conditions such as TMJ dysfunction, tension headache, and FM. They concluded that these types of pain are not due to a structural cycle of pain and spasm; rather, these conditions are mediated by the CNS as hypertonicity of the antagonists and inhibition of the agonists. This muscular imbalance is part of a normal protective adaptation and is not necessarily the cause of the pain. In other words, chronic musculoskeletal conditions are essentially muscle imbalance syndromes elicited in response to a functional pathology.

Chronic Neck Pain and Whiplash

Chronic neck pain (pain lasting more than 1-6 mo) usually is diagnosed without specific structural involvement. Whiplash is the result of a sudden acceleration–deceleration mechanism that transfers energy to the cervical spine (Spitzer et al. 1995). So-called *whiplash-associated disorders* (WAD) have come to encompass any chronic neck pain associated with a motor vehicle accident (MVA). Neck pain without associated trauma typically is diagnosed as mechanical neck pain and often relates to poor posture.

Pathology

The pathological findings of chronic neck pain and WAD generally point to a functional pathology. Pain centralization, altered proprioception, and neuromuscular dysfunction indicate primary involvement of the sensorimotor system.

Pain Centralization Responses

Several researchers have found that patients with chronic neck pain demonstrate global changes in pain response that are evidenced by sensory hypersensitivity throughout the body (Sterling et al. 2002; Sterling et al. 2003; Curatolo et al. 2001; Herren-Gerber et al. 2004; Jull et al. 2007). Using a pain algometer, researchers noted reduced pain pressure thresholds both locally and in other regions of the body. This finding suggests that continued activation of nociception and altered central pain processing occurs well after the initial injury (Sterling et al. 2002). Patients with chronic whiplash demonstrate central hypersensitivity to peripheral stimulation in the neck and lower limb as well as significantly lower pain thresholds (Curatolo et al. 2001).

Proprioceptive Deficits

Cavanaugh and colleagues (2006) demonstrated that pain and altered proprioception result from stretching the mechanoreceptors and nociceptors of the cervical facet joint capsule. Patients with chronic neck pain and WAD demonstrate deficits in local proprioception, including kinesthesia and joint position sense (Heikkila and Astrom 1996; Loudon, Ruhl, and Field 1997; Revel, Andre-Deshays, and Minguet 1991; Sterling 2003; Treleaven, Jull, and Sterling 2003; Treleaven, Jull, and Lowchoy 2005). Heikkila and Wenngren (1998) found that joint position sense does not correlate with pain intensity, concluding that patients with whiplash essentially have a dysfunction of the proprioceptive system.

Patients with chronic whiplash also demonstrate changes in proprioception when compared with control subjects, most notably during gait and task-specific gaze control. Heikkila and Wenngren (1998) found that the change in neck proprioception that occurs with whiplash affects voluntary eye movements. Patients with chronic neck pain (including whiplash) also demonstrate poor postural stability (Karlberg et al. 1995; McPartland, Brodeur, and Hallgren 1997; Madeleine et al. 2004; Sterling et al. 2003; Sjostrom et al. 2003; Treleaven, Jull, and Lowchoy 2005). In addition, Sterling and colleagues (2003) showed persistent motor system dysfunction in patients experiencing whiplash, even after recovery and up to 3 mo beyond. These patients most notably demonstrated increased EMG levels in the cervical spine. These findings, along with global changes in pain response, support the role of the CNS in chronic neck pain.

Neuromuscular Dysfunction

Patients with chronic neck pain exhibit up to a 90% deficit in cervical spine strength (Prushansky et al. 2005; Silverman, Rodriquez, and Agre 1991; Ylinen et al. 2004). Uhlig and colleagues (1995) reported a transformation of fiber type in patients with whiplash, noting a shift from slow-twitch fibers to fast-twitch fibers. Others have found atrophy and fatty infiltration of the suboccipital muscles in patients with chronic neck pain (McPartland, Brodeur, and Hallgren 1997; Hallgren, Greenman, and Rechtien 1994). They postulated that this atrophy may decrease the proprioceptive inhibition of nociceptors at the dorsal horn of the spinal cord, thus causing pain.

Compared with uninjured subjects, patients with chronic whiplash demonstrate increased tension in the trapezius and infraspinatus when performing repetitive upper-extremity tasks (Elert et al. 2001). Superficial muscles (SCM and anterior scalene) in patients with chronic neck pain often fatigue more easily, particularly on the same side of unilateral neck pain (Falla et al. 2004). Similarly, the SCM and upper trapezius have shown increased fatigability in subjects with cervical osteoarthritis (OA).

Recently, the deep neck flexors (longus coli, longus capitis, and rectus capitis anterior) have been implicated in chronic neck pain and whiplash, just as the TrA has been implicated in chronic low back pain. Falla, Jull, and Hodges (2004b) found that the deep neck flexors in particular have reduced EMG activity in patients with neck pain as Janda suggested. Interestingly, 85% of patients with chronic neck pain also have impaired function of the TrA (Moseley 2004).

Researchers have shown that the deep neck flexors are weak (Barton and Hayes 1996; Jull et al. 1999) and have delayed onset in patients with chronic neck pain (Falla, Jull, and Hodges 2004a), findings that indicate a faulty feed-forward mechanism. Jull, Kristjansson, and Dall'Alba (2004) confirmed Janda's suggestion that the SCM is overactivated during head flexion in patients with neck pain. Furthermore, Nederhand and coworkers (2000) found elevated EMG activity of the upper trapezius in patients with whiplash. This accessory muscle is also overactivated when patients with chronic neck pain perform repetitive upper-extremity tasks (Falla, Bilenkij, and Jull 2004).

There is also evidence of peripheral neuromuscular deficits in patients with chronic neck pain. Suter and McMorland (2002) reported significant inhibition of the biceps in these patients. After manipulation of C5, C6, and C7, the patients reportedly improved their biceps strength and neck ROM.

Postural Changes

Patients with chronic neck pain often exhibit a classic cluster of postural dysfunction: forward head, rounded shoulders, and increased thoracic kyphosis. This posture is consistent with that of Janda's UCS (see chapter 4). Patients with chronic neck pain have problems maintaining cervical lordosis (Falla 2004), which is likely due to weakness of the deep neck flexors. In healthy individuals, poor endurance of the deep neck flexors is associated with increased cervical lordosis but not with forward head posture (Grimmer and Trott 1998).

Assessment

Chronic neck pain often affects the sensorimotor system throughout the body. The assessment of patients with chronic neck pain should focus on the upper quarter, including the neck, upper thoracic spine, and shoulder girdle. In addition, the pelvis and trunk stabilizers should be examined to rule out contributing dysfunction. The standard evaluation of chronic neck pain is similar to the evaluation of other cervical dysfunctions discussed later in the chapter. Careful analysis of posture, balance, movement patterns, muscle length, muscle strength, and manual assessment follows the procedures detailed in chapters 5 through 8.

Posture

The patient should be disrobed as much as possible to allow the clinician to visualize the body from head to toe. The clinician should perform a systematic assessment of posture (see chapter 5). Table 12.1 provides key observations in patients with cervical dysfunction. Each finding suggests a possible indication and begins to provide a picture of the root of dysfunction.

Table 12.1   Key Observations in Postural Analysis for Cervical Spine Dysfunction

Postural view	Key observation	Possible indications
Posterior	Shoulder elevation	Tightness of upper trapezius and levator scapula
	Pelvic crest inequality	Leg-length discrepancy; SI rotation
Lateral	Forward head position	Tightness of suboccipitals, SCM, and scalenes; weakness of deep neck flexors
	Altered glenohumeral position	Tightness of pectoralis major; weakness of middle and lower scapular stabilizers
	Deviant chin and neck angle	Hypertrophy of superficial neck flexors
Anterior	SCM hypertrophy	Tightness of SCM; accessory respiration
	Facial scoliosis	Global structural dysfunction

Balance

As noted, poor postural stability has been found in patients with chronic neck pain. The clinician should assess the patient's single-leg balance (see figure 5.19), observing both the quality and quantity of stability as well as noting any compensatory strategies used by the upper body to maintain postural stability. An example of such a strategy is excessive head repositioning.

Gait

In extreme cases of cervical dysfunction, gait patterns can contribute to the problem. The clinician should watch for increased activation of the cervical or shoulder girdle muscles during the entire gait cycle, in particular observing any difference between stance and swing phases. Sometimes, the effect of the stance phase is distributed all the way through the cervical spine, contributing to dysfunction with each step.

Movement Pattern

The three main movement pattern tests for patients with cervical dysfunction are cervical flexion (figure 6.4), CCF (figure 6.7), and shoulder abduction (figure 6.6). Clinicians may also perform the other movement pattern tests from chapter 6 if indicated.

A positive cervical flexion test (chin jutting on head elevation) indicates weakness or fatigue of the deep neck flexors and tightness of the SCM. The CCF endurance test (CCFET) has been shown to be reliable and valid in cases of chronic neck pain (Chiu, Law, and Chiu 2005; Falla, Campbell et al. 2003; Falla, Jull, and Hodges 2004b; Harris et al. 2003) and is more specific to the deep neck flexors when compared with standard neck flexion (Olson et al. 2006). This is likely because the deep neck flexors generally are fatigued (Falla 2004). Variations of the CCFET have been shown to be reliable (Kumbhare et al. 2005; Olson et al. 2006) and valid for patients with whiplash (Kumbhare et al. 2005). Finally, the shoulder abduction movement pattern provides information on the involvement of the upper trapezius and levator scapula with origins on the cervical spine.

In addition to testing these movement patterns, the clinician should observe the patient's breathing pattern while in sitting and in supine positions (figure 6.9). The respiratory pattern may change based on the patient's posture and the relation of the rib cage to gravity. Accessory respiration due to hyperactivity of the SCM and scalenes indicates insufficient stabilization of the rib cage and weakness or inhibition of the diaphragm. Each breath facilitates cervical dysfunction. These patients often have TrPs and tender points throughout the abdominal wall.

To gain a whole-body perspective, clinicians should consider assessing the activation of the trunk stabilizers. This can be done by having the patient perform abdominal hollowing (see figure 6.8). Moseley (2004) found that patients with chronic neck pain who cannot perform abdominal hollowing have an increased risk of also developing low back pain.

Muscle Length and Strength

After postural and movement pattern assessment, the clinician can begin to postulate which muscles are tight or weak. Up until this point in the assessment, the clinician has relied only on careful observation. Now muscle tightness and weakness can be verified and quantified with hands-on techniques, as discussed in chapter 7. In particular, patients with chronic neck pain and whiplash demonstrate tightness of the upper trapezius (Nederhand 2000) and higher activation of the SCM (Barton and Hayes 1996; Jull, Kristjansson, Dall'Alba 2004). The clinician should look for the classic patterns of muscle tightness and weakness to confirm or rule out Janda's UCS.

Manual Assessment

The manual assessment is the final step in the evaluation of the cervical spine. It includes testing for joint mobility and soft-tissue palpation. Janda noted several findings indicative of cervical restrictions:

- Pain at the spinous process of C2 indicates a C1-C2 or C2-C3 restriction.
- A C2 restriction causes pain and TrPs in the levator scapulae and SCM, which then cause pain in the occiput and face.
- A C0-C1 restriction causes pain and spasm of the suboccipital and SCM insertions, along with pain at the transverse processes of C1 and the TMJ.

Patients with chronic cervical pain may also present with pain at the T4 to T8 region. Midthoracic dysfunction (Liebenson 2001) is characterized by increased thoracic kyphosis and prolonged forward head posture, both of which stress the midthoracic vertebrae, causing pain upon spring testing. This dysfunction may be associated with TrPs in the SCM, scalene, masseter, and upper trapezius. Cleland and colleagues (2005) reported that thoracic manipulation in patients with chronic neck pain immediately reduces the pain.

Manual assessment of the cervical region should include evaluation of any scars and other fascial restrictions. TrPs and tender points should also be assessed, particularly in the upper trapezius and levator scapulae. The clinician should also note any evidence of trigger point chains (see chapter 8). Letchuman and colleagues (2005) found that tender points in patients with cervical radiculopathy are more unilateral and are located in muscles innervated by the affected nerve root.

Treatment

Traditional therapy for cervical spine dysfunction focuses on structural approaches such as soft collars, joint manipulation, and modalities. Recent research has shown that exercise is an effective and appropriate intervention in the management of cervical pain. Multimodal treatment including exercise and mobilization or manipulation is more effective than manipulation or modalities alone (Bronfort et al. 2001; Evans et al. 2002; Gross et al. 2002; Gross et al. 2004; Kay et al. 2005; Provinciali et al. 1996). Clinicians should also consider manual therapy for the thoracic spine (Cleland et al. 2005). Meta-analysis suggests that therapeutic exercise for cervical dysfunction is most effective when it includes stretching, strengthening, and proprioceptive exercises for the neck and shoulder (Sarig-Bahat 2003; Kay et al. 2005). Massage alone is of questionable benefit in chronic neck pain (Ezzo et al. 2007; Vernon, Humphreys, and Hagino 2007).

Active Motion and Stretching

While soft-collar immobilization has long been used for early management, new research suggests that soft collars may cause more harm than good. As with treatment for any musculoskeletal injury, active mobilization of the joint and muscles is vital to tissue repair and remodeling. The cervical spine should be no exception to this approach. Active movement to reduce pain after a whiplash injury is more effective than the standard treatment of rest and soft collar (Rosenfeld, Gunnarsson, and Borenstein 2000 2003; Schnabel et al. 2004). In a 2 y follow-up study in Ireland (McKinney 1989), prolonged wearing of soft collars was associated with prolonged symptoms in patients experiencing neck sprains after MVA. Advice to mobilize the neck early after neck injury reduced the number of patients with symptoms after 2 y and was shown to be superior to manipulation (McKinney 1989).

Vassiliou and colleagues (2006) performed a randomized controlled trial of patients with whiplash, comparing physical therapy treatment with a standard soft-collar treatment. The physical therapy included performing active exercises within 14 d after injury as well as completing a home program including Brügger's exercises with Thera-Band resistance (see figure 12.2). The authors noted significant improvements in the physical therapy group after 6 wk and up to 6 mo after the injury when compared with the standard treatment group.

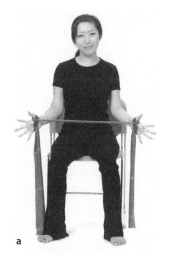 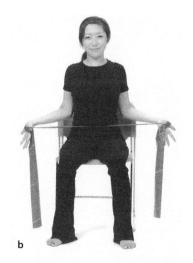 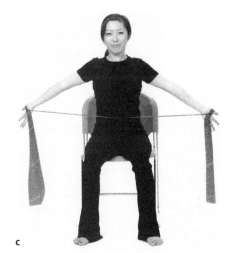

a b c

Figure 12.2 Brügger's exercises.

Patients with neck sprain or whiplash should be encouraged to perform active ROM within pain-free limits as soon after the injury as possible. One simple active exercise is cervical retraction (figure 12.3). Active ROM exercises have been shown to reduce radicular symptoms in the arm (Abdulwahab and Sabbahi 2000) and to improve resting posture (Pearson and Walmsley 1995).

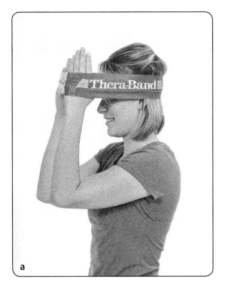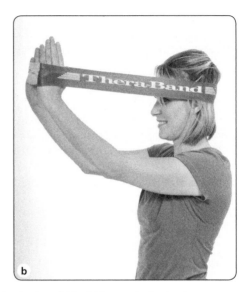

Figure 12.3 Isometric cervical retraction. *(a)* Beginning. *(b)* End. The cervical spine is maintained in neutral as the band is stretched.

Muscle tightness should be addressed through muscle lengthening techniques. Static stretching, contract relax, or PIR can be used (see chapter 10). In particular, contract relax is effective at improving cervical ROM (McCarthy, Olsen, and Smeby 1997). Commonly tight muscles in cervical dysfunction include the upper trapezius, scalenes, SCM, and pectoralis major and minor (the same pattern seen in Janda's UCS). Kinesio taping may be helpful for inhibiting tight muscles (see chapter 10). Ylinen and colleagues (2007) found both stretching and manual therapy to be effective in patients with chronic neck pain.

Another important component of cervical spine treatment is addressing breathing patterns. As stated, chronic neck pain is often associated with tightness of the accessory respiratory muscles (SCM and scalenes). Simply stretching these tight muscles may not be effective. Patients with faulty breathing patterns should be given specific exercises to retrain their breathing.

Strengthening Exercises

Stretching exercises alone are not as effective as well-rounded programs that include muscular flexibility, strength, and endurance training for patients with chronic neck pain (Ylinen et al. 2003). Simple strengthening exercises have been shown to be safe and effective for cervical spine rehabilitation; in fact, low-tech exercises combined with joint mobilization or manipulation produce outcomes similar to those obtained from the more expensive high-tech exercises (Evans et al. 2002; Gross et al. 2002; Randlov et al. 1998). One simple exercise, CCF (see figure 6.7), has been shown to be effective in treating chronic neck pain (Falla et al. 2006). Australian researchers reported that after 6 wk of using the CCF exercise, patients with chronic neck pain significantly improved their posture (Falla et al. 2007). In another randomized controlled trial, performing the CCF exercise for 6 wk significantly improved strength and pain when compared to no exercise (Chiu, Law, and Chiu 2005).

Many times resistance exercises are prescribed to improve posture in patients with cervical dysfunction; however, there is a lack of evidence to support the benefits of resistance training for postural improvement (Hrysomallis and Goodman 2001). Instead, the goal of resistance training should be to improve strength and endurance of postural muscles in supporting normal neck function. Specific strength training of cervical muscles is more effective than general fitness exercises for improving chronic neck pain (Andersen et al. 2008). A simple isometric exercise that targets the deep neck flexors is isometric retraction using an elastic band loop (see figure 12.3).

Both cervical muscles and muscles of the upper thoracic spine and shoulder are strengthened in neck rehabilitation. Strengthening activities include isometrics, dumbbells, elastic resistance, and selectorized machines. Swedish researchers reported that only 12 min of machine-based neck strength training, performed twice a week for 8 wk, increases neck strength by 19% to 35% (Berg, Berggren, and Tesch 1994). In Finland, researchers combined high-intensity (80% 1RM) neck strengthening with elastic bands (figure 12.4) and upper-extremity strengthening with dumbbells for 1 y in women with chronic neck pain (Ylinen et al. 2003). They reported increases in neck strength of 69% to 110% and reduction in pain and disability.

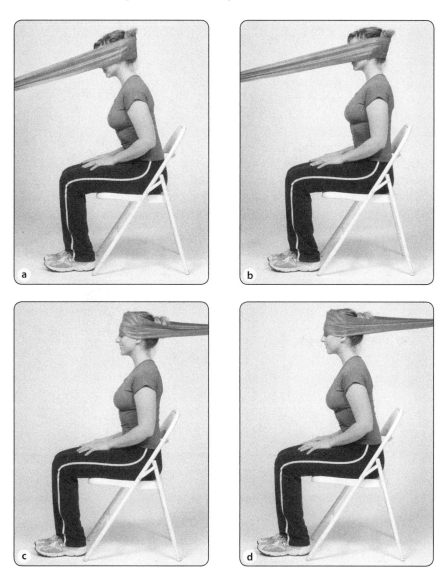

Figure 12.4 A dynamic isometric exercise involving *(a-b)* extension and *(c-d)* flexion of the neck.

Proprioceptive Exercises

As stated previously, the cervical spine is an important region for proprioception due to its high number of mechanoreceptors (Abrahams 1977; McLain 1994). Because of the proprioceptive deficits observed in patients with cervical dysfunction, proprioceptive exercises should be included in rehabilitation. Heikkila and Wenngren (1998) found that deficits in joint position sense improved in patients with whiplash disorders after 5 wk of rehabilitation. Sarig-Bahat (2003) reported strong evidence that both proprioceptive exercises and dynamic resistance exercises benefit the neck and shoulder.

The visual, vestibular, and proprioceptive systems are intimately linked for postural control. Exercises that combine head and eye movement are thought to improve cervical proprioception by utilizing pathways such as occulomotor and vestibulo-ocular reflexes. In a systematic review of exercise for neck pain, French researchers (Revel et al. 1994) noted significant improvements in cervical pain, ROM, and function in patients performing eye–head coupling movements. The authors also noted that kinesthesia improved in patients as symptoms improved. Fitz-Ritson (1995) described phasic eye–head, neck–arm exercises for patients with whiplash that utilize the vestibulo-ocular reflex, such as smooth pursuit, eye–head coupling, and upper-extremity PNF. Jull and colleagues (2007) found that proprioceptive exercises are slightly better than CCF exercise at improving cervical proprioception.

Sensorimotor Training

Since many patients with whiplash and chronic neck pain demonstrate poor balance, SMT (described in chapter 11) should be implemented in cervical rehabilitation to restore postural stability and global movement patterns. Unstable surfaces such as foam pads and balance boards help elicit automatic stabilizing reactions that cannot be trained voluntarily. Specific stabilization training for the cervical spine can also be administered by having the patient use exercise balls while in quadruped and standing positions (see figures 12.5 and 12.6).

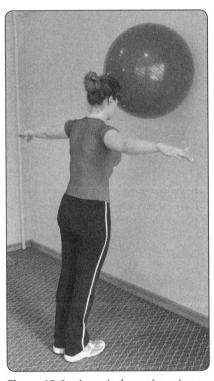

Figure 12.6   A cervical exercise using the exercise ball (with the patient in standing position).

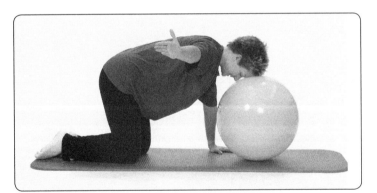

Figure 12.5   A cervical exercise using the exercise ball (with the patient in quadruped position).

Cervicogenic Headache and Facial Pain

Mild headaches are very common and are typically short lived and self-limiting. More severe headaches, such as migraines or cluster headaches, are debilitating and occur more frequently in some individuals. Cervicogenic headaches are assumed to be associated with cervical dysfunction and may include facial pain. Patients with facial pain demonstrate hyperactivity of the masseter and temporal muscles and hypoactivity of the suprahyoid, digastrics, and mylohyoid (Janda 1986b).

Assessment

The assessment for headaches and facial pain mirrors the evaluation for the cervical spine, beginning with postural assessment. Janda recommended screening the cervical spine in all patients with headache or facial pain (Janda 1986b).

Forward head posture in particular corresponds with lower endurance of the deep neck flexors in cervical headache (Watson and Trott 1993). The CCF test can provide valuable information on the strength of the deep neck flexors; patients with cervical headache often exhibit poor strength and endurance of these flexors (Jull 1999; Watson and Trott 1993; Zito, Jull, and Story 2006).

Patients with recurrent headache exhibit imbalance in length and strength of the right and left SCM muscles (Cibulka 2006). Zito, Jull, and Story (2006) noted significantly greater tightness in the muscles implicated in Janda's UCS: the upper trapezius, levator scapulae, scalenes, suboccipital, pectoralis major, and pectoralis minor. Patients with cervicogenic headache also demonstrate increased EMG levels in the upper trapezius when compared with controls (Bansevicius and Sjaastad 1996).

Patients with cervicogenic headache may also experience more upper cervical joint dysfunction. Manual examination provides up to 80% sensitivity in distinguishing patients with cervicogenic dysfunction from patients without headache and patients with migraines (Zito, Jull, and Story 2006).

Treatment

Joint mobilization has been shown to reduce the frequency, duration, and intensity of cervical headaches (Schoensee et al. 1995). A systematic review of physical treatments for cervicogenic headaches concluded that joint manipulation and exercises are effective in both the short and long term (Bronfort et al. 2004); other possibly effective treatments include electrical stimulation (TENS) and stretching. Tricyclic antidepressants are slightly more effective than spinal manipulation in improving headache in the short term, but manipulation provides more long-term sustained benefits and may avoid the side effects of medication (Boline et al. 1995).

In a recent study on exercise for cervicogenic headache (van Ettekoven and Lucas 2006), patients completed a 6 wk treatment of massage, mobilization, and postural exercise. The exercises included elastic-resisted cervical retraction performed twice a day for 10 min (see figure 12.3). Subjects reported significant decreases in the frequency, intensity, and duration of their headaches. These improvements were sustained for 6 mo after the program.

Jull and colleagues (2002) completed a randomized controlled trial of exercise and manual therapy for cervicogenic headache. They found that manipulation was as effective as exercise; combining the two treatments produced slightly better outcomes. Treatment effects were maintained for 12 mo after the intervention.

The treatment for cervicogenic headache should follow the general principles of cervical rehabilitation, including postural correction, joint mobilization and manipulation, local muscle stretching and strengthening, and progression to SMT. Moore (2004) reported on the evaluation and treatment of a patient with cervicogenic headache and Janda's UCS. The patient demonstrated classic postural deviations and muscle imbalances of UCS, and was successfully treated with therapeutic exercise and spinal manipulation.

Temporomandibular Joint Disorders

TMJ dysfunction is often associated with muscle imbalance around the head and neck. While TMJ dysfunction may be isolated in some patients, the incidence of cervical dysfunction is increased in patients with TMJ (Clark et al. 1987).

Pathology

Symptoms of TMJ dysfunction include pain in the joint and face, restricted mouth opening, locking, headache, muscle pain, and joint popping or clicking. This joint noise often is associated with an internal derangement of the cartilaginous anterior disc between the temporal bone and the mandible. Over time, OA develops in the TMJ, sometimes requiring surgery.

Janda observed that patients with TMJ dysfunction demonstrate hyperactivity of the masseter and temporal muscles and hypoactivity of the suprahyoid, digastrics, and mylohyoid (Janda 1986b). Gervais, Fitzsimmons, and Thomas (1989) confirmed Janda's observations, noting increased EMG activity in the masseter and temporalis of patients with TMJ dysfunction. Nishioka and Montgomery (1988) suggested that masticatory hyperactivity is centrally mediated, involving a neurotransmitter imbalance in the basal ganglia.

This primitive pattern of muscle hyperactivity occurs because closing the mouth is more important than opening it. Pterygoid spasm is also often present, although it isn't clear if the pterygoid is prone to tightness or weakness. Pterygoid spasm alters the condyle position, and when coupled with forward head posture, mouth opening may become more difficult. This in turn causes tightness of the SCM, scalene, and suboccipitals, which then increase forces on the mandible and increase masseter activity (Janda 1986b).

Assessment

Evaluation of TMJ dysfunction is similar to the cervical assessment noted previously in this chapter, beginning with postural analysis. Poor posture is postulated to influence TMJ dysfunction (Rocabado, Johnston Jr., and Blakney 1982). Janda (1986b) noted that patients with TMJ disorder often have a forward head posture that is complicated by tightness of the upper trapezii and levator scapulae. This forward head position leads to opening of the mouth with retraction of the mandible; therefore, the jaw protractors and adductors used to close the mouth become tight. The resting position of the lower jaw in relation to the upper jaw is also deviated or protracted or retracted.

Movement assessment specific to the TMJ includes examining the active ROM of the jaw; the clinician should note any deviations or clicking occurring during the movement. In general, patients should be able to open the mouth to a distance equivalent to the combined width of the index and middle fingers. Janda's cervical flexion test may indicate characteristic weakness of the deep neck flexors seen in TMJ dysfunction. Finally, palpation of the TMJ muscles often reveals tightness and TrPs, particularly in the lateral pterygoid, masseter, and temporalis. The SCM, scalenes, suboccipitals, and upper trapezius may also be tight and tender in patients with long-standing dysfunction and poor posture, suggesting the presence of Janda's UCS.

Treatment

Conservative interventions for TMJ dysfunction include anti-inflammatory medications, splinting, and physical therapy involving manual therapy, modalities, and exercise. Arthroscopic surgery is performed sometimes in cases of severe internal derangement or OA. Muscle balance in tight muscles, including muscles with TrPs, is first addressed with spray and stretch (Simons, Travel, and Simons 1999). PIR (see chapter 10) is also effective in addressing latent TrPs in the masseter for improved mouth opening in TMJ patients. Recently, Kashima and coworkers (2006) demonstrated that cervical side bending combined with flexion reduces masseter hardness, but it also increases hardness of the upper trapezius on the ipsilateral side. Manual interventions such as joint mobilization and lateral pterygoid release may also be helpful (Furto et al. 2006). Treatment for patients presenting with TMJ disorders and also Janda's UCS should include strengthening of the deep neck flexors (see page 183) and SMT (see chapter 11).

Two systematic reviews of physical therapy interventions for TMJ dysfunction (McNeely, Armijo Olivo, and Magee 2006; Medlicott and Harris, 2006) suggested that a successful approach is a combination of treatments, including active exercise and manual mobilization, postural training, proprioceptive reeducation, and relaxation and biofeedback training. Furto and colleagues (2006) reported that TMJ dysfunction treated with a combination of manual therapy and exercise significantly improved in as little as 2 wk.

In a series of studies, Austrian researchers administered an exercise protocol to subgroups of patients with craniomandibular disorders and then compared these patients with control subjects on a wait list. Exercises included active and passive jaw movements, posture correction, and relaxation techniques. The four subgroups included (1) patients with anterior disc displacement after reduction (Nicolakis et al. 2000), (2) patients with anterior disc displacement without reduction (Nicolakis, Erdogmus et al. 2001), (3) patients with OA of the TMJ (Nicolakis et al. 2000), and (4) patients without OA but still with TMJ dysfunction (Nicolakis et al. 2002). Each study found exercise helpful, and exercise had up to 75% success in reducing pain and impairment (Nicolakis et al. 2000).

Fibromyalgia and Myofascial Pain

Fibromyalgia (FM) affects about 5 million people in the United States, or roughly 2% of the population. It occurs more frequently in women than in men (Lawrence et al. 2008). The diagnostic criteria for FM were established by the American College of Rheumatology in 1990 (Wolfe et al. 1990). FM is defined as chronic widespread musculoskeletal pain lasting for at least 3 mo that is combined with tender points in 11 out of 18 specific sites on both sides of the body.

Pathology

Some researchers (Häkkinen et al. 2001; Staud 2002; Staud, Robinson, and Price 2005) have suggested that FM has a central neurological basis rather than a peripheral muscular basis, as is commonly believed. Although FM is characterized by widespread muscular pain, there is little evidence to support the role of muscle in its pathophysiology (Simms 1996). Research has shown that pain in FM is not due to muscular tension measured by EMG (Bansevicius, Westgaard, and Stiles 2001; Nilsen et al. 2006; Zidar et al. 1990), suggesting that pain results not from the muscle but from a dysfunctional nociceptive system. Patients with FM experience pain differently than those without FM experience it. FM is most notably characterized by a general increase in pain sensitivity and lowered pain thresholds (Gibson et al. 1994; Mountz et al. 1995), particularly thermal (cold and hot) thresholds (Berglund et al. 2002; Desmeules et al. 2003; Kosek, Ekholm, and Hansson 1996; Lautenbacher and Rollman 1997).

Landmark studies by Gracely and colleagues (2002) used functional MRI to investigate pain processing in the brains of persons with FM. These researchers found that patients with FM experience pain in parts of the brain that are totally different from those parts involved in pain experience in patients without FM; furthermore, brains of patients with FM became active with less-painful stimuli. This finding suggests that FM is augmented by cortical or subcortical pain processing, which is similar to findings in patients with chronic low back pain (Giesecke et al. 2004). Patients with FM demonstrate increased tension in the trapezius and infraspinatus muscle during repetitive upper-extremity tasks when compared with healthy subjects (Elert et al. 2001).

While FM pain is probably CNS mediated, it's also likely that peripheral nociceptive input is necessary to maintain central pain sensitization (Bennett 1996). Kosek, Ekholm, and Hansson (1996) suggested that dysfunctional afferent pathways causing altered pain processing are due to CNS dysfunction. Desmeules and colleagues (2003) demonstrated altered processing of nociceptive input into the CNS in both the brain and the spinal cord of patients with FM, an observation indicating a state of central sensitization and hyperexcitability in the CNS. Excessive activation of muscular nociceptive afferents may contribute to hyperalgesia in FM (Staud, Robinson, and Price 2005). Because FM is influenced by the sensory system and central processing and manifests in the muscular system, it could be considered a dysfunction of the sensorimotor system.

Assessment

A comprehensive assessment of patients with FM should follow the procedures outlined in chapters 5 through 8 to determine the presence of Janda's syndromes, particularly the layer syndrome. Patients with FM exhibit decreased strength and aerobic capacity when compared with healthy individuals (Borman, Celiker, and Hasçelik 1999; Maquet et al. 2002; Mengshoel, Førre, and Komnaes 1990; Nørregaard et al. 1995). Muscular weakness in FM seems to be related more to lack of voluntary effort than to neuromuscular mechanisms (Simms 1996).

TrPs and tender points can be quantified using a pain algometer. Often, this measure is useful in quantifying progress made toward reducing pain levels in patients.

Balance assessment should be included in the evaluation of FM. Because of the sensorimotor component of FM pathophysiology, these patients may exhibit balance deficits.

Treatment

Because of the heterogeneity of FM, treatment programs should be tailored to the individual patient. Pharmacological treatment can be combined with nonpharmacological interventions. Ischemic compression therapy can reduce the pain of myofascial TrPs; this pain can also be addressed with combinations of other treatments including heat, spray and stretch, TENS, interferential current, and active ROM (Hou et al. 2002). Treatment should not focus on reducing TrPs through direct means; rather, exercise to affect the global sensorimotor system may be more effective.

A systematic review in the Cochrane Library (Busch et al. 2002) found that supervised aerobic exercise improves physical capacity and FM symptoms. Another systematic review of FM exercise studies (Mannerkorpi and Iversen 2003) recommended that patients perform low-level aerobic exercise at moderate intensity twice weekly, pool exercises, or strength training at low but adequate loads.

Exercise interventions are helpful but must be started at much lower intensities and progressed much more slowly than the prescriptions given for traditional exercise programs. Several studies have shown improvements in physical fitness, FM status, and pain levels through a well-rounded exercise program including aerobic, flexibility, strength, and balance exercises (Buckelew et al. 1998; Jones et al. 2002; Jones et al. 2008; Martin et al. 1996; Rooks et al. 2007).

Resistance training can be particularly effective and safe for FM when provided appropriately. Jones and colleagues (2002) compared a 12 wk strengthening program with a stretching program in patients with FM. While both groups improved, the strengthening group exhibited more improvements than the stretching group displayed. The strengthening program minimized eccentric contractions, using elastic bands that were on slack between repetitions and keeping exercises near the midline. Exercises were also performed more slowly on the concentric phase than on the eccentric phase.

Häkkinen and colleagues (2001) reported improved strength and EMG activity after a 21 wk strengthening program in patients with FM. The Finnish researchers confirmed through several other studies that women with FM have neuromuscular characteristics and ability to gain strength that are similar to those of women without FM (Häkkinen et al. 2000; Valkeinen et al. 2005; Valkeinen et al. 2006). This finding suggests that fatigability is not a limiting factor in FM. Moderate to high levels of resistance exercise, progressing from 40% to 80% of 1RM, have been safely implemented in patients with FM and have been found to improve strength, muscle cross-sectional area, and neuromuscular activation (Valkeinen et al. 2004; Valkeinen et al. 2005).

Case Study

A female collegiate swimmer 21 y of age competed in middle- and long-distance freestyle events. Her primary complaint was chronic pain in the neck and right shoulder and arm that occurred after swimming for less than 1 h. She was injured approximately 3 y earlier when someone dove on her head while she was in the pool. She underwent two rounds of physical therapy (including modalities, traction, and shoulder and neck strengthening) for her cervical spine over the past year but continued to experience symptoms when attempting to return to swimming.

Examination and Assessment

On physical examination, the patient exhibited generalized hypermobility, bilateral pes planus, and a right anterior SI innominate rotation. She also demonstrated upper-thoracic breathing patterns rather than diaphragmatic breathing. Her cervical and lumbar active ROM were both pain free and within normal limits. Manual evaluation of the cervical spine was unremarkable. She demonstrated a normal upper- and lower-quarter neurovascular examination. She had some tender points in the right upper trapezius. Both upper extremities demonstrated normal strength except for weakness (with a rating of 4/5) in the right lower trapezius. She also had weakness of the right gluteus maximus (4/5) and poor endurance of the deep cervical flexors. Her right scapula demonstrated winging and instability in a quadruped position.

Differential diagnosis included cervical sprain or strain, herniated cervical disc, thoracic outlet syndrome, shoulder instability, and SI rotation. Diagnostic imaging included MRI, which demonstrated sprain of the C1-C2 alar ligament. Dynamic surface EMG revealed decreased and delayed activation of the right gluteus maximus and inhibition of the right lower trapezius (a 61% decrease in activity when compared with the left side).

The athlete was diagnosed with cervical sprain. Upon physical therapy evaluation, she demonstrated several other findings that may have contributed to her chronic pain syndrome. These included an anterior SI rotation, abnormal breathing patterns, and cervical flexor fatigue. She demonstrated unilateral muscle imbalance of the hip and shoulder and instability of the scapulothoracic complex. Immediately upon correction of the right SI rotation with the muscle energy technique (MET), the right gluteus maximus strength returned to 5 out of 5, indicating muscular inhibition rather than weakness.

Treatment and Outcome

The athlete began physical therapy twice a week, with a daily home program. She began with MET self-correction, diaphragmatic breathing, and cervical stretches. Janda's SMT was initiated for progressive dynamic stabilization training of the foot, pelvis, scapulo-thoracic region, and cervical spine. Exercises included stabilization on an exercise ball, muscle activation using elastic resistance, and balance training with dynamic cervical stabilization. Within 1 mo, the athlete was asymptomatic and returned to the pool for a progressive reentry program. Meanwhile, she continued a home exercise program. She also initiated a land-based cardiorespiratory conditioning program. After 2 mo of therapy, she was discharged from physical therapy, demonstrating a normal physical examination and full strength of her hip and shoulder. Two months after discharge, she competed and achieved an A-cut qualifying time for nationals in the 1,650 yd (1,500 m) freestyle event, breaking a school record.

Janda's Approach Versus the Traditional Approach

In this athlete, the traditional approach of localized treatment using modalities and strengthening exercise was not effective in addressing the source of her pain. This case report describes a novel approach to treatment, without the use of modalities, for chronic neck pain in a competitive swimmer with cervical instability. Because the swimmer's cervical examination was normal and pain occurred only during and after swimming, it was postulated that cervical instability and fatigue were contributing to pain and compensations, particularly at the hip. Physical examination and surface EMG assessment demonstrated unilateral muscle imbalances and an SI rotation that may have compensated for cervical and shoulder fatigue, thus causing chronic pain. The Janda approach of SMT was used to increase proprioceptive input into the CNS to encourage stabilization of the entire body. Because the athlete demonstrated unilateral inhibition of her phasic system muscles (cervical flexors, lower trapezius, and gluteus maximus), emphasis was placed on multiple muscle activation, particularly of the phasic system muscles. Dynamic stabilization and endurance, rather than muscular strength, were the focus. Inexpensive home exercise equipment was used to facilitate rehabilitation. A reentry program and land-based conditioning program were also used for her return to competitive swimming. After 3 y of pain, the athlete was able to return to competition within 2 mo of this specialized rehabilitation program.

Summary

The cervical spine is a challenging region for clinicians to evaluate and treat. It is an important area of proprioception, and new research links cervical dysfunction to the sensorimotor system, supporting Janda's approach to chronic cervical pain. Janda's UCS may be present in many patients with chronic neck pain, whiplash, headache, TMJ dysfunction, and FM. Clinicians should be aware of UCS in these patients so appropriate functional interventions can be implemented.

UPPER-EXTREMITY PAIN SYNDROMES

Chronic upper-extremity musculoskeletal pain associated with disability has been reported in 21% of the U.S. population (Gummesson et al. 2003). The complex anatomy of the shoulder plays an important role in positioning the entire upper extremity for hand function, creating a vital kinetic chain for daily living. Because of its versatility in positioning and posture, the shoulder may be predisposed to muscle imbalance syndromes, including impingement, thoracic outlet syndrome, and shoulder and neck pain. Lateral elbow pain (i.e., tennis elbow) may also be associated with muscle imbalances. As with other regional chronic pain syndromes, clinicians must consider neuromuscular factors in managing upper-extremity pain syndromes.

This chapter begins with a review of the regional considerations of the upper extremity, including functional anatomy of the shoulder complex, proprioception, and chain reactions. Next, Janda's functional assessment of the shoulder is discussed. Common functional pathologies are reviewed, including shoulder impingement and rotator cuff tendinosis, shoulder instability, thoracic outlet syndrome, and lateral epicondylitis. Finally, the chapter presents a case study on the evaluation and treatment of functional shoulder pain in a baseball player.

Regional Considerations

The upper extremity includes the shoulder complex, elbow, wrist, and hand. The primary function of the upper extremity is to manipulate the environment. This creates a need for a wide variety of movements and positions to manage everything from personal hygiene and dressing tasks to vocational and leisure activities. Magermans and colleagues (2005) have described the ROM requirements for upper-extremity ADL. Large glenohumeral rotation is necessary for tasks with high elevation angles, while large axial rotation of the humerus is used during dressing and grooming. Large ranges of elbow flexion are necessary for hair combing, eating, and bathing. Obviously, normal function of all joints in the upper extremity is necessary for ADL.

Functional Anatomy of the Shoulder Complex

The shoulder complex comprises four articulations: the glenohumeral, scapulothoracic, acromioclavicular, and sternoclavicular joints. The synovial glenohumeral joint is supported by capsuloligamentous structures. The glenohumeral capsule itself provides little stability in midrange; instead, joint stabilization is provided by dynamic contraction of the rotator cuff during movement (Apreleva et al. 1998; Culham and Peat 1993; Lee et al. 2000; Saha 1971; Werner, Favre, and Gerber 2007; Wuelker et al. 1994; Xue and Huang 1998). The deltoid (Kido et al. 2003; Lee and An 2002) and biceps (Itoi et al. 1994; Kim et al. 2001) also stabilize the glenohumeral joint.

Contrary to the perception that the rotator cuff only performs humeral rotation, the primary role of the cuff is stabilization and elevation in the scapular plane (Liu et al. 1997; Otis et al. 1994; Sharkey, Marder, and Hanson 1994). Only mild contraction of the rotator cuff is necessary for stability (McQua de and Murthi 2004); therefore, rotator cuff strengthening programs do not necessarily have to fatigue the muscles to improve their function. In fact, fatigue of the rotator cuff can cause as much as 0.1 in. (2.5 mm) of unwanted upward migration of the humeral head during abduction (Chen et al. 1999). A decrease in rotator cuff stabilizing force proportionally increases anterior displacement of the humeral head (Wuelker, Korell, and Thren 1998).

While the rotator cuff plays a vital role in maintaining centration of the humeral head, it is the dynamic scapular stabilizers that coordinate the position of the glenoid with the humerus (Belling-Sørensen and Jørgensen 2000; Kibler 1998b). Fatigue of the scapular stabilizers can significantly reduce rotator cuff strength (Cuoco, Tyler, and McHugh 2004). Thus scapular stabilization is critical for glenohumeral function since the rotator cuff originates on the scapula.

Scapulohumeral function is controlled by two main muscular force couples. These are the (1) rotator cuff and deltoid and (2) scapular rotators. Both are described in the following sections.

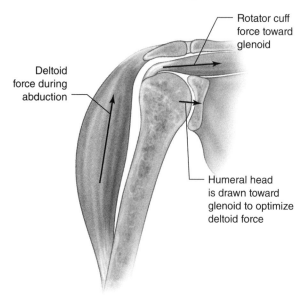

Deltoid force during abduction

Rotator cuff force toward glenoid

Humeral head is drawn toward glenoid to optimize deltoid force

Figure 13.1 Rotator cuff force couples.

Rotator Cuff–Deltoid Force Couple

As stated previously, the primary function of the rotator cuff is not rotation, as commonly defined in anatomy texts; rather, its primary function is dynamic stabilization of the glenohumeral joint. Within the rotator cuff itself, a force couple between the subscapularis and the infraspinatus and teres minor provides a compressive force, drawing the humeral head into the glenoid. This compressive force has been described as a force parallel to the axillary border of the scapula (Inman, Saunders, and Abbott 1944) or as a force perpendicular to the glenoid (Poppen and Walker 1978). The net effect is a depressor force vector that counteracts the elevation force of the deltoid (figure 13.1). This rotator cuff–deltoid force couple is key to shoulder abduction (Lucas 1973; Perry 1978; Sarrafian 1983). In fact, the deltoid force needed for abduction is 41% less when the rotator cuff is activated along with the deltoid contraction (Sharkey, Marder, and Hanson 1994). The supraspinatus is more active at the beginning of ROM, while the middle deltoid is more active near the end (McMahon et al. 1995).

Scapular Rotator Force Couple

The upper and lower trapezius are coupled with the serratus anterior to produce upward rotation of the scapula. Scapular rotation maintains the optimal length–tension relationship of the deltoid during abduction (Doody, Freedman, and Waterland 1970; Lucas 1973; van der Helm 1994; Mottram 1997). The trapezius is more active during abduction than it is during flexion (Moseley et al. 1992; Wiedenbauer and Mortenson 1952) and generally plateaus in EMG activity after 120° (Bagg and Forest 1986).

Different parts of the trapezius have different histological properties that correspond to different functional demands: the lower trapezius is better suited for stabilization, while the upper trapezius is more suited for movement (Lindman, Eriksson, and Thornell 1990). The middle and lower trapezius maintain the vertical and horizontal position of the scapula rather than generate torque (Johnson et al.1994), working at a constant length to resist protraction of the scapula from the serratus anterior.

The lower trapezius relaxes during flexion (Inman, Saunders, and Abbott 1944) and is not active until abduction (Wadsworth and Bullock-Saxton 1997). It becomes more active with shoulder elevation to assist the upper trapezius and serratus anterior in rotating the scapula upward (Bagg and Forest 1988). Proper balance of the trapezius and serratus force couple is believed to reduce the superior migration of the scapula, improve posterior scapular tilt, facilitate optimal glenohumeral congruency, and maximize the available subacromial space (SAS) under the coracoacromial arch to avoid impingement (Ludewig et al. 2004; Mottram 1997). If the lower trapezius is inhibited, the deltoid loses its length–tension relationship and may overwork the infraspinatus (Cram and Kasman 1998). Muscle activation and timing are key to not only proper activation of the force couple but also overall function of the shoulder complex. For example, if the lower and middle trapezius react too slowly in relation to the upper trapezius, the upper trapezius may become overactive, leading to scapular elevation rather than upward rotation (Cools et al. 2003).

Using EMG analysis, several authors have described the sequencing of muscle activation during shoulder movement. Often, muscles are activated before movement in a feed-forward mechanism. This preactivation stabilizes segments before movement initiation. For example, during rotation the rotator cuff and biceps are activated before the deltoid and pectoralis major, a finding that supports the suggested role of the rotator cuff and biceps in stabilizing the glenohumeral joint (David et al. 2000). Cools and colleagues reported that the deltoid is activated before the trapezius, while Wadsworth and Bullock-Saxton (1997) reported that the upper trapezius is activated before abduction.

Shoulder Proprioception

The glenohumeral joint capsule of the shoulder consists mainly of the superior, middle, posterior, and inferior glenohumeral ligaments. All four types of mechanoreceptors (see chapter 2) have been identified in 40% to 50% of human specimens (Guanche et al. 1999). Vangsness and colleagues (1995) noted a higher prevalence of type I and II receptors in the glenohumeral ligaments as well as in the coracoclavicular and coracoacromial joint capsules. Steinbeck and colleagues (2003) specifically identified type I receptors in the inferior glenohumeral ligament (IGHL). The IGHL provides the most stability to anterior dislocation during the throwing motion (O'Brien et al. 1994). The presence of type I Ruffini endings in this ligament is consistent with their function in responding to stretch at the limits of motion and suggests that these specific mechanoreceptors have a role in muscular reflexes used to stabilize the shoulder (Steinbeck et al. 2003).

Glenohumeral mechanoreceptors are thought to prevent dislocation through proprioceptive feedback mechanisms that help control muscular stabilizers (Jerosch et al. 1993). Guanche and colleagues (1995) found a reflex arc between the glenohumeral capsule and the muscles crossing the shoulder joint in cats. They stimulated branches of the axillary nerve terminating in the glenohumeral capsule and noted EMG activity in the rotator cuff muscles. This finding suggests the joint capsule plays an afferent role in controlling muscular reflexes. Because the rotator cuff functions mainly as a dynamic stabilizer rather than a mover, the capsular mechanoreceptors are thought to play an integral role in providing feedback to prevent subluxation or dislocation through the reflex arc. Guanche and colleagues (1995) provided further evidence for a reflexive feedback system through deafferentation of sensory feedback in the joint capsule. They showed that in felines, transection of capsular afferent branches of the axillary nerve ends EMG activity of the shoulder muscles.

As stated previously, the mechanical contribution of glenohumeral capsular ligaments to shoulder stability is minimal; instead, reflexive co-contractions facilitated by afferent capsular feedback are more likely to stabilize the joint (Veeger and van der Helm 2007).

Most capsular mechanoreceptor feedback is provided when the capsule is on tension rather than when it is relaxed during early and midranges of motion (Jerosch et al. 1997).

Further evidence to support the role of capsular mechanoreceptors in maintaining glenohumeral stability has been shown through studies on shoulder proprioception. Shoulder proprioception can be divided into submodalities of kinesthesia and joint position sense (Lephart and Fu 2000). Proprioceptive information seems to be enhanced during external rotation, when the capsule is taut, rather than during internal rotation (Allegrucci et al. 1995; Blasier, Carpenter, and Huston 1994); this is likely due to the prevalence of type I mechanoreceptors in the IGHL (Steinbeck et al. 2003). Shoulder kinesthesia is reduced after damage to the anterior capsule following glenohumeral dislocation (Smith and Brunolli 1989). Lephart and colleagues (1994) also reported a significant difference in kinesthesia and joint position sense between stable and unstable shoulders. They further noted that surgical reconstruction of the anterior capsule restores normal proprioception. These results suggest that the anterior capsule plays an important role in maintaining glenohumeral integrity through proprioceptive mechanisms.

Chain Reactions

The upper extremity forms a single kinetic chain from the upper spine to the fingers. The upper extremity is connected to the axial skeleton by only one true articulation: the sterno-clavicular joint. Therefore, the shoulder complex relies on muscles to begin the kinetic chain to transfer forces from the trunk. The proximal end of the kinetic chain begins in the cervical spine, thoracic spine, and ribs. The upper trapezius and levator scapulae have origins on the cervical spine, while the middle trapezius and rhomboids originate in the thoracic spine. The ribs serve as an origin for the pectoralis major and serratus anterior. The upper thoracic spine extends, rotates, and laterally flexes during elevation in the sagittal and scapular planes (Theodoridis and Ruston 2002). Thus thoracic mobility is important in the upper-extremity kinetic chain.

There are several important muscle slings (see chapter 3) to consider in the upper extremity; these are summarized in table 13.1. Because 50% of the total force in overhand throwing comes from the legs and trunk (Kibler 1995), the entire kinetic chain from the foot to the hand, particularly in athletes, should be considered during assessment of upper-extremity dysnfuction.

Table 13.1 Muscle Slings in the Upper Extremity

Muscle sling	Muscles
Flexor	Anterior deltoid, pectoralis minor, trapezius, biceps hand flexors
Extensor	Posterior deltoid, rhomboids, triceps hand extensors
Anterior	Biceps, pectoralis major, internal oblique, contralateral hip abductors, sartorius
Spiral	Rhomboids, serratus anterior, external oblique, contralateral internal oblique, contralateral hip adductors

Kibler's (1998b, 2006) discussion on the upper-extremity kinetic chain helped revo-lutionize the way clinicians approach evaluation and rehabilitation. According to Kibler (1998b), the scapula provides the following:

- A stable glenohumeral articulation
- Protraction and retraction on the thoracic wall to position the arm
- Elevation of the acromion to avoid impingement

- A base for muscle attachment (rotator cuff and scapular rotators)
- A link for transferring force proximally to distally in throwing

The importance of the kinetic chain is evident when describing the pathomechanics of rotator cuff tendinitis. Poor scapular stabilization increases activity of the upper trapezius for stabilization, which in turn increases scapular elevation. Scapular elevation alters the direction of the axis of the glenoid fossa; this change may be accompanied by increased and constant activity in the rotator cuff, leading to rotator cuff tendinitis.

Motor patterns in both the upper and lower extremity are influenced by the upper extremity. When a person is standing, elevation of the shoulder activates the contralateral erector spinae (Davey et al. 2002) as well as the lower-extremity muscles to maintain postural stability (Mochizuki, Ivanova, and Garland 2004). This activation results from feed-forward motor control used to stabilize the trunk before arm movement begins, regardless of the direction of the arm movement (Hodges et al. 1997b). Again, pathology demonstrates the influence of the kinetic chain; patients with shoulder and neck pain demonstrate poor postural stability (Karlberg et al. 1995). This phenomenon indicates a disruption in the feed-forward mechanism (chapter 2), indicating CNS involvement in mediating chronic shoulder pain.

Assessment

As with other chronic musculoskeletal pain, upper-extremity pain may manifest as global changes throughout the body. Long-standing UCS may be compensated for with LCS; therefore, the entire body should be included in the assessment of upper-extremity chronic pain.

Posture

A cause-and-effect relationship between posture and muscle imbalance has yet to be established; however, it is commonly thought that posture is related to muscle imbalance and function. Poor posture has been described with UCS changes (chapter 4). Griegel-Morris and colleagues (1992) noted common postural deviations in healthy individuals: 66% had forward head posture, 38% had increased thoracic kyphosis, and 73% had rounded shoulders. The authors also noted that forward head posture and increased kyphosis are associated with interscapular pain.

Forward head posture (protraction of the cervical spine) often is increased in patients with shoulder pain (Greenfield et al. 1995). A forward head posture reduces flexion ROM of the shoulder (Bullock, Foster, and Wright 2005). Forward head posture and rounded shoulders change the normal orientation of the plane of the scapula from 30° to 45° anterior to the frontal plane (Doody, Freedman, and Waterland 1970; Johnston 1937; Poppen and Walker 1976). This slouched posture significantly alters the kinematics of the scapula during elevation (Kebaeste, McClure, and Pratt 1999; Finley and Lee 2003). Shoulder protraction also reduces the height of the SAS (Solem-Bertoft, Thuomas, and Westerberg 1993), implicating rounded shoulders in impingement syndrome. Shoulder strength can also be affected by poor posture: Positioning the scapula in protraction or retraction significantly reduces shoulder elevation and rotation strength (Kebaetse, McClure, and Pratt 1999; Smith et al. 2002; Smith et al. 2006). Postural deviations and imbalances consistent with Janda's UCS have been reported in swimmers (Layton et al. 2005), dental hygienists (Johnson et al. 2003), and persons with upper-extremity work-related disorders (Novak 2004).

As described in chapter 5, characteristic postural deviations are seen in UCS due to muscular imbalance; these include forward head posture (tight suboccipitals and weak deep neck flexors), rounded shoulders (tight pectoralis and weak scapular stabilizers), and scapular winging and protraction. Winging of the scapula (prominence of the medial border) is often attributed to weakness of the serratus anterior, but it may also be caused by weakness of the rhomboids or trapezius (Martin and Fish 2008). Mottram (1997) described pseudowinging as prominence of the inferior border (as opposed to the medial border). Pseudowinging is related to tightness of the pectoralis minor. Scapular instability may be evident in postural analysis. Three presentations of scapular instability have been identified:

1. Pronouncement of the inferior medial border due to imbalance in scapular tilt across a transverse axis
2. Prominence of the entire medial border (winging) due to imbalance across a vertical axis
3. Superior translation and prominence of the superior medial border

Recently, Burkhart, Morgan, and Kibler (2003) described the SICK scapula (Scapular malposition, Inferior medial border prominence, Coracoid pain, and dysKinesis of scapular movement). The SICK scapula (figure 13.2) is most commonly seen in athletes with impingement who rely on overhead movements. Typically, the scapula is depressed, protracted, and downwardly rotated.

Janda described a manual test for scapular instability resulting from weakness of the rhomboid or serratus anterior. Using one hand to stabilize the anterior shoulder, the clinician places the other hand, with fingers extended, at the vertebral inferior angle. The clinician then pushes the fingers upward under the scapula. Normally, the fingers should disappear under the scapula only to the distal interphalangeal joints; with scapular weakness and instability, the fingers will progress further (see figure 13.3).

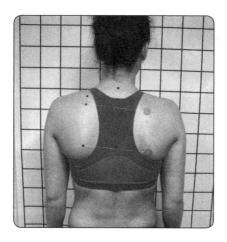

Figure 13.2 The right SICK scapula is protracted, downwardly rotated, and depressed.

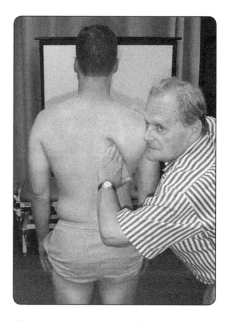

Figure 13.3 Janda's test for scapular instability.

Balance and Gait

Patients with chronic shoulder pain should be assessed for single-leg balance. Subtle compensations are sometimes apparent in the single-leg stance, such as elevation of the contralateral shoulder. Such elevation may indicate an overactive trapezius that is facilitated with every step and lead the clinician to suspect that the source of shoulder pain may be located somewhere else in the kinetic chain.

Movement Patterns

Janda's two primary tests for upper-extremity function are the push-up test and the shoulder abduction test (see figures 6.5 and 6.6). In the push-up test, the scapula normally abducts and upwardly rotates as the trunk is lifted upward. There is no associated scapular elevation. Winging of the scapula, excessive scapular adduction, or inability to complete scapular ROM in the direction of abduction indicates weakness of the serratus anterior. Shoulder shrugging during the push-up indicates overactivity of the upper trapezius and levator scapulae. During the shoulder abduction test, any elevation of the shoulder girdle that occurs before 60° of shoulder abduction is positive for impaired force couples, such as a hypertonic upper trapezius and levator scapulae combined with a weak middle and lower trapezius.

Patients with shoulder pain often exhibit dyskinesis (altered scapular kinematics) and altered muscle activation patterns when compared with healthy individuals (Lin et al. 2005). Dyskinesis is associated with decreased posterior tilt, decreased upward rotation, and increased elevation, which in general are related to an imbalance of scapular rotators that manifests as weakness of the serratus anterior and lower trapezius and tightness of the upper trapezius. These altered kinematics can persist even after pain has resided (Babyar 1996).

Muscle Strength and Length

As described in chapter 4, Janda's UCS includes shoulder muscle imbalance: a tight upper trapezius, levator scapulae, and pectoralis major combined with a weak lower trapezius and serratus anterior. Janda further noted that the posterior rotator cuff and deltoid are prone to weakness, possibly jeopardizing the critical rotator cuff–deltoid force couple. The pectoralis minor is also classified as a muscle prone to tightness; a tight pectoralis minor alters scapular kinematics (Borstad and Ludewig 2006; Mottram 1997). Borstad (2006) reported that the distance between the sternal notch and the coracoid process correlates well with pectoralis minor shortness (figure 13.4) and that this measurement is a better indicator than standard visual assessment in supine. Imbalance of the scapular rotator muscles also affects the trapezius–serratus anterior force couple. Kibler (1998b) agreed with Janda that the lower trapezius and serratus anterior are prone to inhibition that results in scapular instability.

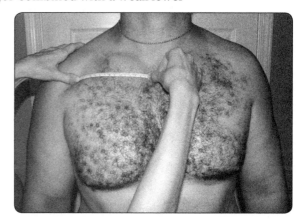

Figure 13.4 Measurement from the sternal notch to the coracoid process can be used as an indicator of pectoralis minor tightness.

Muscle testing with a handheld dynamometer or isokinetic dynamometry provides the most accurate measure of muscle strength. The shoulder complex is vulnerable to muscle imbalance because of its large range of movement and dependence on force couples for dynamic muscular stability. Normal abduction-to-adduction (AB:AD) ratios are between 0.79 and 1.0 (Mayer et al. 2001; Tata et al. 1993). The normal external rotation-to-internal-rotation (ER:IR) concentric isokinetic strength ratio is between 0.74 and 0.87 (Tata et al. 1993; Warner et al. 1990). Athletes who depend on overhead movements typically exhibit lower ER:IR ratios because they need greater internal rotation strength to meet their functional demands.

More recently, functional muscle balance in athletes has been reported as the ratio of eccentric external rotation to concentric internal rotation (Bak and Magnusson 1997). This is because the functional motion of overhead throwing involves concentric firing of the internal rotators followed by eccentric firing of the external rotators after ball release. If eccentric external rotation strength is less than concentric internal rotation strength, there is a significantly greater risk of shoulder injury (Wang and Cochrane 2001). This ratio has been reported in different athletes (Yildiz et al. 2006), including badminton players (Ng and Lam 2002), volleyball players (Wang and Cochrane 2001), and baseball players (Noffal 2003).

Imbalances in ROM and flexibility (typically measured by internal and external rotation) alter shoulder kinematics. Specifically, anterior tightness alters the scapulohumeral rhythm and decreases posterior scapular tilt, while posterior tightness causes more superior and anterior translation of the humeral head (Lin et al. 2006). Posterior capsular tightness, often demonstrated by a loss of internal rotation, may increase anterior translation of the humeral head (Lin et al. 2006; Tyler et al. 1999). This tightness may also cause many functional problems such as decreased ROM for deceleration during follow-through in the throwing motion.

Athletes with shoulder muscle imbalance are more likely to experience shoulder injury (Wang and Cochrane 2001). The mechanics of throwing make athletes susceptible to shoulder imbalances in ROM and strength, particularly external rotation weakness and decreased internal rotation ROM (Baltaci and Tunay 2004). The posterior rotator cuff (infraspinatus and teres minor) provides dynamic restraint to anterior instability during the throwing motion (Cain et al. 1987). In athletes who use overhead throwing, posterior cuff weakness may lead to pain due to a rotator cuff force imbalance of the external and internal rotators (Wilk et al. 1993). Imbalances in both strength and ROM are common in athletes participating in a variety of sports requiring overhead movement.

Baseball players have significantly more external rotation ROM and less internal rotation ROM (Borsa et al. 2005, 2006; Donatelli et al. 2000; Tyler et al. 1999); however, their total ROM in their throwing arm is not significantly different from that of the nondominant arm (Ellenbecker et al. 2002). While most baseball players exhibit greater internal rotation strength and lower ER:IR ratios when compared with nonathletes (Cook et al. 1987; Ellenbecker and Mattalino 1997; Wilk et al. 1993), researchers have also reported normal ER:IR strength ratios in these athletes (Alderink and Kuck 1986; Mikesky et al. 1995 ; Sirota et al. 1997). Elbow extension-to-flexion strength ratios are between 71% and 100% in baseball players (Mikesky et al. 1995).

Swimmers also generally have greater internal rotation strength and lower ER:IR ratios (McMaster, Long, and Caiozzo 1992; Rupp, Berninger, and Hopf 1995; Warner et al. 1990). AB:AD ratios are also reduced in both swimmers and water polo players (McMaster, Long, and Caiozzo 1991, 1992). Volleyball players have greater internal rotation, elbow extension, and wrist extension strength when compared with nonathletes (Alfredson, Pietilä, and Lorentzon 1998; Wang et al. 1999; Wang and Cochrane 2001).

Over time, tennis players demonstrate significantly less internal rotation ROM as well as less total ROM on their dominant side (Ellenbecker et al. 1996; Kibler et al. 1996). Tennis players often have significantly more strength in wrist extension (Ellenbecker, Roetert, and Riewald 2006; Strizak et al. 1983). Ellenbecker and colleagues also showed that female tennis players have significantly more forearm pronation strength and less supination strength on their dominant side, demonstrating a functional muscle imbalance.

Common Pathologies

There are several common chronic pain syndromes of the upper extremity. These include impingement, instability, thoracic outlet syndrome, shoulder and neck pain, and lateral elbow pain. The imbalance and chronic pain in these conditions are generally mediated by the CNS and manifested in the muscular structures; therefore, clinicians should consider a functional approach rather than a structural approach in managing these conditions.

Shoulder Impingement and Rotator Cuff Tendinosis

Shoulder impingement was first described as a clinical entity by Neer in 1972 (Neer 1972). Impingement is caused by narrowing of the SAS either due to bony growth (primary impingement) or superior migration of the humeral head caused by weakness or muscle imbalance (secondary impingement; Brossman et al. 1996; Hallström and Kärrholm 2006; Jerosch et al. 1989; Ludewig and Cook 2002). The result is inflammation or damage to the rotator cuff tendons; therefore, chronic impingement can lead to rotator cuff tendinosis. As secondary impingement is related to glenohumeral instability (Jobe 1989), it is sometimes described as *functional instability;* it occurs mostly in athletes less than 35 y of age who use overhead throwing motions (Belling Sørensen and Jørgensen 2000).

Pathomechanics of Impingement

The pathomechanics of secondary impingement may involve one or both of the shoulder force couples: the deltoid and rotator cuff or the scapular rotators. Alterations in deltoid and rotator cuff coactivation and rotator cuff imbalances are evident in patients with impingement (Burnham et al. 1993; Leroux et al. 1994; McClure, Michener, and Karduna 2006; Myers et al. 2003; Warner et al. 1990). Weakness or damage of the rotator cuff leads to an inability to control the upward shear of the humeral head into the SAS after activation of the deltoid during abduction (Jerosch et al. 1989; Weiner and Macnab 1970). Throwing athletes with shoulder pain exhibit delayed activation of the subscapularis when compared with those without pain (Hess et al. 2005). In addition, impingement is associated with deltoid weakness (Michaud et al. 1987) and atrophy and a decrease in Type II muscle fibers (Leivseth and Reikerás 1994; Kronberg and Baström 1997).

Imbalance in the scapular rotator force couple leads to weakness and altered activation of the middle and lower trapezius and serratus anterior in impingement (Cools et al. 2003, 2004, 2005; Ludewig and Cook 2000; Moraes, Faria, and Teixeria-Salmela 2008; Wadsworth and Bullock-Saxton 1997). These alterations are often seen bilaterally (Cools et al. 2003; Cools, Declercq et al. 2007; Røe et al. 2000; Wadsworth and Bullock-Saxton 1997), a finding that suggests a central mechanism of chronic tendinosis pain, consistent with Janda's theories.

Patients with impingement demonstrate altered kinematics, including less upward rotation and external rotation as well as increased anterior tilt (Borstad and Ludewig 2002; Cole, McClure, and Pratt 1996; Endo et al. 2001; Hébert et al. 2002; Ludewig and Cook 2000; Lukasiewicz et al. 1999; McClure, Michener, and Karduna 2006). The change in scapular kinematics changes the orientation of the glenoid and is thought to reduce the SAS, thus compressing the rotator cuff and biceps tendon (Brossmann et al. 1996; Flatow et al. 1994; Ludewig and Cook 2000; Solem-Bertoft, Thuomas, and Westerberg 1993); these changes also progress with age (Endo et al. 2001).

Kibler (2006) described scapular dyskinesis as a loss in scapular retraction and external rotation with altered timing and magnitude of upward scapular rotation. This leads to an anterior tilt of the glenoid and subsequent reduction in rotator cuff force.

Compared with uninjured individuals, athletes with impingement have significantly more EMG activity in the upper trapezius (74% and 94% maximum voluntary isometric contraction [MVIC], respectively) and significantly less EMG activity in the lower trapezius (56% and 48% MVIC, respectively; Cools, Declercq et al. 2007). Athletes with impingement also demonstrate trapezius muscle imbalance on both the injured and uninjured shoulders, showing upper-to-lower-trapezius (UT:LT) ratios of 1.56 to 2.19, which are significantly higher than ratios observed in uninjured controls (1.23-1.36 UT:LT).

In addition to weakness and muscle imbalance, muscle fatigue alters both glenohumeral and scapulothoracic kinematics. Rotator cuff fatigue allows the humerus to migrate superiorly by up to 0.1 in. (2.5 mm; Chen et al. 1999), while scapular fatigue leads to less posterior tilt and external rotation of the scapula (Ebaugh, McClure, and Karduna 2006a, 2006b).

Muscle tightness has also been implicated in secondary impingement. A tight pectoralis minor limits upward rotation, external rotation, and posterior tilt and reduces SAS (Borstad and Ludewig 2005). Athletes with impingement who use overhead movements often have a tight posterior capsule and decreased humeral internal rotation (Myers et al. 2006; Tyler et al. 2000).

There is some debate whether static posture plays a role in impingement. Some researchers have reported altered scapular position in patients with impingement (Burkhart, Morgan, and Kibler 2003; Kibler 1998b; Kugler et al. 1996); other researchers have shown no significant difference in scapular posture between subjects with and subjects without impingement (Greenfield et al. 1995; Hébert et al. 2002; McClure, Michener, and Karduna 2006). As discussed previously, however, a cause-and-effect relationship of posture and impingement has yet to be established. Posture should be considered as one of many factors in chronic musculoskeletal pain (Lewis, Green, and Wright 2005; Sahrmann 2002b).

The term *swimmer's shoulder* is used to describe impingement in swimmers. This condition is found in 26% to 50% of competitive swimmers (McMaster and Troup 1993; Richardson et al. 1980; Rupp, Berninger, and Hopf 1995). Muscle imbalances in the rotator cuff and scapula have been identified in swimmers with impingement (Bak and Magnusson 1997; Pink et al. 1993; Rupp, Berninger, and Hopf 1995; Ruwe et al. 1994; Scovazzo et al. 1991; Warner et al. 1990). Swimmer's shoulder also correlates with glenohumeral instability (McMaster, Roberts, and Stoddard 1998). Carson (1999) noted the value of early identification of muscle imbalances in swimmers. He described the use of rebalancing techniques in the rehabilitation of a competitive swimmer exhibiting an asymmetrical stroke with dysfunction in the contralateral hip and shoulder.

Rehabilitation of Impingement

Rehabilitation rather than surgery is recommended for secondary impingement (Brox and Brevik 1996; Kronberg, Németh, and Broström 1990; Michener, Walsworth, and Burnet 2004; Morrison, Frogameni, and Woodworth 1997). Patients with primary impingement (type II and III acromion), however, have only a 64% to 68% success rate with conservative treatment (Morrison, Frogameni, and Woodworth 1997). While rehabilitation and arthroscopic surgery improve impingement symptoms equally (Haarh et al. 2005; Haarh and Andersen 2006), rehabilitation is less costly (Brox et al. 1993).

In a systematic review, Michener, Walsworth, and Burnet and colleagues (2004) found strong support in the literature for therapeutic exercise of the rotator cuff and scapular muscles as well as for stretching of the anterior and posterior shoulder. Furthermore, exercise is more effective when combined with joint mobilization (Michener, Walsworth, and Burnet 2004; Senbursa, Baltaci, and Atay 2007). The following are impingement rehabilitation recommendations with evidence-based rationale:

- **Integrate the entire upper-extremity chain during exercise.** This facilitates the kinetic chain from the hand to the spine (Burkhart, Morgan, and Kibler 2003; Kibler 1998b, 2006; McMullen and Uhl 2000). Figure 13.5 illustrates exercises that integrate the whole kinetic chain.

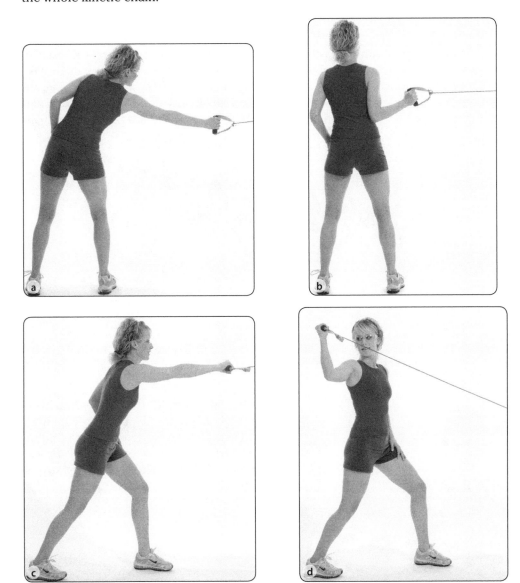

Figure 13.5 Exercises integrating the upper-extremity kinetic chain. *(a)* Exercise 1, start; *(b)* exercise 1, end; *(c)* exercise 2, start; *(d)* exercise 2, end.

- **Include hip and trunk stabilization exercises.** This facilitates force transmission and proximal stabilization between the upper extremity and the trunk (Burkhart, Morgan, and Kibler 2003; Kibler 1998b, 2006; McMullen and Uhl 2000).
- **Isolate the rotator cuff and scapular stabilizers first, before performing multijoint movements.** Performing multijoint shoulder movements does not increase the strength of smaller single-joint muscles such as the rotator cuff (Giannakopoulos et al. 2004). Strengthening exercises isolating the rotator cuff should be performed first (Jobe and Pink 1993; Malliou et al. 2004).

- **Exercise in the scapular plane.** The scapular plane offers the most balanced position of the capsule and provides ideal joint centration during elevation (Borsa, Timmons, and Sauers 2003).

- **Exercise both shoulders.** Abnormal muscle activation often occurs in both the involved and the uninvolved shoulder (Cools et al. 2003; Cools, Declercq et al. 2007; Wadsworth and Bullock-Saxton 1997).

- **Include neuromuscular exercises such as closed kinetic chain exercises and PNF.** Patients with impingement demonstrate reduced proprioception (Machner et al. 2003) and so require proprioceptive rehabilitation (Ginn and Cohen 2005; Kamkar, Irrgang, and Whitney 1993; Smith and Burnolli 1989). Figure 13.6 illustrates a closed kinetic chain shoulder exercise for improving proprioception (Naughton, Adams, and Maher 2005).

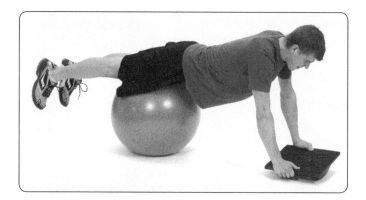

Figure 13.6   A closed kinetic chain exercise performed on a wobble board and an exercise ball.

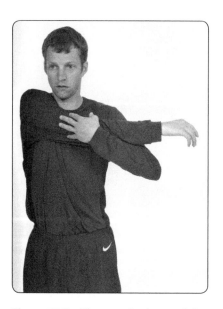

Figure 13.7   The cross-body stretch for posterior shoulder tightness.

- **Stretch the posterior shoulder when internal rotation is limited.** The posterior capsule is often tight in athletes with impingement, limiting internal rotation and follow-through (Myers et al. 2006; Tyler et al. 2000). The cross-body stretch (see figure 13.7) improves internal rotation in subjects with posterior shoulder tightness (McClure et al. 2007).

- **Balance the lower trapezius with the pectoralis minor.** Weakness of the lower trapezius is often opposed by tightness of the pectoralis minor. Mottram (1997) described an exercise that sets the scapula by cuing the lower trapezius opposite the pectoralis minor (see figure 13.8). A standing door stretch increases pectoralis minor length (see figure 13.9; Borstad and Ludewig 2006).

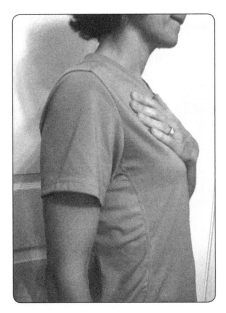

Figure 13.8 Cuing the lower trapezius against the pectoralis minor.

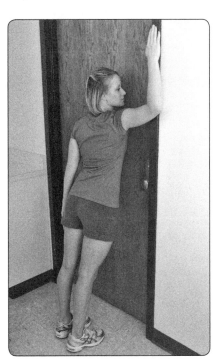

Figure 13.9 The standing door stretch for the pectoralis minor.

- **Strengthen the lower trapezius while avoiding impingement.** Traditional strengthening of the lower trapezius uses isotonic prone overhead flexion, which may contribute to impingement. Exercises with elastic resistance (figure 13.10) can activate the lower trapezius in a position free of impingement (McCabe et al. 2001).

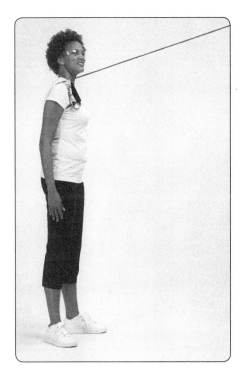

Figure 13.10 Lower trapezius facilitation and strengthening.

- **Use scapular and proprioceptive taping.** Several impingement studies have found shoulder taping to be effective (Lewis, Green, and Wright 2005; Page and Stewart 1999; Schmitt and Snyder-Mackler 1999; Selkowitz et al. 2007; Wang et al. 2005). Figure 13.11 illustrates kinesio taping that inhibits the upper trapezius and facilitates the lower trapezius.

- **Use the full can rather than the empty can exercise.** The full can exercise is effective for supraspinatus activation (Takeda et al. 2002), while the empty can exercise reduces the SAS and alters scapular kinematics more than the full can does (see figure 13.12; Thigpen et al. 2006).

- **Include exercises for scapular depression.** Shoulder depression can increase the SAS (Hinterwimmer et al. 2003). The shoulder sling exercise facilitates shoulder depression and abduction (figure 13.13).

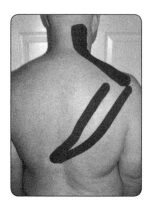

Figure 13.11 Kinesio taping for shoulder impingement imbalance.

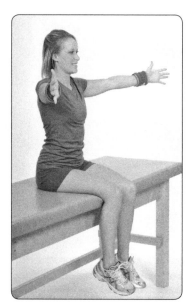

Figure 13.12 The full can exercise.

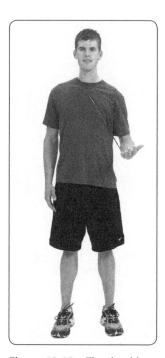

Figure 13.13 The shoulder sling exercise.

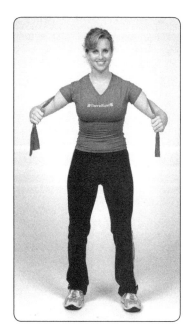

Figure 13.14 The dynamic hug exercise.

- **Incorporate oscillation exercise for muscle balance.** Oscillation exercise with a Flexbar (see figure 11.14 on page 169) activates phasic upper-extremity muscles more than it activates tonic upper-extremity muscles (Page et al. 2004).

- **Include biceps and deltoid exercises.** The biceps and deltoid are important secondary stabilizers (Itoi et al. 1994; Kido et al. 2003; Lee and An 2002), and the deltoid is often atrophied and weak (Kronberg, Larsson, and Broström 1997; Leivseth and Reikerás 1994).

- **Strengthen the serratus anterior.** The dynamic hug exercise (figure 13.14) is more effective than the serratus punch in activating the serratus anterior (Decker et al. 1999).

• **Incorporate exercises that balance the upper and lower trapezius.** Cools and coworkers (2007) recommended four exercises with favorable UT:LT ratios: side-lying external rotation (figure 13.15), side-lying forward flexion (figure 13.16), prone horizontal abduction with external rotation (figure 13.17), and prone extension (figure 13.18).

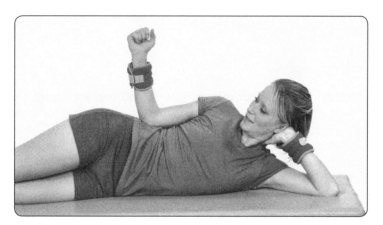

Figure 13.15 External rotation in the side-lying position.

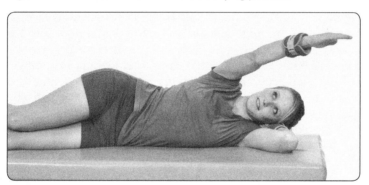

Figure 13.16 Forward flexion in the side-lying position.

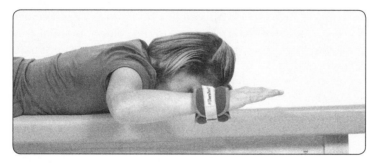

Figure 13.17 Prone horizontal abduction with external rotation.

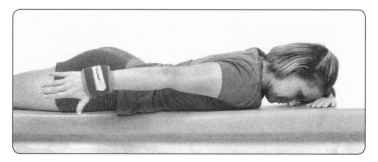

Figure 13.18 Prone extension.

- **Include the push-up plus.** Additional protraction at the end of a traditional push-up not only activates the serratus but also has a favorable ratio of upper trapezius and serratus anterior activation (Ludewig et al. 2004).

- **Progress to plyometrics in athletes who use overhead movements.** Plyometric training performed by tossing weighted balls can significantly improve the ER:IR ratio in baseball pitchers (Carter et al. 2007).

Shoulder Instability

Shoulder instability can result from a number of factors, including altered glenoid position or hypoplasia, humeral retroversion, and rotator cuff weakness (Saha 1971). Glenohumeral instability is classified by the direction of instability. The most common directions are anterior and inferior; instability in these directions is often due to capsular deficiency in the inferior glenohumeral ligament. Multidirectional instability describes a more global instability of the glenohumeral capsule, one that involves multiple planes.

Instability is classified as either traumatic or atraumatic in origin. Traumatic instability generally involves unilateral dislocation in one direction (usually anterior and inferior) and usually requires reconstructive surgery. Atraumatic instability is often multidirectional, evident in both shoulders, and treated conservatively with rehabilitation.

As discussed earlier, impingement is related to instability. The term *functional instability* (activity-related symptoms with or without clinically detectable laxity) is often used to describe the phenomenon of instability leading to impingement (Belling Sørensen and Jørgensen 2000). Mild instability increases the demands on the rotator cuff for stabilization, causing fatigue, anterior subluxation, and subsequent impingement (Belling Sørensen and Jørgensen 2000). Functional instabilities can occur in other joints (such as the ankle) and are related to sensorimotor dysfunction. Regardless of the joint, functional instabilities often exhibit altered muscle activation patterns and muscle imbalances in strength and flexibility.

As stated previously, the glenohumeral joint provides important proprioceptive information to the surrounding muscles that provide dynamic stability (Guanche et al. 1995). Persons with a traumatic shoulder dislocation often have decreased proprioception (Smith and Brunolli 1990), which is restored after reconstructive surgery (Lephart et al. 1994; Pötzl et al. 2004). Damage to the glenohumeral ligaments disrupts the capsular mechanoreceptors, thus reducing feedback to the dynamic stabilizing muscles (Jerosch et al. 1993).

The rotator cuff provides primary dynamic stabilization (Apreleva et al. 1998; Culham and Peat 1993; Lee et al. 2000; Saha 1971; Werner, Favre, and Gerber 2007; Wuelker et al. 1994; Xue and Huang 1998), while the biceps (Kim et al. 2001; Itoi et al. 1994) and deltoid (Kido et al. 2003; Lee and An 2002) provide secondary stabilization. Any imbalance in strength or activation of the dynamic stabilizers can contribute to functional instability (Barden et al. 2005; Belling Sørensen and Jørgensen 2000; Wuelker, Korell, and Thren 1998). For example, weakness of the infraspinatus decreases the compressive forces of the rotator cuff, while tightness of the pectoralis major increases anterior shear forces, promoting anterior instability (Labriola et al. 2005).

Several researchers have demonstrated altered muscle activation patterns in patients with shoulder instability (Illyés and Kiss 2006, 2007; Kim et al. 2001; Kronberg, Broström, and Németh 1991; Kronberg and Broström 1995; McMahon et al. 1996; Morris, Kemp, and Frostick 2004). In general, activation of the serratus anterior, deltoid, and supraspinatus is decreased, while biceps activation is sometimes increased. Scapular kinematics are also altered in patients with instability in patterns similar to those with impingement: decreased posterior tilt and decreased upward rotation (von Eisenhart-Rothe et al. 2005; Matias and Pascoal 2006; Ogston and Ludewig 2007). Scapular position is highly correlated with centering of the humeral head on the glenoid (von Eisenhart-Rothe et al. 2005), a finding that highlights the important role dynamic scapular stabilization plays in instability.

Athletes who perform overhead movements are particularly vulnerable to functional instability. Swimmers with instability often have impingement, a condition otherwise known as *swimmer's shoulder* (Bak and Faunø 1997; Rupp, Berninger, and Hopf 1995). Throwing athletes with shoulder instability demonstrate altered EMG patterns during throwing, including increased activity in the biceps and supraspinatus and decreased activity in the internal rotators and serratus anterior in order to avoid anterior instability (Glousman et al. 1988).

There is some debate about the relationship between the shoulder capsule and imbalances in shoulder ROM. Glenohumeral instability has been associated with imbalances in ROM, most notably an increase in external rotation and a decrease in internal rotation (Warner et al. 1990). Excessive external rotation (Mihata et al. 2004) or a tight posterior capsule (Lin, Lim, and Yang 2006; Tyler et al. 1999), commonly seen in athletes performing overhead movements, is thought to increase anterior and inferior translation of the humerus, thus leading to instability. Recently, however, Borsa and colleagues (2005) suggested that capsular length is not associated with the characteristic imbalance of increased external rotation and decreased internal rotation found in baseball pitchers. They discovered that pitchers have significantly more posterior translation of the glenohumeral joint in both shoulders when compared with anterior translation, a finding that suggests laxity rather than tightness of the posterior capsule. It is possible, therefore, that the lack of internal rotation seen in pitchers is related to muscular tightness rather than capsular tightness.

The principles of rehabilitation for instability are very similar to those of rehabilitation for impingement, which were discussed earlier. Strengthening exercises for the scapula and rotator cuff can improve functional instability and reduce the recurrence of shoulder dislocation (Aronen and Regan 1984; Burkhead and Rockwood 1992; Ide et al. 2003). Closed kinetic chain exercises are also beneficial for shoulder instability (Naughton, Adams, and Maher 2005).

Shoulder and Neck Pain

Shoulder and neck pain (described as *cervicobrachial pain syndrome* or *trapezius myalgia*) is characterized by muscular pain in the upper trapezius and levator scapulae. It is often related to repetitive overhead work activities and prolonged postures and is most often observed in females. Novak (2004) noted that work-related upper-extremity pain syndromes are characterized by muscle imbalances similar to those described in Janda's classification.

The ratio of UT:LT EMG activation may be useful in quantifying shoulder and neck pain; the normal ratio is 1:1 (Cram and Kasman 1998). Patients with shoulder and neck pain often have elevated UT:LT ratios due to an overactive upper trapezius. Menachem, Kaplan, and Dekel (1993) described pain over the upper medial angle of the scapula that radiates into the neck and shoulder in females. Of these patients with levator scapulae syndrome, 60% had normal radiographs and notable warmth in the area that was possibly related to inflammation of a bursa (Menachem, Kaplan, and Dekel 1993).

Larsson and colleagues (1998) reported significantly lower microcirculation on the painful upper trapezius of patients with shoulder and neck pain. Patients with work-related shoulder and neck pain also have altered EMG patterns (Larsson et al. 1998; Madeleine et al. 1999; Schulte et al. 2006; Szeto, Straker, and O'Sullivan 2005; Voerman, Vollenbroek-Hutten, and Hermens 2007; Westgaard, Vasseljen, and Holte 2001) that sometimes precede pain (Szeto, Straker, and O'Sullivan 2005). The EMG patterns of the upper trapezius in patients with shoulder and neck pain are similar to those in patients with other types of chronic neck and shoulder pain (Voerman, Vollenbroek-Hutten, and Hermens 2007), suggesting similar neuromuscular dysfunction. Schulte and colleagues (2006) reported decreased activity of the biceps in subjects with work-related pain of the upper trapezius, a finding that indicates change in the central control strategies. Experimental pain created by injecting the upper trapezius reduced EMG activity of the upper trapezius and increased EMG activity of the lower extremity, demonstrating a CNS response from local nociceptive afferents to reorganize and coordinate activation of the trapezius (Falla, Farina, and Graven-Nielsen 2007).

Patients with shoulder and neck pain also demonstrate altered processing of the somatosensory system. They have increased pain pressure thresholds (PPT) and decreased sensitivity to light touch when compared with patients without pain (Leffler, Hansson, and Kosek 2003). While the source of the pain is structural, clinicians must remember to treat the cause of pain functionally through the sensorimotor system.

Exercise programs including stretching and strengthening of muscle imbalances can be beneficial to shoulder and neck pain (Ahlgren et al. 2001; Randlov et al. 1998; Vasseljen et al. 1995; Waling et al. 2000), although the long-term benefits are questionable (Waling et al. 2002). Work-related muscle imbalance syndromes require workplace and ergonomic modifications as well as specific exercises to correct the imbalances (Novak 2004). Biofeedback training may decrease overactivation of the upper trapezius in patients with shoulder and neck pain (Madeleine et al. 2006). Six weeks of inhibitory taping of the upper trapezius combined with strengthening of the lower trapezius can improve the UT:LT ratio (Wang et al. 2005).

Thoracic Outlet Syndrome

Thoracic outlet syndrome (TOS) is characterized by compression of the neurovascular structures between the neck and the shoulder—specifically, between the scalenes and the first rib or between the pectoralis minor and the coracoid process. Symptoms include paresthesia, numbness, and pain in the upper extremity. Obviously, muscle tightness and imbalance play a role in TOS.

Poor posture and repetitive overhead work may contribute to TOS (Mackinnon 1994). Abnormal posture and compensated work patterns cause an imbalance in muscle tightness and weakness in the upper back, neck, and shoulder, contributing to increased mechanical pressure around the nerves (Mackinnon, Patterson, and Novak 1996; Novak, Collins, and Mackinnon 1995).

Hajek and colleagues (1978) described the postural deviations resulting from muscle imbalance in TOS. Tightness of the SCM leads to a forward head position; tightness of the upper trapezius and levator scapulae causes elevation and protraction of the shoulder girdle, along with altered movement patterns. Tightness of the pectoralis minor and major also contributes to shoulder protraction. The authors recommended stretching tight muscles with the assumption that the phasic muscles would easily recover their strength.

Novak, Collins, and Mackinnon (1995) reported improvement in 60% of patients with TOS at 1 y following a program that included patient education, activity modification, postural correction, and therapeutic exercise. Exercises included stretching for the upper trapezius, levator scapulae, scalene, SCM, and suboccipitals. Strengthening exercises were performed for the middle and lower trapezius and serratus anterior. Interestingly, these are the same muscles that Janda identified as being prone to tightness and weakness, respectively.

Lateral Epicondylalgia

Lateral epicondylalgia (LE) is better known as *tennis elbow* and is a common cause of elbow pain. Lateral pain is more common than medial pain (Pienimäki, Siira, and Vanharanta 2002). Recently, tennis elbow was classified as a tendinosis or tendinopathy rather than a tendinitis because of its chronicity (Nirschl and Ashman 2003; Stasinopoulos and Johnson 2006). The term *tendinitis* refers to an acute inflammation of the tendon, while *tendinosis* refers to chronic inflammation, typically due to overuse.

The pathomechanics of LE seem to be related to the proximal tendons of the extensor carpi radialis (ECR) and extensor digitorum (ED). Anatomical studies have shown that the ECR is subject to increased stress, particularly with wrist activities involving power (Briggs and Elliott 1985). Dynamic analysis with EMG has shown increased acti-

vation of the ECR and ED in patients with LE compared with patients without LE (Bauer and Murray 1999; Finsen et al. 2005; Morris et al. 1989). More recently, however, other authors have noted decreased EMG activity in the ECR (Alizadehkhaiyat et al. 2007; Rojas et al. 2007). The supinator muscle may also play a role in lateral elbow pain (Erak et al. 2004); therefore, clinicians should rule out radial tunnel syndrome when evaluating a patient with LE.

These biomechanical findings suggest an imbalance of the wrist extensors and flexors in the pathology of LE. Muscular imbalance is not confined to the elbow; in fact, imbalance has been demonstrated in the entire upper extremity (Alizadehakhaiyat et al. 2007). As shown with other chronic muscle imbalance syndromes (such as chronic neck pain and FM described in chapter 12), patients with chronic LE exhibit lowered PPT and larger referred pain patterns compared to control subjects' TrPs (Fernández-Carnero et al. 2007); these observations suggest central sensitization of pain. Thus chronic lateral elbow pain in some patients may be mediated by the CNS and may require focus on muscle balance rather than the traditional focus on the pain itself. This is perhaps why systematic reviews and meta-analyses of clinical trials in LE often report a lack of evidence to support treatments other than exercise (Bisset et al. 2005).

Because LE is a tendinosis, anti-inflammatory medication may not be as effective as controlled exercise (Kraushaar and Nirschl 1999). In particular, resistive exercise is an important component in rehabilitation. Therapeutic putty shows the highest EMG levels of the extensor carpi radialis brevis when compared with two other hand exercises (Landis et al. 2005). A novel exercise using a Flexbar (see figure 13.19) may be effective at managing tennis elbow. The exercise focuses on eccentrically loading the wrist extensors, which is thought to be more effective than concentric exercises for tendinosis (Woodley, Newsham-West, and Baxter 2007). The patient begins the exercise by grasping the Flexbar with both wrists extended. The

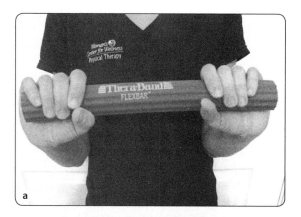

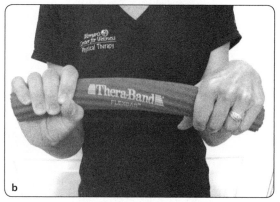

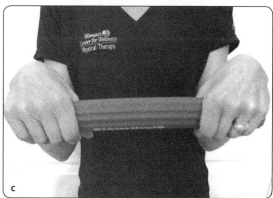

Figure 13.19 Eccentric elbow exercise with the Flexbar.

unaffected wrist then flexes to rotate the Flexbar while the affected wrist remains extended. The patient then slowly flexes the affected wrist against the resistance of the Flexbar, creating an eccentric contraction of the wrist extensors.

Tendon rehabilitation should involve balancing opposing muscle groups (such as the wrist flexors and extensors) as well as the entire kinetic chain of the shoulder (Kibler et al. 1992). Clinicians must consider continued strengthening of the entire upper kinetic chain, even after the patient's elbow pain has subsided. Residual weakness of the entire upper extremity has been demonstrated after recovery from LE (Alizadehkhaiyat et al. 2008); therefore, emphasis should be placed on strengthening the rotator cuff and scapular stabilizers during and after recovery.

Poor body mechanics may also play a role in LE. In a study of tennis players, Kelley and coworkers (1994) reported greater EMG levels of the wrist extensors and pronator teres during ball impact and early follow-through as well as poor mechanics during backhand strokes. Simply instructing tennis players to use a double-hand backstroke may reduce the incidence and severity of their LE (Giangarra et al. 1993).

Elbow braces and taping have shown some reduction of pain (Ng and Chan 2004; Struijs et al. 2004, 2006; Vicenzino et al. 2003). These interventions may affect proprioception through stimulation of the skin. Recently, a wrist brace applying external wrist extension was shown to reduce the elevated EMG levels of wrist extensors during grip by patients with tennis elbow (Faes et al. 2006).

Case Study

A right-handed male baseball pitcher aged 17 y was diagnosed with right shoulder tendinitis. Pain began 2 wk earlier, when he pitched a game and threw 150 pitches; he developed right posterior shoulder pain after the game. He rated the pain in his right posterior shoulder 7 out of 10, but pain occurred only during throwing. He experienced the pain just before ball release and not during deceleration. He denied any cervical or elbow pain. He didn't have any night pain, and the pain did not fluctuate. He denied any significant medical history or previous shoulder, elbow, back, or leg injuries.

Examination and Assessment

On examination, he demonstrated right shoulder depression, mild to moderate bilateral scapular winging, and a right scapula that was protracted +1.2 in. (+3 cm) when compared with the left. He demonstrated prominent bilateral acromioclavicular joints. He had decreased spinal curves and no evidence of scoliosis. On visual inspection, he appeared to have normal arthrokinematics. He had tenderness over his right posterior rotator cuff, just inferior to the angle of the acromion.

He had full active ROM that was pain free and equal bilaterally with the exception of internal rotation at 90°, 55° versus the left internal rotation, 80° (25° deficit on right). Horizontal adduction was also reduced on the right, 35° versus 55° on the left. He demonstrated increased external rotation at 90° bilaterally. He had a –3.5 in. (–9 cm) difference on right internal rotation with Apley's scratch test.

He demonstrated full, pain-free MMT throughout the shoulder and scapular stabilizers with the exception of some pain occurring with resisted internal and external rotation at a 90°/90° position. Serratus strength appeared normal during the push-up. Isokinetic testing revealed smooth curves for internal and external rotation. He demonstrated a 13% deficit for external rotation and an 8% deficit for internal rotation. His ER:IR ratio was 54%. He demonstrated moderate weakness (5/10) of his lower abdominal muscles; otherwise, his trunk strength was within normal limits (WNL). He had mildly decreased bilateral hamstring length.

All special tests for the shoulder were unremarkable for the rotator cuff, impingement, labrum, and biceps. He did report right posterior shoulder pain in the apprehension position, which was relieved with relocation or horizontal adduction into the scapular plane. He also had right posterior shoulder pain with a posterior humeral glide. He had some pain and tightness of the posterior capsule with overpressure.

It was postulated that the athlete had a tight posterior capsule that may have caused the humeral head to migrate anteriorly, thus stressing the anterior capsule. Subsequently, the posterior rotator cuff had to stabilize the anterior translation more than usual during the pitcher's prolonged outing. This led to an overuse tendinitis of the posterior rotator cuff.

Treatment and Outcome

A 4 wk treatment plan was initiated. It included the following three components:

1. A home exercise program of Thera-Band resistance exercises for the rotator cuff and scapular stabilizers, stretching for the right shoulder posterior capsule and hamstrings, and strengthening exercises for the lower abdominal muscles

2. Three sessions of physical therapy for posterior capsule mobilization, scapular and rotator cuff strengthening, shoulder stretching, dynamic stabilization activities, plyometrics, isokinetic strengthening, and trunk strengthening

3. An interval throwing program with progression to the mound

In 4 wk, the athlete returned to throwing at 100% without pain. He continued the stretching and Thera-Band routine as a daily maintenance program. Impingement in athletes who rely on overhead movement is common because of the demands placed on the shoulder during functional activities. Posterior capsular tightness must be addressed in addition to scapular stabilizer strength and dynamic rotator cuff strength.

Janda's Approach Versus the Traditional Approach

This case demonstrates the importance of understanding a functional approach to shoulder pain. The traditional structural signs of primary SA impingement were not apparent in the evaluation; however, signs of shoulder instability and muscle imbalance were apparent. While no apparent signs of UCS were present in this athlete, there were some initial signs of pelvic dysfunction, including weakness of the lower abdominal muscles and tight abdominal muscles, which are possible precursors to LCS. By evaluating the entire kinetic chain, the trunk, and the lower extremities of a patient with a shoulder complaint, clinicians may find dysfunction elsewhere in the system; however, it is impossible to determine which came first in this case. A simple, focused exercise program targeting both the shoulder and the pelvis helped this athlete quickly return to baseball. Ruling out structural causes of shoulder impingement helps clinicians develop appropriate treatment of functional pathology for a quick return to activity.

Summary

The shoulder demonstrates an intricate balance of structure and function. By understanding the functional pathology of shoulder dysfunction, clinicians can perform an appropriate assessment and can initiate effective interventions. Several evidence-based exercises are effective in functional shoulder rehabilitation. Other upper-extremity syndromes, including shoulder instability, TOS, and LE, can be assessed and treated quickly once a functional pathology has been identified.

LUMBAR PAIN SYNDROMES

Management of low back pain remains a challenge due to a lack of specific diagnosis and a lack of consensus on its proper management among the various health professions. Back injury can begin with damage to one tissue, which may then alter the biomechanical function of the joint. Damage to tissue in the low back may have a cascading effect on other tissues, leading to pain as well as intolerance of certain activities. Nevertheless, there is increasing evidence that trunk muscle function plays an important role in the management of patients with low back pain. Impairments of trunk muscle function may compromise the structural integrity of the spinal complex, lending it susceptible to further injury, prolonged recovery, or chronicity of pain. Management of low back pain requires a better understanding of the sensorimotor control mechanisms utilized for trunk stabilization and postural control (Ebenbichler et al. 2001; Radebold et al 2001).

This chapter begins by reviewing key anatomical structures and their functional interdependence. Understanding this functional interdependence lays the foundation for a deeper appreciation of the complexities involved in the management of chronic low back pain. This chapter discusses the role that muscle imbalances, postural control, and altered CNS pain processing play in lumbar pain syndromes. Assessment and management strategies using Janda's global approach to the sensorimotor system are presented and then illustrated by a case study.

Regional Considerations

The spine is stabilized by bone, discs, ligaments, and muscle restraints; this stabilization system maintains the spine in a neutral zone within the physiological threshold to avoid functional instability (Panjabi 1992b). The spine is affected by reactive forces placed on it through the multisegmental nature of muscle contraction that is necessary for spinal stability. It has been shown that in the absence of muscle contraction, the lumbar spine buckles under compressive loads of as little as 4.5 lb (2 kg; Morris, Lucas, and Bresler 1961). Significant microtrauma of the lumbar spine can occur with rotation of as little as 2°, indicating the importance of neuromuscular control of the spine (Gracovetsky, Farfan, and Helleur 1985). Mounting evidence points to the vital functional contribution of the various trunk muscles to postural stability (Cholewicki and McGill 1995; Gardner-Morse and Stokes 1998; McGill 2002; Hodges and Richardson 1996, 1997b; 1998; O'Sullivan et al. 1997). Subsequently, specific training regimens addressing the functional recovery of these various trunk muscle groups have been developed (McGill 1998; Cordo and Nashner 1982; Grenier and McGill 2007; Janda et al. 2007; Bullock-Saxton, Janda, and Bullock 1993; Richardson and Jull 1993; Richardson, Hodges, and Hides 2004; O'Sullivan 2005; Sterling, Jull, and Wright 2001; Sahrmann 2001; Radebold et al. 2001; Kolar 2007, 1999).

Sensorimotor control of spinal stability ensures the precise interaction of all the muscles of the trunk. The following sections summarize the key muscle groups that contribute to spinal stability.

Paravertebral Muscle Group

From a functional perspective, the paravertebral muscles are subdivided into two groups: (1) the short, deep muscles of the spine that span one or few segments, such as the rotatores, intertransversarii, multifidus, and interspinales (see figure 14.1), and (2) the long erector spinae that span multiple segments (see figure 14.2). Traditionally, it was believed that the rotators and intertransversarii, collectively known as the deep rotators of the spine, create axial twisting torque for rotation of the spine. However, these muscles are rich in muscle spindles (Nitz and Peck 1986) and have been shown to function as position sensors or transducers at every joint in the thoracic and lumbar spine. (McGill 2002). The rotator muscles produce no EMG during isometric rotation of the spine in either direction. However, significant EMG activity is recorded when spinal rotation changes direction. There is strong evidence that these deep muscles of the back function as position sensors in the spinal proprioception system rather than as torque generators; hence, they play an important role in the control of posture.

Contraction of the long erector spinae muscles balances the opposing activity of the abdominal muscles. The line of action of these long multisegmental muscles produces a large extensor moment while placing a minimum of compressive forces on the spine. In addition, the lumbar sections of the longissimus and iliocostalis muscles produce

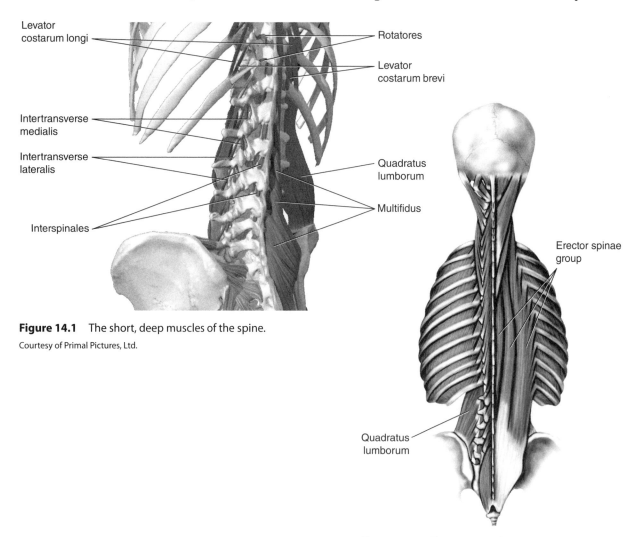

Figure 14.1 The short, deep muscles of the spine.

Courtesy of Primal Pictures, Ltd.

Figure 14.2 The erector spinae.

Reprinted from R.S. Behnke, *Kinetic anatomy*, 2nd ed. (Champaign, IL: Human Kinetics), 134.

large posterior shear forces to counter the anterior shear forces generated when the upper body is flexed forward as in lifting. However, these muscles lose their oblique line of action with lumbar flexion, so that a flexed spine is vulnerable to damaging shear forces. Thus fully flexing the spine during exercise or assuming a posterior pelvic tilt during flexion movements disables these posterior shear protectors and should not be recommended to patients (McGill 1998, 2002; McGill, Hughson, and Parks 2000).

Abdominal Muscles

The abdominal fascia contains the rectus abdominis and connects laterally to the aponeurosis of the external obliques, internal obliques, and TrA (see figure 14.3). The rectus abdominis has been shown to be the major trunk flexor and is most active during sit-ups and curl-ups (Juker et al. 1998). In addition to contributing to trunk flexion, the obliques are involved in spinal rotation and lateral flexion (McGill 1991, 1992). They appear to play an important role in lumbar stabilization when the spine is placed under pure axial compression (McGill 1991, 1992, 1996, 1998; McGill, Hughson, and Parks 2000, 2002). The obliques have also been shown to be involved in challenged lung ventilation, assisting in active expiration (Henke et al. 1998). The obliques and rectus abdominis demonstrate direction-specific activation patterns with respect to limb movements, providing postural support before actual limb movement begins (Hodges and Richardson 1997, 1999). The close interlinking of these muscles contributes to the control of trunk stability and movements of the spine.

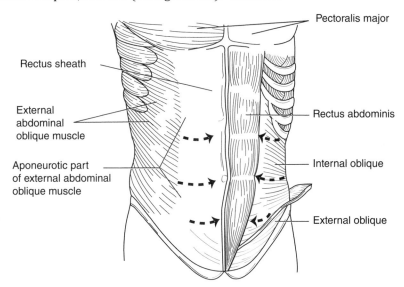

Figure 14.3 The abdominal fascia contains the rectus abdominis and connects laterally to the aponeurosis of the external obliques, internal obliques, and TrA.

Reprinted, by permission, from S. McGill, 2002, *Low back disorders* (Champaign: Human Kinetics), 69.

Hodges and Richardson (1997b) have shown that postural activation of the TrA occurs independently of the direction of limb movements. It has been proposed that the TrA plays a functional stabilization role different from that of the rectus abdominis and oblique abdominal muscles. As a result, training the TrA forms a cornerstone of many stabilization programs. However, its central focus in treatment programs is debatable. Grenier and McGill (2007) demonstrated little mechanical rationale for low-load exercise programs for the TrA. Kavcic, Grenier, and McGill (2004) found that no single trunk muscle played a dominant role in spinal stability, as the roles of individual muscles changed across tasks. Contraction of the entire abdominal wall has been hypothesized to enhance spinal stabilization through the production of hooplike forces around a rigid cylinder in the abdominal cavity (see figure 14.4). These hooplike forces increase stiffness of the lumbar spine and hence stability of the spine (Porterfield and DeRosa 1998).

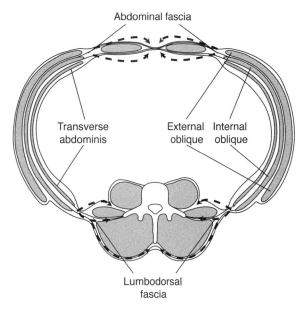

Figure 14.4 Hooplike forces around a rigid cylinder in the abdominal cavity.

Reprinted, by permission, from S. McGill, 2002, *Low back disorders* (Champaign: Human Kinetics), 81.

Intra-Abdominal Pressure

There is increasing evidence that an increase in intra-abdominal pressure (IAP) contributes to spinal stability. Contraction of the abdominal muscles, pelvic floor, and diaphragm correlate closely with increased IAP in a variety of postural tasks. (Cresswell, Grundström, and Thorstensson 1994; Hodges and Richardson 1997, 1999; Hodges, Martin Eriksson, Shirley, and Gandevia 2006; Hodges, Sapsford, and Pengel 2007; McGill and Norman 1994; Ebenbichler et al. 2001). While it is well accepted that the diaphragm is the primary muscle of inspiration, several researchers have hypothesized that it is also involved in the postural control of the trunk (Cresswell, Grundström, and Thorstensson 1994; Hodges and Richardson 1999; Hodges and Gandevia 2000; Hodges, Martin Eriksson, Shirley, and Gandevia 2006). Contraction of the diaphragm increases IAP by taking advantage of the hooplike geometry of the abdominal muscles and precedes initiation of limb movement (Hodges 1999). This contraction of the diaphragm occurs simultaneously with activation of the TrA (Hodges 1999) and independently of phase of respiration. In addition, the pelvic floor muscles help control IAP and stiffness of the lumbopelvic region (Hodges 2007). Furthermore, as IAP is modulated during respiration, it is likely to be accompanied by changes in pelvic floor activity.

Reflexive activation of the lumbopelvic musculature plays an important role in dynamic stability and function of the spine (Hodges 1996, 1997; Janda 1978, Janda et al. 2007; Jull and Janda 1987). The ability of the intrinsic spinal muscles in this region to provide sufficient spinal stiffness in coordination with IAP contributes to the dynamic stability of the spine. Researchers have demonstrated an impaired feed-forward mechanism (a delayed onset of TrA activation) in anticipation of extremity movement in patients with chronic low back pain (Hodges 1997, 1999, 1998). Additionally, multifidus atrophy has been shown to occur soon after acute episodes of low back pain despite early symptom reduction or resolution (Hides, Richardson, and Jull 1994).

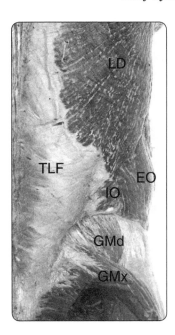

Figure 14.5 The thoracolumbar fascia, TrA, internal oblique, and latissimus dorsi.

Thoracolumbar Fascia

The thoracolumbar fascia is a very strong tissue with a well-developed lattice of collagen fibers. It covers the deep muscles of the back and trunk. The bony attachments of the fascia span from the spinous processes of the lumbar spine to the PSIS. The TrA and internal oblique muscles are intertwined with the posterior fascia, in the same way the latissimus dorsi is intertwined with the thoracolumbar fascia, forming part of the hoop around the abdomen (see figure 14.5). Contraction of these muscles contributes to the stiffening and stabilization of the lumbar spine via the thoracolumbar fascia (Porterfield and DeRosa 1998; Ebenbichler et al. 2001; McGill 2002).

Common Pathologies

Low back pain is often a vague and nonspecific diagnosis. While chronic low back pain may have several etiologies, clinicians should be aware of several neuromuscular pathologies found in low back pain syndromes that may provide clues about the specific etiology. These neuromuscular factors include muscle imbalance, poor postural control, minimal brain dysfunction, and SI joint dysfunction.

Muscle Imbalances in Low Back Pain

Chronic low back pain is often associated with imbalances in hip muscle length, strength, and endurance rather than with structural factors (Nourbaksh and Arab 2002). Imbalances in hip ROM have also been implicated in low back pain (Ellison, Rose, and Sahrmann 1990; van Dillen et al. 2000). Janda first noted weakness of the gluteal muscles in patients with low back pain (1964). Subsequent studies by Nadler and colleagues (2000, 2001) confirmed the association of hip extensor weakness and low back pain in female athletes; interestingly, however, the researchers did not find such an association in male athletes. Nadler (2002) also reported hip abductor weakness as a factor in low back pain in female athletes.

Postural Control and Chronic Low Back Pain

Precise control of posture and balance is essential for ADL and higher levels of physical activity as well as for the prevention of musculoskeletal injuries. Afferent input from the visual, vestibular, and proprioceptive systems is channeled into the CNS, resulting in motor output. External perturbations trigger APRs that are necessary to maintain equilibrium. These postural responses are specific to the magnitude, type, and direction of the perturbation and include responses that merely stiffen the trunk for stabilization and responses that are needed to restore equilibrium, particularly when the COG moves outside of the BOS.

Several researchers have demonstrated that patients with chronic low back pain have poor postural control (Byl and Sinnot 1991; Luoto et al. 1998; Radebold et al. 2001). This finding suggests a sensorimotor dysfunction in these patients. Byl and Sinnot (1991) found that patients with chronic low back pain use the hip strategy rather than the normal ankle strategy when they have their eyes closed. These patients also exhibit delayed or altered reaction times of the trunk and pelvic muscles (Luoto et al. 1998; Radebold et al. 2000; Wilder et al. 1996; Hodges 1996, 1997; Bullock-Saxton, Janda, and Bullock 1993; Hungerford, Gilleard, and Hodges 2003; Richardson and Hodges 1996). Postural control was found to be significantly worse in patients with lumbar discectomy than in subjects without discectomy when their eyes were closed but not when their eyes were open (Bouche et al. 2006). The authors postulated that patients with lumbar discectomy who experience pain develop visual compensations for sensorimotor deficits.

Minimal Brain Dysfunction in Low Back Pain

Patients with idiopathic chronic low back pain exhibit altered pain processing throughout their body (Giesecke et al. 2004; Giesbrecht and Battié 2005). Janda's neurological paradigm was further strengthened by his findings of minimal brain dysfunction in patients with chronic low back pain (Janda 1978). He found a lack of coordinated behavior in all areas of function, including psychological (intellectual and stress adaptation) as well as neuromuscular (motor and sensory deficits) dysfunction. He concluded that the minimal brain dysfunction symptoms found in 80% of patients with chronic low back pain supported the theory of an organic CNS lesion with maladaptation of the system as a functional pathology (Janda 1978). Thus he supported a biopsychosocial approach to low back pain.

Sacroiliac Dysfunction

Vleeming and colleagues (1995) noted that the gluteus maximus and contralateral latissimus dorsi provide a perpendicular force to stabilize the SI joint. When stimulated, the SI joint activates the gluteus maximus, quadratus lumborum, and multifidus (Holm, Inhahl, and Solomonow 2001). Hence, the SI joint provides lumbopelvic stabilization for locomotion and posture. Changes in the loading of the SI joint may alter the activation of stabilizing muscles. Contraction of the TrA has been shown to increase SI joint stability (Richardson et al. 2002). Preactivation of the multifidus and internal oblique muscles contributes to compression of the SI joint necessary for lumbopelvic stabilization during load transfer from double- to single-leg stance (Hungerford, Gilleard, and Hodges 2003).

In his 1964 thesis, Janda (1964) reported that the gluteal muscles are inhibited in patients with SI joint dysfunction, even in the absence of pain. Janda noted that patients with SI joint dysfunction have concurrent spasms of the iliacus, piriformis, and quadratus lumborum and inhibition of the gluteus maximus on the blocked side. They also demonstrate inhibition of the gluteus medius on the contralateral side. Patients with SI joint dysfunction also display an increased shift of the pelvis toward the nonblocked side during stance.

Janda suggested that spasm of the piriformis pulls on the sacrotuberous ligament, causing SI joint pain. Piriformis spasm is also related to hamstring tightness due to the insertion of the long head of the biceps femoris on the sacrotuberous ligament. Inhibition of the gluteus maximus and medius is sometimes seen on the contralateral side, as is tightness of the lower rectus abdominis.

Patients with SI joint pain have different motor control strategies compared with controls. Hungerford, Gilleard, and Hodges (2003) reported that in patients with SI joint pain who assumed a single-leg stance, the internal obliques, multifidus, and gluteus maximus were significantly delayed on the symptomatic side, while the biceps femoris was activated significantly sooner. Furthermore, the onset of EMG activity differed between the painful and nonpainful sides. The authors postulated that the delayed activation of the internal obliques and multifidus altered the feed-forward strategy and thus diminished their effectiveness in stabilizing the lumbopelvic region. Additionally, the early onset of biceps femoris activation may have compensated for a delay in the gluteus maximus for hip extension or for augmenting force closure across the SI joint via the sacrotuberous ligament and posterior thoracolumbar fascia. Page and Stewart (2000) found hamstring muscle imbalances in patients with SI joint pain, noting weaker hamstring muscles on the anteriorly rotated side.

Assessment

Chronic low back pain affects the entire sensorimotor system. The assessment of patients with chronic low back pain includes the upper quarter and lower quarter. Careful analysis of posture, balance, movement patterns, muscle length, and muscle strength as well as manual assessment follows the procedures detailed in chapters 5 through 8.

Posture

The patient should disrobe as much as possible so that the clinician can visualize the body from head to toe. The clinician should perform a systematic assessment of posture (see chapter 5). Table 14.1 provides key observations in patients with lumbar dysfunction. Each key observation suggests a possible indication and helps to provide a picture of the root of dysfunction. Patients with LCS often exhibit one of two types of posture (see chapter 4). LCS type A posture (figure 4.3b) is characterized by more of an anterior pelvic tilt, slight hip flexion and knee flexion, lumbar hyperlordosis limited to the lumbar spine, and hyperkyphosis in the upper lumbar and thoracolumbar segments. LCS type B posture (figure 4.3c) is characterized by a minimal lumbar lordosis that extends into the thoracolumbar segments with compensatory kyphosis in the thoracic area. The head is protracted. The COG is shifted backward, and the knees are in recurvatum.

Table 14.1 Key Observations in Postural Analysis for Lumbar Spine Dysfunction

Postural view	Key observations	Possible indications
Posterior	Iliac crest inequality	Leg-length discrepancy or SI rotation
	Flattened gluteal muscles	Weak gluteal muscles with associated ipsilateral SI joint dysfunction
	Asymmetrical and hypertrophied paraspinals	Impaired deep stabilization of the spine, in particular the abdominal muscles
	Lateral shift of pelvis	Weakened gluteus medius on the side that the pelvis is shifted toward
Lateral	Increased lordosis	Tight hip flexors or weak gluteal muscles
	Glenohumeral medial rotated position	Tightness of pectoralis major or weakness of middle and lower scapular stabilizers
	Chin and neck angle	Hypertrophy of superficial neck flexors; weakness or inhibition of deep neck flexors
Anterior	SCM hypertrophy	Tightness of SCM; accessory respiration
	Deep abdominal creases	Impaired coordination of abdominal muscles
	Lower rib cage angle flaring	Impaired respiration and deep spinal stabilizing system

Balance

As noted earlier, poor postural stability is found in patients with chronic low back pain. The clinician should asses the quality and timed response of single-leg balance (see page 71) while also noting the compensatory strategies used to maintain postural stability, such as the ankle, hip, or step strategy. Single-leg balance can discriminate those with chronic back pain from those without pain (Luoto et al. 1998) and can be used to screen for risk of injury (Tropp, Ekstrand, and Gillquist 1984b; Tropp and Odenrick 1988).

Gait

Adequate balance, timing, and recruitment of the musculature are imperative for smooth and efficient gait. Any imbalance or impaired recruitment or coordination in any part of the kinetic chain will manifest with each step, appearing as faulty patterns and inefficient energy expenditure. In short, gait assessment provides an overall picture of the dynamic function of the sensorimotor system. Attention is directed toward the pelvis and trunk in the sagittal, frontal, and transverse planes. The following are the most commonly observed gait faults in patients with chronic low back pain:

- Inadequate apparent hip hyperextension during the terminal stance phase of gait. This finding indicates gluteal weakness or inhibition that overstresses the lumbar segments.

- Increased lateral pelvic shift on the stance leg, a contralateral pelvic drop, or excessive pelvic rotation. This finding indicates inadequate lateral pelvic and trunk stability and control. The muscles primarily supporting the lateral pelvic brace are the gluteal and abdominal muscles. Functioning gluteal muscles, in particular the gluteus medius, are necessary to counter the adduction moment and to control the femoral medial rotation during the early stance phase of the gait cycle. Excessive hip adduction during gait has been shown to result from gluteus medius weakness (Reischl et al. 1999).

Movement Patterns

In functional pathology, observing the quality of movement is more important than testing for muscle strength. The clinician should focus on the quality, sequencing, and degree of activation of the muscles involved in the movement pattern in order to evaluate the coordination of the synergists. The quality and control of the movement pattern are imperative, as an improper pattern may cause or perpetuate adverse stresses on the spine and other joint structures. The three movement pattern tests for patients with lumbar pain are the hip extension (page 79), the hip abduction (page 80), and the curl-up (page 82). Clinicians may also perform other movement pattern tests described in chapter 6 if indicated.

A positive hip extension test often indicates inadequate stabilization of the trunk or weakness of the gluteus maximus. Delayed recruitment or weak activation of the gluteus maximus induces compensatory overload stresses on the lumbar spine and simultaneous overactivity of the thoracolumbar erector spinae. Lewis and Sahrmann (2005) showed that patients with anterior hip pain have delayed onset of the gluteus maximus. Other studies (Hungerford, Gilleard, and Hodges 2003; Voigt, Pfeifer, and Banzer 2003; Hodges and Richardson 1996, 1998, 1999; McGill, Hughson, and Parks 2000, 2002; Radebold et al. 2001) have shown the importance of the feed-forward mechanism (activation of the abdominal muscles and lumbar erector spinae in the premovement phase of hip extension) in stabilizing the trunk to control the pelvis during limb movement.

A positive hip abduction test provides valuable information about the quality of the lateral pelvic brace and indirect information about the stabilization of the pelvis in the frontal plane during gait. A delayed recruitment or weak activation of the gluteus medius is often associated with tightness of the TFL-IT band and quadratus lumborum and concomitantly inadequate spinal stabilization by the abdominal wall.

A positive trunk curl-up test reveals a dominance of the hip flexors over weakened abdominal muscles. If the curl-up is performed with adequate abdominal contraction, flexion or kyphosis of the upper trunk is observed. However, if the movement is performed primarily with the hip flexors, curling of the upper trunk is minimal and an anterior tilt of the pelvis may be observed.

A routine examination of the neuromuscular system must also include an evaluation of the respiration pattern, especially for patients with chronic musculoskeletal pain symptoms that had limited response to previous therapies. The clinician should observe the breathing pattern while the patient is in sitting and supine positions (see page 88). The respiratory pattern may change as the patient's posture and the relation of the rib cage to gravity change. Accessory respiration due to hyperactivity of the SCM and scalenes indicates insufficient stabilization of the rib cage by the abdominal muscles and weakness or inhibition of the diaphragm. These patients often have tender points or TrPs throughout the diaphragm and abdominal wall.

Muscle Length and Strength

Following careful assessment of posture and movement patterns, the clinician can begin to postulate which muscles are tight or weak. At this time, muscle tightness and weakness can be verified and quantified with the hands-on muscle length and strength tests described in chapter 7. The clinician should look for the classic patterns of muscle tightness and weakness to confirm or rule out Janda's LCS.

Manual Assessment

The manual assessment, including joint mobility testing and soft-tissue palpation, is the final step in the evaluation. Janda described several findings of the manual assessment that may indicate lumbar dysfunction:

- Pain and tenderness at the spinous processes of the lumbar segments, particularly L4-L5 and L5-S1, due to overstress at these segments
- Hypomobility with or without pain in the upper lumbar or lower thoracic segments due to dominance and overactivation of the thoracolumbar paraspinals
- TrPs and hypertonicity in the hip flexors, quadratus lumborum, and thoracolumbar paraspinals secondary to the dominance of these muscles over the inadequate or weakened gluteal and abdominal muscles

Management of Low Back Pain Syndromes

Lumbar pain syndromes are best treated with a combination of approaches. Multimodal nonsurgical management of low back pain may include manual passive mobilization of joints and soft tissue, neuromuscular reactivation, exercise prescription, sensorimotor training, posture correction, movement or ergonomic reeducation, and conditioning exercises. A comprehensive rehabilitation program should stress enhancement of motor patterns and functional tasks rather than focus on specific muscles (Standaert and Herring 2007).

The management strategy should be dynamic in nature, meaning that it should alter according to changes in the patient's condition. The clinician should always avoid a cookbook mentality in the management and rehabilitation of the patient and so should design a strategy that meets the specific needs of each individual patient. Emphasis should be placed on patient education regarding the value of fitness and the safety of resuming activities. Appropriate patient education may prevent fear and avoidance and promote better coping strategies for pain management.

Respiration

Correcting a faulty respiratory pattern is integral to the success of any rehabilitation program that addresses the movement system. Treatment must be directed at restoring normal subcortical motor programs through motor training. For respiratory training to be effective, however, the new motor program must be practiced repeatedly under a variety of conditions until it becomes the program of choice. In circumstances where voluntary motor training is unsuccessful, reflex therapy as described by Vojta and Peters(1997) and Kolář (1999, 2007) is necessary to activate postural reactions including physiological respiration. Lewit (1999, 1980) contends that no other movement can be normalized if the breathing pattern is not ideal.

Dynamic Spinal Stabilization

After respiration has been addressed, training the patient in the proper abdominal brace is essential for any spinal stabilization training, whether static or dynamic. Contraction of the closely interlinked abdominal wall muscles and posterior fascia produces hoop stresses and elevates IAP, contributing to the stiffening and stabilizing forces acting on the lumbar spine. The patient has to be instructed to breathe normally while maintaining the abdominal brace without going into a posterior pelvic tilt or lumbar flexion. Once the patient has mastered the abdominal brace in the supine position, extremity movements are introduced to challenge the CNS to maintain the co-contraction and IAP in order to achieve spinal stability during movement. The challenge of the exercise can then be progressed by adding various postures; reciprocal extremity movements; resistance; labile surfaces; dynamic functional movements such as squatting, lifting, reaching, pulling, or pushing; and finally functional activities that the patient needs or desires.

Much more research is needed on the efficacy of dynamic stabilization exercises. There is controversy among researchers and clinicians as to whether isolated muscle activation (the TrA and multifidus viewpoint) or simultaneous contraction of all abdominal muscles (the bracing viewpoint) is better (Standaert and Herring 2007). The rehabilitation program should be tailored to the patient's primary dysfunction and goals. In any case, the clinician should monitor each exercise to ensure that the patient maintains the abdominal brace and avoids compensatory movements at the spine. It is essential to educate the patient on good alignment and form for the purpose of self-correction during the home exercise program, which is performed without supervision.

Sensorimotor Training

SMT, described in chapter 11, utilizes labile and unstable surfaces to stimulate the afferent system to facilitate more effective motor programs on a subcortical level. Doing so improves dynamic stability, posture, and movement patterns.

SMT has been shown to improve muscle reaction time (Luoto et al. 1998) in as little as 2 wk (Wilder et al. 1996). Janda (1992) reported on the results of a neck and low back rehabilitation program using SMT, noting that 75% of patients had improved motor performance and 91% had improved pain. Significant improvement in gluteal muscle EMG activity was shown in patients with chronic low back pain who walked on balance sandals for 1 wk (Bullock-Saxton, Janda, and Bullock 1993). Balance sandals used in functionally closed kinetic chain activities are an effective means of increasing lower-extremity muscle activity (Troy Blackburn, Hirth, and Guskiewicz 2003).

SMT should be initiated early in the rehabilitation process (see chapter 11). Particular attention should be given to ensure that the patient maintains a neutral position of the lumbar and cervical spine during each exercise. The challenge of the exercise should allow the patient to balance comfortably on the labile tool without having to raise the arms or hold onto an external support. Perturbations can be introduced in various ways to facilitate APRs at the subcortical level.

Case Study

S.M. is a 46 y old computer programmer. He has a 10 y history of intermittent low back pain punctuated with periodic episodes that prevent him from going to work or participating in recreational soccer and basketball. The most recent flare-up in symptoms occurred when he was picking up a lounge chair. He felt a sharp, stabbing pain in his low back and referred pain in his left buttock. The symptoms eased after 3 to 4 d of staying home from work and taking over-the-counter anti-inflammatory medications. Upon returning to work, where he spends most of his day sitting at the computer, he started to develop a constant deep, throbbing pain (varying from 2-6 on a scale of 10) in the lumbar region and intermittent referred symptoms to the left buttock. Symptoms were aggravated after sitting for more than 30 min, bending over to pick up items on the floor, putting his pants or socks on, getting in and out of the car, taking his shirt off, and participating in sport activities. Symptoms were eased with medications and assuming a supine hook-lying position.

MRI of the lumbar spine revealed disc dessication with a 0.2 in. (4 mm) broad-based disc bulge encroaching on the inferior recess of the left neural foramina with foraminal narrowing. There was also mild to moderate canal stenosis with hypertrophic facet degenerative changes. There were no red flags in his past medical or family history. S.M.'s goals were to prevent future flare-ups and return to his recreational soccer and basketball games.

Examination and Assessment

The following are the findings of S.M.'s initial evaluation:

- Posture and muscle analysis
  - Narrow base of support and anterior center of mass with compensatory posterior sway of thoracic spine
  - Asymmetrical hypertrophy of thoracolumbar paraspinals from T7 to L2, with increased muscle bulk on the right compared with the left
  - Hypertrophy of left hamstrings with concurrent hypotrophy of bilateral gluteal muscles
  - Thickening of right Achilles tendon; when questioned, patient reported recurrent chronic ankle sprains in his younger days
- Active trunk movements
  - Limited trunk movements secondary to muscle guarding
- Single-limb stance
  - Increased lateral pelvic shift that is worse on left than right
- Neurological tests
  - All negative
- MMT
  - Gluteus medius: right 4/5, left 4 minus/5
  - Gluteus maximus: 4/5 bilaterally

- Respiratory pattern
  - Decreased lateral rib cage excursion with inspiration
  - Decreased caudal shift of the rib cage with expiration
- Movement pattern tests
  - Prone hip extension
    - Right: excessive lumbosacral extension with delayed gluteus maximus recruitment
    - Left: hamstring dominance with excessive lumbosacral extension and pelvic rotation; delayed gluteus maximus recruitment
  - Hip abduction
    - Compensatory hip flexion indicating TFL dominance over synergist gluteus medius; concurrent increase in pelvic posterior rotation indicating inadequate stabilization from the trunk stabilizers
  - Prone knee flexion
    - Increased lumbar rotation and extension secondary to stiff and short two-joint hip flexors
- Muscle length tests
  - One-joint hip flexors: WNL
  - Two-joint hip flexors: stiff bilaterally, neither leg hangs perpendicular to the floor (knee flexion to 75°)
  - Hamstrings: right 55°, left 50° with passive straight-leg raise
- Passive joint mobility (posterior–anterior pressures)
  - Hypomobile and painful on right L5-S1
  - Painful on left L4-L5
  - Hypomobile central T8-T9 and T9-T10
- TrP palpation
  - TrPs in left quadratus lumborum, left psoas major, bilateral adductor longus and pectineus, and left hamstrings

Treatment and Outcome

The typical and traditional treatment approach to a patient with these findings would most likely entail manual joint or soft-tissue mobilizations and muscle length or strength restoration. Minimal attention would be given to correcting respiration or movement patterns or addressing SMT. In this case scenario, the initial treatment stage focused on educating the patient and restoring proper respiratory patterns. Abdominal bracing techniques were instructed and the patient practiced abdominal bracing with various functional movements such as getting in and out of bed or a chair or a car, rolling in bed, bending, and reaching. S.M. noticed a big difference in pain level when he engaged his abdominal muscles and when he did not. Abdominal bracing was a powerful tool he used for controlling and managing his own symptoms. He was also advised to frequently change his positions and to avoid a sustained flexed or rotated trunk position when he was sitting at work. He was also instructed to widen his BOS and shift his center of mass slightly toward his heels when standing so that his weight was more evenly distributed on his feet. This reduced tissue stresses on his lumbar segments from excessive paraspinal activity and hence reduced his pain level.

Initial Stage

Treatment and exercises during the initial stage also included the following:

- Active prone knee flexion without any compensatory pelvic rotation or lumbar extension (this exercise also aimed at elongating the tight two-joint hip flexors)
- Passive hip flexor stretch in a modified Thomas test position or half-kneeling position
- Gentle knee extension performed with hips flexed to 90° in supine position to elongate the hamstrings as well as improve gliding of perineural structures
- PIR techniques for hamstrings and two-joint hip flexors to inhibit the tone of these muscles with spontaneous reduction of the TrPs and subsequent improvement in recruitment and strength of the gluteal muscles

After the third visit, S.M.'s symptoms significantly changed from a constant pain to an intermittent pain, depending on the type of activities he engaged in. Referred symptoms to his left buttock were infrequent. He reported that he was now able to sit for greater than an hour but changed position every 30 to 40 min for preventative measures. He still had trouble with reaching overhead and bending his trunk, all necessary movements for his recreational sports.

Intermediate Stage

The intermediate stage of rehabilitation consisted of the following:

- PIR for the quadratus lumborum and adductors followed by facilitation of the gluteus medius
- Gluteal (medius and maximus) strengthening exercises with focus on proper form
- Abdominal bracing concurrent with bilateral arm elevation in supine position to prepare S.M. for overhead reaching activities in ADL or soccer and basketball
- Abdominal bracing concurrent with unilateral hip flexion in supine position to prepare S.M. for independent lower-extremity movements while maintaining spinal stability
- Hip hinge exercises in the sagittal and transverse planes to encourage a neutral spine posture (i.e., movement from the hips rather than flexion and rotation at the lumbar segments)
- SMT

After the sixth visit, S.M.'s symptoms were very much under control. S.M. rarely experienced low back pain except for the times when he sat longer than normal. He returned to treadmill walking and slow running for 30 min without aggravation of symptoms. His next goal was to gradually return to recreational soccer and basketball.

Final Stage

The final stage of the rehabilitation was to return the patient to his previous activity level. This stage consisted of the following:

- Further SMT with increasing challenge using elastic resistance, free weights, proprioceptive tools, and plyometrics
- Putting S.M. in positions that troubled his back and training proper motor patterns, such as overhead throwing, kicking a soccer ball, shooting a basket, and dribbling a ball, to spare his back
- Continued patient education on the importance of proper and ideal ergonomics and postural balance

The entire rehabilitation process for S.M., from initial evaluation to discharge, entailed 12 sessions spread over 3 mo. In the beginning rehabilitation focused on pain management and patient education; it then progressed to restoring muscle length and recruitment balance and finally to designing a specific exercise program to return the patient to his desired activity goals. Emphasis was placed on proper movement patterns to ensure ideal motor programs in the CNS were enhanced. In summary, a comprehensive rehabilitation program should focus on enhancing motor patterns and functional tasks rather than focus on specific muscles.

Janda's Approach Versus the Traditional Approach

The traditional treatment approach often attempts to reduce pain and dysfunction of the musculoskeletal system through various modalities such icing, applying heat, taping, external bracing, and joint or soft-tissue mobilization. The Janda approach includes all of these modalities, especially in the early stages, but also includes a careful analysis of muscle imbalance and its role in the perpetuation of the dysfunction. The muscular system lies at a functional crossroads since it is influenced by stimuli from both the CNS and the musculoskeletal systems. Muscles that tend to get weak often go hand in hand with muscles that tend to get tight. The traditional approach of strengthening a weak muscle entails progressive overload during exercise training in order to increase muscular strength, power, hypertrophy, and endurance. However, strengthening of a weak muscle in the presence of a tight or hypertonic muscle may be less than effective because the tight muscle is recruited first due to its lowered irritability threshold. Janda'a approach hypothesized that a weak muscle may merely be one that is inhibited because of a tight or hypertonic antagonist (Sherrington's law of reciprocal inhibition). He hypothesized that restoring muscle tension or the length of a tight muscle might spontaneously facilitate a weak antagonist. In the case scenario of S.W., PIR techniques to inhibit the hypertonic hip flexors caused spontaneous improvement of gluteal recruitment. The normalization of muscle tone and length should be followed by specific strengthening, SMT, movement reeducation, and endurance training.

Summary

Lumbopelvic muscle function plays an important role in the management of patients with low back pain. Impairments of lumbopelvic muscle function may compromise the structural integrity of the spinal complex, making it susceptible to further injury, prolonged recovery, or chronicity of pain. Management of low back pain requires an understanding of the sensorimotor mechanisms utilized for trunk stabilization and postural control.

CHAPTER 15

LOWER-EXTREMITY PAIN SYNDROMES

Pain syndromes of the lower extremity are often related to adaptive pathogenic changes that occur over time, such as muscle imbalances and asymmetrical strength deficits. These adaptive changes become painful or are a result of trauma for which poor compensation has taken place. Being bipedal, humans do not have much room for compensatory or strategic redistribution of forces; their ability to function while resting an injured lower limb is severely limited. This chapter begins by discussing regional considerations of the lower extremity such as functional anatomy and so on. This is followed by a brief review of the kinetic chain reactions of the extremity. Assessment and common pathologies are described. The chapter ends with a case study.

Regional Considerations

The lower extremities are a complex set of joints and muscles that work together, often as one functional unit. While gait and balance are the primary functions of the lower extremities, these extremities are also important components in functional tasks such as lifting or running. Lower-extremity function is heavily influenced by chain reactions, which often can be linked to chronic musculoskeletal syndromes throughout the body.

Functional Anatomy

Undoubtedly, the lower extremities are important to human gait and function. The lower-extremity skeleton includes the hemipelvis, femur, tibia, fibula, and bones of the foot, and the lower-extremity joints are the hip, knee, and ankle. The antigravity role played by the lower extremity demands several functions of the musculoskeletal system, including muscular, biomechanical, proprioceptive, and transfer functions.

- **Muscular function.** Powerful muscles capable of significant eccentric function include pennate and multipennate fiber arrangements to allow for significant force production during short arcs of ROM with long levers. The large bulk of the antigravity muscles used for power generation and transfer is evident in the size of the gluteal muscles, quadriceps, adductors, hamstrings, gastrocnemius, and soleus. An oblique and transverse arrangement of muscle groups such as the gluteus maximus, hamstrings, popliteus, and peroneus longus allows for efficient transverse motion during normal function.

- **Biomechanical function.** Biomechanically, the lower extremity requires a rapidly changeable lever system that allows for alternating flexibility and rigidity during the gait cycle. In addition, the lower extremity requires the ability to control its segments in space on a stable lumbopelvic unit; this is referred to as an *open chain function*. The ability to support the more proximal segment of the lower extremity on a stable weight-bearing tripod of the foot with the ideal control of mass by the hip and pelvic musculature (sometimes referred to as the *reverse open chain function)* is also necessary for proper function. In particular, control of pronation and supination are important for gait (Ker et al. 1987).

• **Proprioceptive function.** The lower extremity also plays a role in proprioceptive function. As described in chapter 2, afferent information from the foot is important for controlling posture and gait (Freeman 1965). The phenomenon of biped ambulation in humans is characterized by an intricate timing of biomechanical events presided over by subcortical programs and reflex reactions that can be modulated depending on the circumstances under which movement occurs. Walking on a gravel surface or slowly scaling a hilly terrain requires different strategies of feed-forward planning and feedback adjustments as opposed to sprinting, during which there is little time for feedback and subsequent adjustments. Even during normal uninterrupted gait, the system runs on autopilot. It is thought that supraspinal pathways integrated with spinal cord CPGs are responsible for adult locomotory gait, rhythm, and perpetuation (Leonard 1998).

• **Energy transfer function.** A network of ligaments and tendons that store and release energy creates a system of force transmission from distal to proximal segments of the lower extremity. This system is intimately linked to the trunk and upper body. The pelvic stabilizers, the stabilizing core of abdominal muscles, the respiratory and pelvic diaphragms, and the axial spinal musculature and fascia are also crucial to lower-extremity function (Dalstra 1997; Vleeming et al. 1995; Lee 1997; Cholewicki, Juluru, and McGill 1999). The transfer of energy from the lower body to the trunk to the upper body is an excellent example of chain reactions occurring in the lower extremity.

Kinetic Chain Reactions

The erect posture adopted by humans can have significant consequences for the overload and deterioration of the lumbopelvic region. It is not unusual for patients in their late 30s or 40s to begin displaying signs of breakdown in lumbopelvic function. The region has a rich and intricate concentration of nerves from the two major plexuses serving the pelvis and lower extremity. The muscular arrangement is complex, and muscles of the region serve multiple roles to support the axial skeleton and the viscera as well as act as a crossroads for force transference between the lower extremities and the torso and upper extremities.

The entire lower extremity should be considered as a whole rather than as individual joints and segments because of the complex chain reactions occurring throughout. These complex motions are often evident during gait. A detailed description of gait is beyond the scope of this chapter; however, a brief review will demonstrate the complex chain reactions occurring during ambulation.

Ambulation consists of cyclical and alternating swing and stance phases. A full gait cycle lasts approximately 1 s, about 38% of which is swing phase and 62% of which is stance phase (see figure 15.1; Root, Orion, and Weed 1997). Pronation and

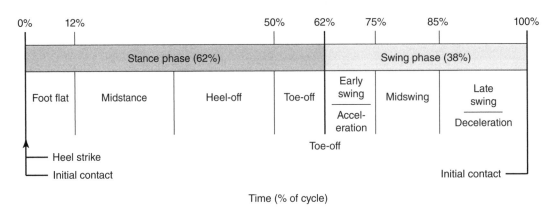

Figure 15.1 Phases of the gait cycle.

Adapted, by permission, from P. Houglum, 2005, *Therapeutic exercise for musculoskeletal injuries,* 2nd ed. (Champaign, IL: Human Kinetics), 358.

supination are the two main aspects of kinetic and arthrokinematic movement during the stance phase. The stance phase is initiated by a chain reaction of calcaneal eversion and subsequent talar motion through inertia of the leg and ground friction at heel strike. The swing phase is a true open chain, the goal of which is to transform ground reaction forces into forward momentum. This momentum assists in supination of the contralateral stance limb, clearing the ground, and preparing the swing limb for the ensuing stance phase. Since the swing phase of gait is governed only by muscular effort and is free of the ground reaction constraints that govern the stance phase, a milder and altered form of pronation and supination occur in the foot, and talar involvement is minimal.

Pronation of the foot allows for energy storage, shock absorption, terrain adaptation, and balance maintenance. Supination, on the other hand, is more active, requiring concentric muscle activity and momentum of the swing leg combined with arthrokinematic mechanisms that force the foot toward osseous stability and predominantly concentric muscle activity for propulsion. If the timing, the degree of pronation and supination, or the strength of the involved muscles changes, the coordinated alignment of the bones becomes inefficient and the achievement of stability on demand becomes impossible. For example, weakness of the hip may lead to an inability to externally rotate the femur. This may in turn lead to an inability to achieve ideal resupination of the foot. Thus the screw-home mechanism (the coupled arthrokinematic relationship of extension and external rotation of the tibial plateau on the femur) needed for knee stability is compromised and patellofemoral pain may result (Ireland et al. 2003).

As described in chapter 3, several obligatory motions are seen in the closed kinetic chain reactions of the lower extremity. These reactions can occur distally to proximally or proximally to distally, and their obligatory motions include (1) pronation that leads to tibial internal rotation that leads to knee valgus and flexion that leads to hip internal rotation and (2) supination that leads to tibial external rotation that leads to knee varus and extension that leads to hip external rotation. Because these movements are obligatory, any deficit in motion at one segment must be compensated for by another segment. Without compensation, the deficit may prevent necessary motions. For example, increased pronation in the foot during the foot-flat phase of gait facilitates femoral internal rotation; however, terminal extension of the knee before push-off requires external rotation to complete the screw-home mechanism.

Assessment

A review of Janda's principles highlights the great insight and predictive thought process that brought him many admirers within the fields of rehabilitation and medicine. The assessment and intervention for lower-extremity musculoskeletal pathologies follows the processes described in parts II and III of this text. As stated previously, the entire lower extremity should be evaluated regardless of the diagnosis or the location of pain. Chapters 5 and 8 detail the specific progression of musculoskeletal evaluation.

- **Posture and alignment.** Assessment begins with an evaluation of posture and alignment, particularly of the lower extremity but also throughout the body. The structural variations observed in both limb and foot may lead to compensatory patterns that cannot be accommodated throughout a lifetime. For example, forefoot and rear-foot varus, valgus deformities, Morton's foot, genu recurvatum, or genu valgus may lead to pronated or supinated feet. This change in foot position can affect postural stability (Cote et al. 2005), increase postural fatigue over time (Rothbart 2002), and eventually lead to repetitive strain injury or an increased risk for traumatic injury from an external source.

- **Balance and gait.** Balance and gait are evaluated next. The clinician assesses the efficiency of the movement and the control of the support (foot) or suspension (pelvis and hip) structures. Single-leg stance is an easy test to perform. When administering this test, the clinician notes the patient's duration and quality of balancing with eyes open and eyes closed (Janda and VáVrová 1996); normative data on duration and age are available (Bohannon et al. 1984); see chapter 5. A videotaped review of gait is very helpful in identifying deviations from expected function, such as the utilization of the rocker mechanism at the ankle and MTP (metatarsal phalangeal) joints. Excessive pronation during gait and running is associated with a variety of conditions including ACL injury, plantar fasciitis, medial tibial stress syndrome, and stress fractures (Beckett et al. 1992; Delacerda 1980; Giladi et al. 1985; Smith et al. 1997; Viitasalo and Kvist 1983). The effect that subtalar pronation, which is measured by static anatomical foot alignment, has on the impact forces or the rate of loading when landing from jumping, during which the sequence of heel-to-toe action is reversed, has been questioned (Hargrave et al. 2003). In fact, the neuromuscular component of shock absorption may be more important than the biomechanical components, which are the components currently measured for assessment. The intrinsic joint stability provided by the muscles, the distribution of forces within the kinetic chains as organized by the CNS, and the tensile properties of tendons and ligaments may play a more important role than the one pronation or supination or any other joint angle plays during dynamic movement.

- **Movement patterns.** The most common movement pattern tests performed for lower-extremity dysfunction are the prone leg raise and side-lying hip abduction (see chapter 6). Despite the tendency of phasic muscles to become inhibited with lower-extremity injury (Bullock-Saxton et al. 1994), there is no hard and fast rule as to which muscle and to what degree inhibition may occur in; that is to say, spraining an ankle does not automatically lead to an inhibited gluteus maximus. Lehman (2006) questioned the validity of the prone leg extension for assessment based on a single case of a runner with an ankle sprain who showed no delay in gluteus maximus activation. The prone leg extension is more sensitive to functional chronic sensorimotor dysfunction than to acute or subacute structural lesions such as an ankle sprain; therefore, Lehman's findings are not surprising.

- **Muscle length and strength testing.** Gross ROM and bilateral comparison can indicate muscle imbalances and areas of tightness or inhibition. MMT can be used to quantify muscle weakness. Asymmetrical stress factors should be eliminated in order to decrease biomechanical overload and compromise. Clinicians can then begin to determine biomechanical causes of pain based on muscle imbalance. At this time, muscles can be palpated for tender points or TrPs; the possible patterns and chains of these points are established.

- **Neurological screening.** It is always important to rule out neurological compromise of the lower extremity that might result from spinal pathology or functional instability. Entrapment of nerves from the lumbosacral plexus, most notably the sciatic nerve, can cause pain and dysfunction in the lower extremity. The subclinical presentation of such lumbar pathology can include diverse symptoms such as apparent hamstring strain, Achilles tendinitis, trochanteric bursitis, knee pain, adductor pain, plantar fasciitis, and metatarsalgia.

- **Functional movement patterns.** Functional movement analysis is often helpful in lower-extremity pain syndromes. Functional movements include single-leg squatting, stepping up, stepping down, lunging, and single-leg standing rotation.

A rather important aspect that is often overlooked clinically is torsional deviation in the compensatory overload of the lower extremity. These variations in the transverse plane depend on increased or decreased version of the hip and tibial torsion. The result is misalignment between the hip and knee, the knee and foot, or the hip, knee, and foot and increased muscular system load. It is hypothesized that the musculoskeletal system does not easily tolerate transverse plane and coronal plane faults (such as pelvic obliquity or rotated pelvis), as it does sagittal plane faults (such as increased or decreased lumbar lordosis), because the effects of asymmetric loading on rotational movements are more pronounced with these types of faults.

Intervention

Once the assessment has been completed, the clinician summarizes the findings and prioritizes a treatment plan based on the principles described in chapters 9 through11. First and foremost, the patient's activities are restricted if necessary to allow for tissue recovery and healing. Local modalities are used to reduce pain and inflammation. Intervention follows Janda's three stages of rehabilitation: (1) normalization, (2) restoration of muscle balance, and (3) SMT and training of skilled movements.

1. Normalization. First, CNS input from the peripheral proprioceptors is normalized. Manual therapy, including soft-tissue mobilization to improve soft-tissue mobility where restricted, may be applied to joints and tissues throughout the lower extremity, from the hip to the metatarsals. External devices such as orthotics, wedges, or supports can be helpful at restoring normal biomechanical position for optimal proprioceptive input. Taping of the feet, legs, hips, and thighs using rigid taping or kinesio taping in combination with other modalities of choice may help with soft-tissue unloading and pain relief.

2. Restoration of muscle balance. When restoring muscle balance, muscle tightness is addressed first. The clinician attempts to normalize tone in muscles that display hypertonicity or spasm and then to facilitate inhibited muscles. The techniques described in chapter 10 are used to normalize abnormal tone and eliminate TrPs or tender points in the intrinsic and extrinsic muscles. Origin–insertion stimulation, along with isometric exercises and submaximal eccentric exercises (Umphred 2001), can be introduced to facilitate inhibited pelvic and lower-extremity muscles and prepare them for further loading and complex exercises. As stated earlier, the patterns of imbalance may or may not follow traditional patterns described by Janda, depending on the chronicity of the injury. For example, the clinician may find that the vastus lateralis is inhibited and fails MMT (rather than the vastus medialis obliquus, which is more commonly inhibited).

3. SMT and training of skilled movements. The use of SMT to improve hamstrings-to-quadriceps strength ratios has been demonstrated (Heitkamp et al. 2001). Weight-bearing femoral control is retrained based on the altered ROM findings. The clinician assesses the need for SMT to improve strength control and coordination with emphasis of either distal–proximal or proximal–distal control. Next, intervention progresses to movement synergies for the lower quarter, such as stepping, lunging, hopping, jumping, and twisting, with particular attention given to the dysfunctional movements noted in the assessment. Next is retraining of movement control and top-down or bottom-up stability. The goal is to slowly increase endurance and load of the motor system via microprogression while maintaining phasic–tonic balance in exercise choices. This progresses to repetitive qualitative training of fundamental movements in order to establish these patterns centrally and to increase endurance in these skilled movements. Gradually the patient returns to normal activities with a reentry program consisting of microprogressions.

Muscle Balance and Imbalance in the Lower Extremity

As noted in chapter 4, imbalance in muscle strength is sometimes necessary for functional activities such as sports. For example, soccer players playing different positions exhibit different hamstrings-to-quadriceps strength ratios (Oberg et al. 1984). Runners have tighter hamstrings and soleus muscles than nonrunners have (Wang et al. 1993), and indoor track runners develop invertor-to-evertor strength imbalances after training (Beukeboom et al. 2000). While these functional muscle imbalances are not associated with pain or pathology, they can lead to injury.

In in older adults, reduced ROM in hip extension during gait (possibly due to hip flexor tightness or gluteus maximus weakness) has been associated with an increased risk of falls (Kerrigan et al. 2001). In addition, older adults have significantly weaker hip abduction and adduction, which may also contribute to lateral instability and falls (Johnson et al. 2002).

Several researchers have described the role of muscle imbalance in sport injuries. Knapik and colleagues (1991) reported a higher risk of injury in athletes with imbalances in knee flexor strength or hip extension flexibility greater than 15% between the right and left sides. Female athletes with hip extensor weakness are more prone to lower-extremity injury (Nadler et al. 2000); similarly, female athletes demonstrating global hip weakness, particularly in hip abduction and external rotation, tend to develop anterior knee pain (Cichanowski et al. 2007). Hip external rotation and abduction weakness is associated with lower-extremity injury in athletes (Leetun et al. 2004). Soccer players with flexibility imbalances have a higher incidence of musculoskeletal injury (Ekstrand and Gillquist 1982, 1983; Witvrouw et al. 2003).

Common Pathologies

Janda's LCS is sometimes seen in lower-extremity pathology, although it is not as prevalent as it is in patients with chronic low back pain. Nonetheless, evidence suggests that muscle imbalance and altered function play a significant role in the musculoskeletal pathologies commonly seen in the lower extremity. These imbalances can reflect strength asymmetry between limbs, agonist–antagonist strength asymmetry in a single limb, or altered firing patterns (Knapik et al. 1991; Nadler et al. 2000; Tyler et al. 2001; Lewis and Sarhmann 2005). When addressing lower-extremity pathology, the strong relationship between limited motion and decreased strength (and therefore muscle inhibition) cannot be overstressed (Ireland et al. 2003). Supporting Janda's observation that gluteus maximus weakness occurs in lower-extremity pathology, Nadler and colleagues (2000) found significant differences in side-to-side symmetry of maximum hip extension strength between female athletes with lower-extremity injury and female athletes without injury. Precipitating factors other than direct trauma may include fatigue, postural stresses, leg-length discrepancy, nutritional deficiencies, and muscle constriction (Travell and Simons 1992; Brunet et al. 1990; Friberg 1983; Gofton and Trueman 1971; Morscher 1977). Janda noted that patients with discrepancies tend to shift toward the longer side. He also suggested that the significance of leg-length disparity (see figure 15.2) varies among individuals and depends on a person's choice of compensation through the sensory motor system. Arbitrary definitions of what constitutes pathological leg-length discrepancy are not clinically helpful.

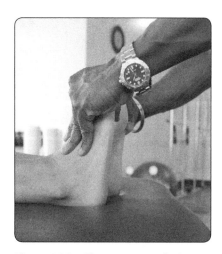

Figure 15.2 The assessment for leg-length discrepancy.

Hip and Thigh Pain

When considering a musculoskeletal cause for symptoms arising from the hip, thigh, and groin, it is important to rule out gastrointestinal and genitourinary causes as well as possible compression or entrapment of the neurovascular tissues. Symptoms can arise out of local trauma, but when the etiology is insidious and gradual, the diagnostic algorithm can be difficult and obscure. For example, sport hernia (a tear of the transverse fascia of the posterior aspect of the inguinal canal, sometimes involving the fascial attachment of the rectus abdominis or external and internal oblique muscles) may display pain patterns and symptoms similar to those of osteitis pubis and athletic pubalgia (Gerhardt, Brown, and Giza 2006). Chronic musculoskeletal pain associated with muscle imbalance includes groin pain and injury, hamstring strain, iliotibial band syndrome, and hip arthritis.

Groin Pain and Injury

Groin strains are quite common in sports that require multiple changes of direction during running. The groin area consists of the hip adductor group, which is prone to tightness per Janda's classification, possibly predisposing the area to strain. The adductors originate on the pubis and insert on the medial posterior aspect of the femur (see figure 15.3). Researchers have shown that the cause of groin injury may not be the groin area itself but rather the supporting areas of the abdominal core and hip.

Athletes with chronic groin pain demonstrate delayed activation of the TrA compared with controls (Cowan et al. 2004). Researchers found that hockey players are 17 times more likely to be injured when their strength ratios of hip abductors to adductors are inadequate (< 80%), whereas flexibility is not a significant factor in predicting injury (Tyler et al. 2001).

Hölmich et al. (1999) utilized a successful gradual strengthening and conditioning program for weak abdominal muscles and hip adductors in athletes with chronic groin pain. Furthermore, a preventive strengthening program for the hip adductors was utilized to forestall likely injuries in at-risk ice hockey players (Tyler et al. 2001).

Hamstring Strains

Hamstring strains are common in sports requiring frequent starts and stops and changes of direction. Chronic and repetitive hamstring strains are very difficult to manage during a sport season. Hamstring strains have been associated with muscle imbalances, although there

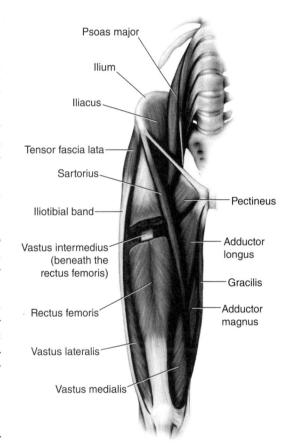

Psoas major

Ilium

Iliacus

Tensor fascia lata

Sartorius

Iliotibial band

Vastus intermedius
(beneath the
rectus femoris)

Rectus femoris

Vastus lateralis

Vastus medialis

Pectineus

Adductor
longus

Gracilis

Adductor
magnus

Figure 15.3 The hip adductors (groin area).

Reprinted from R.S. Behnke, 2006, *Kinetic Anatomy*, 2nd ed. (Champaign: Human Kinetics), 198.

is some discrepancy in the literature. While some researchers report that strength imbalances rather than flexibility imbalances are factors in hamstring strain (Orchard et al. 1997), others report the exact opposite, finding flexibility imbalances rather than strength imbalances to be the causative factors (Worrell et al. 1991). Still other researchers report both (Jönhagen et al. 1994). Sprinters with previous hamstring injury have tighter hamstrings and lower eccentric torque than uninjured sprinters have (Jönhagen et al. 1994). A low hamstrings-to-quadriceps strength ratio (<60%) and low side-to-side hamstrings strength ratio (<90%) have been associated with hamstring injury

(Cameron, Adams, and Maher 2003; Orchard et al. 1997). Some authors have suggested that hamstring injuries due to muscle imbalances can be reduced with eccentric training programs (Croisier et al. 2002). A recent study reported that a progressive agility training program with trunk stabilization exercises is more effective than an isolated hamstring stretching and strengthening rehabilitation program (Sherry and Best 2004).

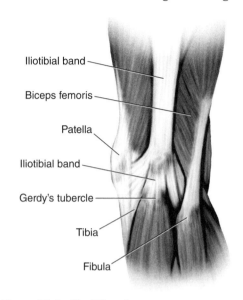

Iliotibial band

Biceps femoris

Patella

Iliotibial band

Gerdy's tubercle

Tibia

Fibula

Figure 15.4 The IT band.

Reprinted from R.S. Behnke, 2006, *Kinetic anatomy*, 2nd ed. (Champaign: Human Kinetics), 193.

Iliotibial Band Syndrome

The IT band originates as the TFL, becoming a thick, fibrous fascial band running down the side of the thigh and inserting on the lateral condyle of the tibia (see figure 15.4). The IT band also has fascial insertions into the lateral aspect of the patellar retinaculum. Iliotibial band syndrome (ITB syndrome) is often related to running and is a relatively common symptom among athletes. Incidental palpation may reveal a tender IT band on many individuals even though it may not be a cause for complaint. Clinically, a tight IT band is a secondary response to increased stability demands; therefore, it is important to find out why this strategy has been adopted and if the inappropriate stresses can be redistributed and the symptoms eliminated. Often, patients with a tight IT band exhibit hip abductor weakness and adductor tightness. Hip abductor tightness may occur as a result of poor stabilization of the pelvis (from weak gluteus medius) in the frontal plane, which facilitates the TFL as a secondary hip stabilizer. Fredericson et al. (2000) found significant gluteus medius weakness in runners with ITB syndrome. After 6 wk of rehabilitation, 90% of the athletes returned to running pain free. Kinesio taping to inhibit a tight adductor may also be helpful in reducing ITB syndrome (see figure 15.5).

Hyperpronation or hypopronation can cause excessive lateral heel strike or excessive medial translation and rotation of the femur, both of which have been associated with ITB syndrome. A sudden increase in activity volume can also precipitate symptoms. It is questionable whether the IT band itself is the true culprit or whether the muscles that attach to it and lie underneath it are to blame for the apparent tightness. Sometimes the symptomatic limb displays no apparent tightness during Ober's test (see figure 15.6), and sometimes the nonsymptomatic side is tighter. In many cases, release of the IT band and normalization of vastus lateralis tone can improve ROM

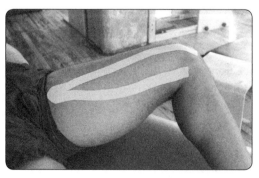

Figure 15.5 Kinesio taping to inhibit the hip adductors in the ITB syndrome.

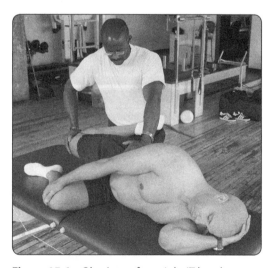

Figure 15.6 Ober's test for a tight IT band.

and reduce pain levels so dramatically that a true contracture of the IT band must be called into question. The number of failed lateral release surgeries must also cause the clinician to ponder the logic of a purely structural solution that ignores neuromuscular considerations. There are anecdotal reports that stretching the IT band harvested from cadavers is impossible.

Gait analysis may give insight into compensation or cause for the symptoms in ITB syndrome. Loss of proximal or distal control and weakness should be identified and treated both manually and with exercise; however, proper function of the local musculature and tone normalization are key to relieving symptoms.

Hip Pain and Arthritis

While the hip is one of the most stable joints in the body, it is also one of the most load bearing. Chronic hip pain can be caused by tendinitis of the iliopsoas or IT band (as already discussed) or by degenerative arthritis. Janda identified the gluteus maximus and medius as being prone to weakness and the iliopsoas as being prone to tightness. Lewis and Sahrmann (2005) demonstrated that altered firing patterns might be the cause of anterior hip pain.

Hip OA is a degenerative process that sometimes leads to total joint replacement. Arthritic joints exhibit arthrogenous muscle inhibition (AMI; Hurley and Newham 1993), in which the muscles surrounding an arthritic joint become weak and inhibited. AMI is most likely due to a loss of normal proprioceptive input from intact joint mechanoreceptors (see figure 15.7). While cause has not been established, muscle imbalances similar to those in Janda's LCS have been identified in patients with hip OA. Long and colleagues (1993) reported inhibition of the gluteus maximus and medius as well as facilitation of the TFL, rectus femoris, and adductors in hip OA. Patients with hip OA also exhibit altered muscle activation patterns (Long et al. 1993; Sims et al. 2002) and impairments in balance (Majewski et al. 2005) and gait (Watelain et al. 2001).

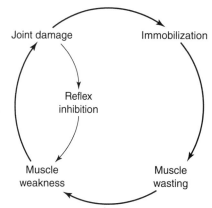

Figure 15.7 The cycle of arthrogenous muscle inhibition.

While total hip replacement (THR) may provide pain relief and improve general function, significant strength deficits of up to 80% loss remain up to 2 y postoperation (Long et al. 1993; Horstmann et al. 1994; Horstmann et al. 2002; Reardon et al. 2001; Shih et al. 1994). These deficits remain consistent with Janda's observations in knee extension, hip abduction, and hip extension. Patients who have undergone THR also demonstrate impaired postural control and motor strategies (Majewski et al. 2005; Nallegowda et al. 2003; Trudelle-Jackson et al. 2002). Patients with abnormal gait patterns resulting from muscle imbalance often need revision (Long et al. 1993); therefore, a second phase of rehabilitation conducted 4 mo after THR is recommended in patients with residual deficits (Trudelle-Jackson et al. 2002).

Knee Pain and Injury

Because the primary extensors of the knee are the quadriceps (of which the vasti muscles are prone to weakness) and hamstrings (prone to tightness), the knee may be predisposed to muscle imbalance syndromes. Common knee dysfunctions associated with muscle imbalance include anterior knee pain, ACL injury, and knee OA.

Anterior Knee Pain

Anterior knee pain (AKP), also known as *patellar tendinitis* or *patellofemoral pain syndrome* (PFPS), is a common symptom associated with physical activity over time. It is often acquired gradually and insidiously and is experienced during activity such

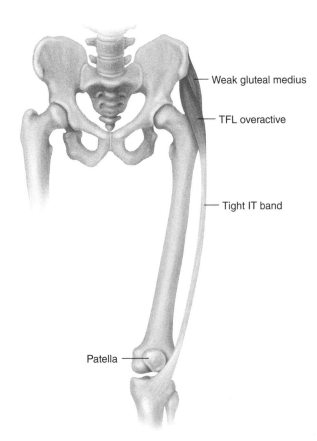

— Weak gluteal medius

— TFL overactive

— Tight IT band

Patella —

Figure 15.8 Biomechanical cause of AKP from muscle imbalance.

as running, going up or down stairs, or squatting or even when resting, when the knee is passively flexed for prolonged durations such as in sitting. The pain may be felt in the soft tissue surrounding the knee or under the patella or both.

Consistent with Janda's pattern of imbalance in the LCS, weakness of the vasti and hip muscles is associated with AKP (Cichanowski et al. 2007; Ireland et al. 2003; Moller et al. 1986; Robinson and Nee 2007). Patients with AKP may demonstrate 25% to 50% reductions in hip abduction, extension, and external rotation. Another possible mechanism for hip weakness that causes knee pain is the IT band acting as a stabilizer for hip stability in the frontal plane (due to gluteus medius weakness). In this case, shortened fascial connections with the distal IT band and the lateral patellar retinaculum could alter patellar tracking, causing AKP (see figure 15.8; Page 2001).

Piva and colleagues (2005) noted poor flexibility in the hamstrings, quadriceps, and gastrocsoleus as well as a significant decrease in hip abductor strength in patients with PFPS. Witvrouw and colleagues (2001) also noted poor flexibility of the hamstrings and quadriceps but found no strength deficits in athletes with patellar tendinitis.

In addition to strength and flexibility, an important consideration in the assessment of AKP is the timing of muscle activation relative to other muscle groups. Voight and Wieder (1991) described a motor control deficit in patients with AKP, noting a reversal of the normal order of firing between the vastus medialis (VM) and the vastus lateralis (VL) in which the VL fired earlier. Depite this observed assymetry in VM and VL activation, it seems that strengthening the muscles that control the patella directly may not be as effective as improving the muscle imbalance at the hip. As little as 6 wk of rehabilitation to improve strength and flexibility of the hip can reduce patellofemoral pain (Tyler et al. 2006).

Recently, researchers in Finland demonstrated that home exercises alone are as effective as home exercises plus arthroscopic surgery for patients with PFPS (Kettunen et al. 2007). Clinically, great emphasis has been placed on strengthening the VM versus the VL in an attempt to improve patellar tracking and control relative to the trochlear groove. The EMG evidence has not supported this idea (Grabiner et al. 1986; Taskiran et al. 1998; Mirzabeigi et al. 1999). With the use of EMG biofeedback, selctive and preferential recruitment of the VM during voluntary activities is possible; however, it does not reduce pain any more so than exercising without biofeedback reduces pain (Zhang and Ng 2007). This apparent lack of effect may be because the major strength imbalance does not occur at the knee but possibly occurs more proximally or even distally.

Biomechanical causes of PFPS can be addressed by evaluating femoral control throughout knee flexion and extension during reversed open chain actions performed with the foot fixed, especially in weight bearing. Grazing and pathological overload of the patella can arise from the relative movement between the femur and the tibia and the lateral displacement of the patella tendon insertion at the tibial tuberosity relative to the femoral trochlear groove. As observed clinically, there is often a loss of transverse control of the femur behind the patella (Gray 1996). This loss of control is due either to excessive or inadequate femoral rotary range or control or to uncoordinated femoral rotation relative to patella position during activity.

Secondary aggravating complications can arise from changes in soft tissue and muscle tone, such as tightening of the IT band and lateral retinaculum, hypertonicity of the VL, spasm of the popliteus, and VM weakness. The vasti muscles can be a source of referred pain to the knee (Travell and Simons 1983), and the VM may be as sensitive as the popliteus to abnormal internal and external rotary stresses at the knee. Weakness of the VM often causes overload of the popliteus as it assists in terminal knee extension through the screw-home mechanism.

Knee Arthroscopy

In addition to the knee injury and its effects on the sensorimotor system, further trauma—albeit skilled and intentional—results from surgery in the athlete. The resulting effect on muscle balance and strength makes it imperative that some form of rehabilitation is carried out after surgery. As suggested by Janda, reflex muscle inhibition occurs after surgery in the quadriceps (Morrisey 1989), not only locally at the surgical site but also at the hip (Jaramillo, Worrell, and Ingersoll 1994) and even in the absence of pain after meniscectomy (Shakespeare et al. 1985). As to be expected, the degree of reflex inhibition can be linked to the degree of joint damage (Hurley 1997). A detailed clinical examination of the patient can reveal a considerable number of inhibited muscles, some of which may be critical for successful rehabilitation. If these inhibitions are not discovered during the clinical examination, the rehabilitation process may be delayed or fail. Scar tissue treatment in terms of pain, nociception, and mobility is critical for postsurgical rehabilitation success.

Anterior Cruciate Ligament Injury

ACL tears are common among athletes in sports requiring quick changes in direction, such as basketball and football. Female athletes are more prone to ACL injury, possibly due to poor control of dynamic knee stability when landing from a jump.

This lack of control may be due to a muscle imbalance involving weak hip extension, abduction, and external rotation (Ireland et al. 2003) that prevents females from counteracting the valgus-adduction-internal-rotation mechanism of ACL injury (see figure 15.9).

The hamstrings counteract the anterior tibial shear and excessive internal tibial rotation of the quadriceps near full extension (Aagaard et al. 2000). Stretch to the ACL inhibits the quadriceps but simultaneously stimulates the hamstrings (Solomonow et al. 1987). Hamstring weakness in female athletes has also been implicated as a factor for ACL injury (Buckley and Kaminski 2003). Some authors recommend specific hamstrings-to-quadriceps strength ratios to prevent ACL injury (Moore and Wade 1989), while others report no relationship between knee strength imbalances and injuries (Grace et al. 1984). Baratta and colleagues (1988) reported that athletes with hypertrophied quadriceps had inhibited hamstrings unless they actively included hamstring strengthening in their programs. These authors suggested that failing to exercise the antagonist hamstrings increases the risk of ligamentous damage.

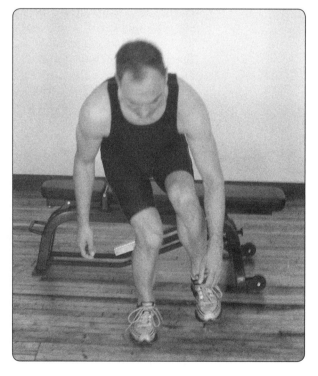

Figure 15.9 The mechanism of ACL injury.

The ACL is thought to play an important proprioceptive role in knee stability; when it is damaged or absent, there is a loss of afferent information necessary for ideal muscle function (Barrack et al. 1989; Pitman et al. 1992). Single-leg balance can also decline (Zätterstrom et al. 1994) as a result of ACL deficiency (ACL-D).

Patients with ACL-D are at a higher risk of developing knee OA due to chronic instability and loss of afferent input from the ACL (O'Connor et al. 1992); therefore, surgical reconstruction of the ACL is often necessary. A significant degree of proprioception can be restored by sensory reinnervation of the ACL graft postsurgery (Ochi et al. 2002). After ACL injury, strength and balance can be improved with training, especially with SMT as described in chapter 11 (Beard et al. 1994; Chmielewski et al. 2005; Fitzgerald et al. 2000; Ihara and Nakayama 1986; Risberg et al. 2007; Zätterstrom et al. 1994). SMT has been found to be more effective than strength training in restoring neuromuscular function after ACL injury (Beard et al. 1994; Ihara and Nakayama 1986; Risberg et al. 2007).

Postoperative complications associated with muscle imbalance may hinder rehabilitation. Page (2001) reported that 79% of patients with ACL reconstruction and AKP have a tight IT band and weak hip abductors. The incidence of OA among patients with reconstructed knees is very high: Up to 78% of injured knees had degenerative changes (von Porat et al. 2004). This is not surprising in the light of the following findings in patients who previously underwent ACL reconstruction:

- Altered muscle activation, often with increased EMG activity of the hamstrings and quadriceps inhibition (Williams et al. 2005)

- Altered quality of the chondral and ligamentous knee restraints (Vasara et al. 2005)

- Elevated cartilage metabolic markers for up to 2 y after surgical repair, suggesting abnormal cartilage metabolism (Beynnon et al. 2005)

Knee Osteoarthritis

As stated previously, Janda's muscle imbalance patterns are seen clinically in OA. Interestingly, quadriceps weakness has been identified as a cause of knee OA (Becker et al. 2004; Hootman et al. 2004; Slemenda et al. 1997; Slemenda et al. 1998), a finding that connects muscle imbalance and OA. In fact, there is a 64% less risk of developing knee OA when the quadriceps is strong (Hootman et al. 2004). Fitzgerald and colleagues (2004) suggested that quadriceps activation failure is a possible neuromuscular mechanism for knee OA. In this case the muscle is not weak so much as it is not able to contract efficiently.

While strength and ROM deficits in patients with knee OA are obvious, a less obvious but important factor that often goes unappreciated is the loss of proprioception as a result of the physical changes within the joints. This loss can lead to a decreased awareness of body position and increased postural sway (Hassan et al. 2001; Wegener et al. 1997). Reduced proprioception in older adults may be responsible for the initiation or advancement of knee degeneration (Barrett et al. 1991). This may be due to a process termed *neurogenic acceleration of osteoarthrosis* by O'Connor and colleagues (1992). Neurogenic acceleration is the loss of afferent proprioceptive input combined with joint instability that speeds up the arthritic process.

The use of elastic knee bandages was found to increase the proprioceptive ability of joint position sense by 40% (Barrett et al. 1991). This finding indicates that external supports or tape may be useful in giving proprioceptive feedback by allowing the patient to access afferent information from other receptors or to use existing proprioception more efficiently.

Foot and Ankle Injury and Pain

When viewed as part of a kinetic chain, the distal end of the lower extremity can be an important instigator in the development and maintenance of pathology throughout the body. As noted in chapter 2, the foot is a very important area for proprioception as well as for posture and balance. Two common foot and ankle pathologies involving muscle imbalance and sensorimotor dysfunction are chronic ankle sprains and plantar fasciitis.

Chronic Ankle Sprains

A significant amount of research has been done on the etiology, consequences, and rehabilitation of ankle sprains. Acute lateral ankle sprains have been associated with muscle imbalances, particularly weakness of the dorsiflexors and invertors (Baumhauer et al. 2001; Wilkerson et al. 1997), as well as impairments in balance (Goldie et al. 1994). In many cases, acute ankle sprains heal without incident and leave no noticeable deficits; however, ankle sprains may also lead to impairments such as chronic instability, pain and swelling, and increased risk for reinjury.

Chronic ankle sprains are also referred to as *functional ankle instability* (FAI). They have been associated with arthrogenic muscle weakness (McVey et al. 2005; Tropp 1986), including inhibition of the peroneals (Hopkins and Palmieri 2004; Santilli et al. 2005) and even the hip abductors (Nicholas et al. 1976; Bullock-Saxton 1994). However, contradictory evidence stating that weakness is not a factor has also been given (Kaminski et al. 2001; Lentell et al. 1990; Ryan 1994). Rather than weakness, altered muscle activation patterns have been found in patients with FAI. Onset latency in several muscle groups is altered in the ankle (Delahunt et al. 2006; Konradsen and Ravn 1990) as well as in the hip abductors and hip extensors (Beckman and Buchanan 1995; Bullock-Saxton et al. 1994).

FAI is most likely due to a sensorimotor dysfunction rather than a strength deficit (Tropp, Askling, and Gillquist 1985). More than 30 years ago, Freeman and colleagues (1965) described functional instability as a loss of afferent proprioceptive input with a resulting loss of dynamic muscular stabilization in soldiers with chronic ankle sprains and normal strength. More recently, Ryan (1994) confirmed their findings, reporting normal strength but significant impairments in single-leg balance in patients with FAI. Deafferentation (the loss of afferent proprioceptive input) has been considered to be a factor limiting the ability of recovery after injury (Cornwall and Murrell 1991; Freeman 1965; Nicholas et al. 1976; Lentell et al. 1990). It is quite possible that due to the varied circumstances, degree of damage, and individual sensory motor responses involved during and after injury, different compensatory factors may occur at different times with different individuals. Hence the apparent conflicting evidence.

Clinically the importance of proprioception from the lower leg has long been acknowledged. Fitzpatrick and colleagues (1994) found that the most critical factor in maintaining upright stance and determining postural sway was afferent input from the lower legs. O'Connell (1971) had long ago demonstrated the effect of impaired proprioception on the positive support reaction or extensor thrust reaction that arises from stimulation of the cutaneous, muscle, and joint mechanoreceptors of the foot. This input, combined with other complex stimuli, is necessary for maintaining upright posture and gait. Several authors (Cornwall and Murrell 1991; McGuire et al. 2000; Payne 1997; Tropp et al. 1984) have found evidence supporting the role that proprioception plays in maintaining balance and proper function of the lower extremity and limiting the risk for ankle injury. The compensatory postural changes and reliance on hip stability and strategies for balance seen in FAI (Brunt 1992; Perrin et al. 1997; Pinstaar et al. 1996; Tropp and Odenrick 1988) may predispose the individual to further injury or pain.

The rehabilitation approach at present favors the use of unstable surfaces and SMT (see chapter 11) to aid the individual in regaining strength, eliminating inhibition, or compensating more efficiently for deafferentation. In 1965, Freeman described the use of unstable rocker and wobble boards to restore the automatic sensorimotor functions of the ankle and lower extremity in soldiers with FAI. Many authors have demonstrated that SMT for 4 to 8 wk has very positive effects on improving proprioception, functional stability, balance, and postural control (Clark et al. 2005; Eils and Rosenbaum 2001; Freeman et al. 1965; Gauffin et al. 1988; Linford et al. 2006; Hale et al. 2007; Holme et al. 1999; Kidgell et al. 2007; Osborne et al. 2001; Tropp et al. 1984; Wester et al. 1996). More recently, Osborne and colleagues (2001) found that SMT in patients with chronic ankle sprain improves muscle activation speed in both ankles, suggesting a possible training effect on the entire CNS.

In the 1970s, Janda developed balance sandals (see figure 11.13 on page 168) for use in SMT. These sandals increase the level of activation and reduce the onset activation time in the lower leg (Blackburn et al. 2003; Lanza et al. 2003) and hip (Bullock-Saxton et al. 1993; Myers et al. 2003). SMT can also be prophylactic in reducing the risk for injury (Clark et al. 2005; Holme et al. 1999; McHugh et al. 2007; van der Wees 2006; Verhagen et al. 2005; Wester et al. 1996). While full recovery and ideal kinematics may not be attainable, a well-rounded and specific rehabilitation plan coupled with a sensible choice of future activities may allow the patient many years of pain-free function and a high quality of life.

Plantar Fasciitis

This condition is a common pathology of the plantar foot for both sexes. It reaches a peak among women 40 to 60 y old and is not uncommon among athletes. The origin of the fascial and muscle tissue (Forman and Green 1990) at the medial calcaneal tubercle is the classic location for pain, although lateral fascial foot pain is sometimes present. Pain is often more intense upon loading the foot after significant rest, such as when rising in the morning. It can also result from a sudden increase in load or prolonged standing or walking. Other exacerbating factors include pes planus and weight gain (Prichasuk and Subhadrabandhu 1994).

Plantar fasciitis is thought to be caused by excessive overload of the plantar fascia and foot intrinsic muscles due to improper biomechanics (Root, Orion, and Weed 1977; Valmassey 1996). The increased tendo-osseous strain resulting from compromise of the windlass mechanism (the tightening of the plantar fascia and increase in foot arch height and stability via dorsiflexion of the hallux by virtue of the fascia's attachment to the hallux; Hicks 1954) due to loss of functional stability either within the foot or within the proximal hip and pelvic area leads to inflammation and sometimes tears within the tissue. Failure of the pelvis to perform its suspension function and the proximal musculature to help supinate and lock the foot or control the rate of load onto the foot from proximally to distally (top-down) often contributes to this etiology.

While muscle imbalance has been found in plantar fasciitis, more research is needed to determine if muscle imbalance is a cause or effect of plantar fasciitis. Increased tension on the Achilles tendon increases the strain on the plantar fascia (Cheung et al. 2006). Not surprisingly, Achilles tightness and lack of ankle dorsiflexion are associated with plantar fasciitis (Kibler et al. 1991; Riddle et al. 2003). Weakness around the ankle and in the intrinsic foot muscles has also been reported (Allen and Gross 2003; Kibler et al. 1991).

Loss of intrinsic muscle function is often overlooked. If left untreated, it can lead to an unresolved condition of plantar fasciitis. For example, loss of strength in the flexor hallucis brevis may lead to an unstable first ray. In turn, the control of the foot into pronation and the effectiveness of the windlass mechanism can both be compromised as the first ray becomes unstable and elevates during load bearing. Given the numerous steps taken during an average day, the repetitive strain on the passive restraining structures such as the plantar fascia can cumulate and eventually lead to symptoms.

Conservative treatments such as stretching, taping, orthotics, and night splints have been used successfully in the treatment of plantar fasciitis; however, a review of treatment strategies for plantar fasciitis did not deem any definitive approach as being more efficacious due to a lack of randomized controlled trials (Atkins et al. 1999; Crawford and Thomson 2003). Recently, a non-weight-bearing stretch of the first metatarsophalangeal joint and foot was shown to be more effective than traditional weight-bearing Achilles stretches in reducing chronic heel pain (see figure 15.10; DiGiovanni et al. 2003). Elastic band taping to unload the plantar fascia may also be useful. Massage of the plantar fascia before getting out of bed in the morning is also helpful (see figure 15.11).

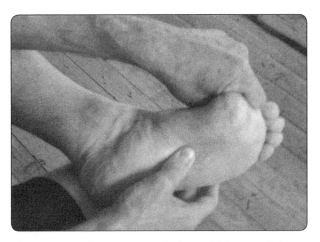

Figure 15.10 First metatarsophalangeal joint stretch for plantar fasciitis.

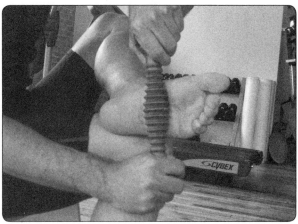

Figure 15.11 Massage for morning plantar fasciitis pain.

Case Study

A young male aged 32 y presented with left foot pain diagnosed as plantar fasciitis. He had been experiencing symptoms for the past 3 wk and described significant pain (5/10), especially upon rising and initial weight bearing and ambulation. The symptoms decreased with continued ambulation. Running provoked symptoms after several minutes. So far, rest and decreased activity had not improved his symptoms, and the patient was eager to return to his activities, such as playing basketball and running 2 or 3 times a week.

Examination and Assessment

On physical examination, the patient's posture was grossly unremarkable. He exhibited no signs of significant UCS, LCS, or layer syndrome. However, he did present with bilateral forefoot varus and increased midfoot pronation on the left in standing and during gait. Decreased active and passive internal rotation of the left hip was noted (see figure 15.12). There was also decreased dorsiflexion ROM at the left talocrural joint. There was local tenderness at the medial calcaneal tuberosity and along the medial aspect of the plantar fascia. There were also TrPs located in the plantar intrinsics such as the quadratus plantae, medial gastrocnemius, external hip rotators, and lumbar paraspinal musculature (see figure 15.13).

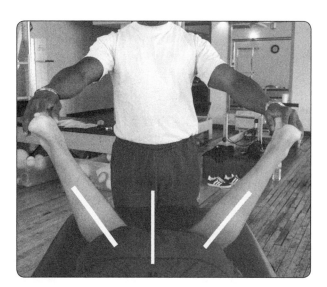

Figure 15.12 Limited internal rotation in the case study patient.

MMT for inhibition demonstrated decreased strength (4/5) and inhibition of the tibialis anterior, flexor hallucis longus, VM, gluteus medius and maximus, and short external rotators of the hip. Tightness of the hip adductors (especially the one-joint adductors) was noted. Single-leg balance was poor, with the patient displaying qualitative and quantitative deficits on both sides. He could balance for only about 10 s with increased hip sway and high activity of the lower-extremity muscles.

Gait assessment revealed poor ability to control the leg in the transverse plane and increased internal rotation excursion during the stance phase on the affected side. There was a loss of hip extension at heel rise and toe-off. This diminished when the patient walked while carrying a lightweight book overhead. This observation indicated a coordination deficit that responded to neural challenging for balance.

The breathing stereotype was also assessed for signs of inefficient use of the diaphragm and therefore possible compromise of torso stability. In this case it was not pathological.

The clinical evaluation aims to document not only the postural presentation but also data pertaining to the tone changes and nociceptive and pain distribution patterns that represent the level of compensation within the system. In addition, balance deficits can be related to functional deficits that affect the patient's ability to control his body spatially. The pattern of muscle inhibition and overactivation, along with the aforementioned data, provides insight into CNS function and dysfunction. It is from this viewpoint that the clinician must engage the rehabilitation process and its principles.

1-Minute Nociceptive Exam™　　　　**Client Name** _____

LEFT	RIGHT
☐　Coccyx	☐　Coccyx
☒　SI joint	☐　SI joint
☒　L4/5/S1	☐　L4/5/S1
☐　L1	☐　L1
☒　11th & 12th ribs	☐　11th & 12th ribs
☒　Diaphragm	☐　Diaphragm
☒　Costosternal junction	☒　Costosternal junction
☒　Upper th spine	☒　Upper th spine
☐　C7/Th1	☒　C7/Th1
☐　1st & 2nd ribs	☒　1st & 2nd ribs
☐　Levator scapulae	☒　Levator scapulae
☐　Infraspinatus	☒　Infraspinatus
☐　Ligamentum nuchae	☒　Ligamentum nuchae
☐　Splenius capitis	☒　Splenius capitis
☐　Rectus capitis posterior minor	☒　Rectus capitis posterior minor
☐　Occipitalis	☐　Occipitalis
☐　Sphenoid/zygomatic arch	☒　Sphenoid/zygomatic arch
☐　Masseter	☒　Masseter
☐　Anterior digastric	☐　Anterior digastric
☐　Omohyoid	☐　Omohyoid
☒　Flexor policis brevis	☒　Flexor policis brevis
☒　Medial gastrocnemius	☐　Medial gastrocnemius
☒　Short hip adductors	☐　Short hip adductors
☒　Foot intrinsics	☐　Foot intrinsics

Figure 15.13　Diagram of TrP locations in the case study patient.

Treatment and Outcome

Physical therapy was initiated twice a week. The patient was treated with PRRT (see chapter 9), which significantly reduced palpatory discomfort along the entire TrP chain and increased hip and ankle ROM. Origin–insertion facilitation and brushing of the quadratus plantae, flexor hallucis longus, tibialis anterior, VM, short external rotators, and gluteus medius were implemented. Isometric exercises were also used to assist in muscle facilitation. Teaching of the short foot and SMT for balance and coordination was introduced with bilateral and later unilateral stance positions during both the static and dynamic phases (see figure 15.14). The functional phase, including step-ups, step-downs, and lunges, was added as tolerated. The quality of control in three dimensions, absence of pain, and maintenance of normal muscle function were the criteria for progression. Retro walking on a treadmill was used to help facilitate hip extension with lumbopelvic stability and to challenge respiration while maintaining stability. Since the patient displayed no true contractures within the musculature, no aggressive stretching was administered. He performed full-ROM exercises as part of his routine. He was taught PIR techniques for the plantar intrinsics and hold relax for the gastrocnemius and soleus complex for postactivity release. Elastic resistance was introduced toward the end of the rehabilitation process to provide added load to his workouts as he progressed to jumping, hopping, and cutting drills used to prepare him for a return to his usual ADL.

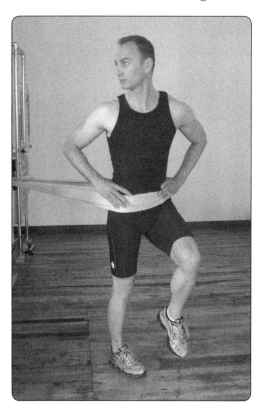

Figure 15.14 Standing external and internal hip rotation.

The patient responded well and within six visits was pain free and able to start running again. He was limited at first to alternating walking and running as he increased his distances. His single-leg balance increased to 17 s per side, and he required less muscle activity to maintain his position. His ROM became symmetrical in the ankle and hips. The left foot appeared to be controlled better during loading. The patient also returned to basketball 5 wk later, working on jumping and landing and improving the endurance strength for this activity through exercise drills and microprogression of activities.

Janda's Approach Versus the Traditional Approach

The Janda approach is an attempt to define the process of rehabilitation through the evaluation and treatment of the sensory-motor system and CNS as an indivisible unit. The traditional approach with its Cartesian divisions and isolation of treatment to specific areas alone while ignoring the interrelationships that exist between different parts of the the body and the CNS is becoming obsolete. Table 15.1 is a brief overview of some of these differences.

Table 15.1 Comparison of Janda Approach and Traditional Approach for Rehabilitation in Case Study

Rehabilitation process aspects	Janda approach	Traditional approach
Emphasis on breathing stereotype	Yes	No
Assessment for LCS, UCS, or layer syndrome	Yes	No
Qualitative gait analysis	Yes	No
Breathing assessment	Yes	Seldom
Use of short foot	Yes	No
Cognitive challenge	Yes	Not usually
SMT for initial and continued strengthening	Yes	Not usually
Use of traditional machine-based exercise	No	Common

Summary

Assessment and treatment of muscle imbalances may have a role in reducing lower-extremity injuries by identifying individuals at increased risk (Knapik et al. 1991). While more prospective studies are needed to establish a cause-and-effect relationship between muscle imbalances and injury, imbalances associated with injury risk have been identified in the groin (Tyler et al. 2001) and knee (Witvrouw et al. 2001). Quadriceps weakness has also been identified as a risk factor for developing knee OA (Hootman et al. 2004).

Assessment of postural stability and proprioception may also help prevent ankle injuries (Payne 1997; Tropp et al. 1994) by identifying individuals who may benefit from preventive SMT. SMT, including the use of balance boards and foam stability trainers, has been shown to reduce the risk for ACL injury (Caraffa et al. 1996; Cerulli et al. 2001; Myklebust et al. 2003) and ankle sprains (Clark et al. 2005; McHugh et al. 2007; Sheth et al. 1995; van der Wees 2006; Verhagen et al. 2005). SMT can also be used in preseason and in-season sport training programs to reduce injuries in soccer, handball, and volleyball (Ekstrand et al. 1983; Emery et al. 2005; Knobloch et al. 2005; Malliou et al. 2004; Petersen et al. 2005; Wedderkopp et al. 1999; Wedderkopp et al. 2003). It is therefore necessary to perform a comprehensive global exam of the patient to assess for sensorimotor deficits that may lead to possible injury. A program of general strengthening is a poor substitute for proper evaluation.

REFERENCES

Aagaard, P., E.B. Simonsen, J.L. Andersen, S.P. Magnusson, F. Bojsen-Møller, and P. Dyhre-Poulsen. 2000. Antagonist muscle coactivation during isokinetic knee extension. *Scand J Med Sci Sports* 10(2): 58-67.

Aarås, A, M.B. Veierød, S. Larsen, R. Ortengren, and O. Ro. 1996. Reproducibility and stability of normalized EMG measurements on musculus trapezius. *Ergonomics* 39(2): 171-85.

Abdulwahab, S.S., and M. Sabbahi. 2000. Neck retractions, cervical root decompression, and radicular pain. *J Orthop Sports Phys Ther* 30(1): 4-9.

Abrahams, V.C. 1977. The physiology of neck muscles; their role in head movement and maintenance of posture. *Can J Physiol Pharmacol* 55(3): 332-8.

Agabegi, S.S., R.A. Freiberg, J.M. Plunkett, and P.J. Stern. 2007. Thumb abduction strength measurement in carpal tunnel syndrome. *J Hand Surg [Am]* 32(6): 859-66.

Ahlgren, C., K. Waling, F. Kadi, M. Djupsjöbacka, L.E. Thornell, and G. Sundelin. 2001. Effects on physical performance and pain from three dynamic training programs for women with work-related trapezius myalgia. *J Rehabil Med* 33(4): 162-9.

Akalin, E., O. El, O. Peker, O. Senocak, S. Tamci, S. Gülbahar, R. Cakmur, and S. Oncel. 2002. Treatment of carpal tunnel syndrome with nerve and tendon gliding exercises. *Am J Phys Med Rehabil* 81(2): 108-13.

Alderink, G.J., and D.J. Kuck. 1986. Isokinetic shoulder strength of high school and college-aged pitchers. *J Orthop Sports Phys Ther* 7(4): 163-72.

Alexander, K.M., and T.L. LaPier. 1998. Differences in static balance and weight distribution between normal subjects and subjects with chronic unilateral low back pain. *J Orthop Sports Phys Ther* 28(6): 378-83.

Alexander, R. 2008. Functional fascial taping for lower back pain: A case report. *J Bodyw Mov Ther* 12(3): 263-4.

Alfredson, H., T. Pietilä, and R. Lorentzon. 1998. Concentric and eccentric shoulder and elbow muscle strength in female volleyball players and non-active females. *Scand J Med Sci Sports* 8(5 Pt. 1): 265-70.

Alizadehkhaiyat, O., A.C. Fisher, G.J. Kemp, and S.P. Frostick. 2007. Strength and fatigability of selected muscles in upper limb: Assessing muscle imbalance relevant to tennis elbow. *J Electromyogr Kinesiol* 17(4): 428-36.

Alizadehkhaiyat, O., A.C. Fisher, G.J. Kemp, K. Vishwanathan, and S.P. Frostick. 2008. Assessment of functional recovery in tennis elbow. *J Electromyogr Kinesiol* [In press].

Alizadehkhaiyat, O., A.C. Fisher, G.J. Kemp, K. Vishwanathan, and S.P. Frostick. 2007. Upper limb muscle imbalance in tennis elbow: A functional and electromyographic assessment. *J Orthop Res* 25(12): 1651-7.

Alkjaer, T., E.B. Simonsen, S.P. Peter Magnusson, H. Aagaard, and P. Dyhre-Poulsen. 2002. Differences in the movement pattern of a forward lunge in two types of anterior cruciate ligament deficient patients: Copers and non-copers. *Clin Biomech (Bristol, Avon)* 17(8): 586-93.

Alkjaer, T., E.B. Simonsen, U. Jorgensen, and P. Dyhre-Poulsen. 2003. Evaluation of the walking pattern in two types of patients with anterior cruciate ligament deficiency: Copers and non-copers. *Eur J Appl Physiol* 89(3-4): 301-8.

Allegrucci, M., S.L. Whitney, and J.J. Irrgang. 1994. Clinical implications of secondary impingement of the shoulder in freestyle swimmers. *J Orthop Sports Phys Ther* 20(6): 307-18.

Allegrucci, M., S.L. Whitney, S.M. Lephart, J.J. Irrgang, and F.H. Fu. 1995. Shoulder kinesthesia in healthy unilateral athletes participating in upper extremity sports. *J Orthop Sports Phys Ther* 21(4): 220-6.

Allen, R.H., and Gross, M.T. 2003. Toe flexors strength and passive extension range of motion of the first metatarsophalangeal joint in individuals with plantar fasciitis. *J Orthop Sports Phys Ther.* Aug;33(8): 468-78.

Alpert, S.W., M.M. Pink, F.W. Jobe, P.J. McMahon, and W. Mathiyakom. 2000. Electromyographic analysis of deltoid and rotator cuff function under varying loads and speeds. *J Shoulder Elbow Surg* 9(1): 47-58.

Al-Shenqiti, A.M., and J.A. Oldham. 2005. Test-retest reliability of myofascial trigger point detection in patients with rotator cuff tendonitis. *Clin Rehabil* 19(5): 482-7.

Alum, J.H., B.R. Bloem, M.G. Carpenter, M. Hulliger, and M. Hadders-Algra. 1998. Proprioceptive control of posture: A review of new concepts. *Gait Posture* 8(3): 214-42.

Andersen, L.L., M. Kjaer, K. Søgaard, L. Hansen, A.I. Kryger, and G. Sjøgaard. 2008. Effect of two contrasting types of physical exercise on chronic neck muscle pain. *Arthritis Rheum* 59(1): 84-91.

Anderson, K. and D.G. Behm. 2005. Trunk muscle activity increases with unstable squat movements. *Can J Appl Physiol.* 30(1): 33-45.

Andersson, E.A., J. Nilsson, Z. Ma, and A. Thorstensson. 1997. Abdominal and hip flexor muscle activation during various training exercises. *Eur J Appl Physiol Occup Physiol* 75(2): 115-23.

Aniss, A.M., S.C. Gandevia, and D. Burke. 1992. Reflex responses in active muscles elicited by stimulation of low-threshold afferents from the human foot. *J Neurophysiol.* 67 (5): 1375-84.

Apreleva, M., C.T. Hasselman, R.E. Debski, F.H. Fu, S.L. Woo, and J.J. Warner. 1998. A dynamic analysis of glenohumeral motion after simulated capsulolabral injury. A cadaver model. *J Bone Joint Surg Am* 80(4): 474-80.

Arokoski, J.P., M. Kankaanpaa, T. Valta, I. Juvonen, J. Partanen, S. Taimela, K.A. Lindgren, and O. Airaksinen. 1999. Back and hip extensor muscle function during therapeutic exercises. *Arch Phys Med Rehabil* 80(7): 842-50.

Arokoski, J.P., T. Valta, O. Airaksinen, and M. Kankaanpaa. 2001. Back and abdominal muscle function during stabilization exercises. *Arch Phys Med Rehabil* 82: 1089-98.

Aronen, J.G., and K. Regan. 1984. Decreasing the incidence of recurrence of first time anterior shoulder dislocations with rehabilitation. *Am J Sports Med* 12(4): 283-91.

Aruin, A.S., and M.L. Latash. 1995. Directional specificity of postural muscles in feed-forward postural reactions during fast voluntary arm movements. *Exp Brain Res* 103(2): 323-32.

Arwert, H.J., J. de Groot, W.W. Van Woensel, and P.M. Rozing. 1997. Electromyography of shoulder muscles in relation to force direction. *J Shoulder Elbow Surg* 6(4): 360-70.

Ashton-Miller, J.A. 2004. Thoracic hyperkyphosis in the young athlete: A review of the biomechanical issues. *Curr Sports Med Rep* 3(1): 47-52.

Ashton-Miller, J.A., E.M. Wojtys, L.J. Huston, and D. Fry-Welch. 2001. Can proprioception really be improved by exercises? *Knee Surg Sports Traumatol Arthrosc* 9(3): 128-36.

Atkins, D., Crawford, F., Edwards, J., and Lambert, M. 1999. A systematic review of treatments for the painful heel. *Rheumatology (Oxford).* Oct;38(10): 968-73. Review.

Azevedo, D.C., T. de Lima Pires, F. de Souza Andrade, and M.K. McDonnell. 2008. Influence of scapular position on the pressure pain threshold of the upper trapezius muscle region. *Eur J Pain* 12(2): 226-32.

Babyar, S.R. 1996. Excessive scapular motion in individuals recovering from painful and stiff shoulders: Causes and treatment strategies. *Phys Ther* 76(3): 226-38.

Backman, E., A. Bengtsson, M. Bengtsson, C. Lennmarken, and K.G. Henriksson. 1988. Skeletal muscle function in primary fibromyalgia. Effect of regional sympathetic blockade with guanethidine. *Acta Neurol Scand* 77(3): 187-91.

Bagg, S.D., and W.J. Forrest. 1986. Electromyographic study of the scapular rotators during arm abduction in the scapular plane. *Am J Phys Med* 65(3): 111-24.

Bagg, S.D., and W.J. Forrest. 1988. A biomechanical analysis of scapular rotation during arm abduction in the scapular plane. *Am J Phys Med Rehabil* 67(6): 238-45.

Bahr, R., O. Lian, and I.A. Bahr. 1997. A twofold reduction in the incidence of acute ankle sprains in volleyball after the introduction of an injury prevention program: A prospective cohort study. *Scand J Med Sci Sports* 7(3): 172-7.

Bak, K. 1996. Nontraumatic glenohumeral instability and coracoacromial impingement in swimmers. *Scand J Med Sci Sports* 6(3): 132-44.

Bak, K., and P. Faunø. 1997. Clinical findings in competitive swimmers with shoulder pain. *Am J Sports Med* 25(2): 254-60.

Bak, K., and S.P. Magnusson. 1997. Shoulder strength and range of motion in symptomatic and pain-free elite swimmers. *Am J Sports Med* 25(4): 454-9.

Ballantyne, B.T., S.J. O'Hare, J.L. Paschall, M.M. Pavia-Smith, A.M. Pitz, J.F. Gillon, and G.L. Soderberg. 1993. Electromyographic activity of selected shoulder muscles in commonly used therapeutic exercises. *Phys Ther* 73(10): 668-77.

Balogun, A., C.O. Adesinasi, and D.K. Marzouk. 1992. The effects of a wobble board exercise training program on static balance performance and strength of lower extremity muscles. *Physiother Can* **44**: 23-30.

Balogun, J.A., A.A. Olokungbemi, and A.R. Kuforiji. 1992. Spinal mobility and muscular strength: effects of supine- and prone-lying back extension exercise training. *Arch Phys Med Rehabil* 73(8): 745-51.

Baltaci, G., and V.B. Tunay. 2004. Isokinetic performance at diagonal pattern and shoulder mobility in elite overhead athletes. *Scand J Med Sci Sports* 14(4): 231-8.

Bandholm, T., L. Rasmussen, P. Aagaard, B.R. Jensen, and L. Diederichsen. 2006. Force steadiness, muscle activity, and maximal muscle strength in subjects with subacromial impingement syndrome. *Muscle Nerve* 34(5): 631-9.

Bansevicius, D., and O. Sjaastad. 1996. Cervicogenic headache: The influence of mental load on pain level and EMG of shoulder-neck and facial muscles. *Headache* 36(6): 372-8.

Bansevicius, D., R.H. Westgaard, and T. Stiles. 2001. EMG activity and pain development in fibromyalgia patients exposed to mental stress of long duration. *Scand J Rheumatol* 30(2): 92-8.

Baratta, R., M. Solomonow, B.H. Zhou, D. Letson, R. Chuinard, and R. D'Ambrosia. 1988. Muscular coactivation. The role of the antagonist musculature in maintaining knee stability. *Am J Sports Med* 16(2): 113-22.

Barden, J.M., R. Balyk, V.J. Raso, M. Moreau, and K. Bagnall. 2005. Atypical shoulder muscle activation in multidirectional instability. *Clin Neurophysiol* 116(8): 1846-57.

Barker, P.J., and C.A. Briggs. 1999. Attachments of the posterior layer of lumbar fascia. *Spine* 24(17): 1757-64.

Barker, S., M. Kesson, J. Ashmore, G. Turner, J. Conway, and D. Stevens. 2000. Guidance for pre manipulative testing of the cervical spine. *Man Ther* 5: 37-40.

Barrack, R.L., H.B. Skinner, and S.L. Buckley. 1989. Proprioception in the anterior cruciate deficient knee. *Am J Sports Med* 17(1): 1-6.

Barrett, D.S., A.G. Cobb, and G. Bentley. 1991. Joint proprioception in normal, osteoarthritic and replaced knees. *J Bone Joint Surg Br* 73(1): 53-6.

Barton, P.M., and K.C. Hayes. 1996. Neck flexor muscle strength, efficiency, and relaxation times in normal subjects and subjects with unilateral neck pain and headache. *Arch Phys Med Rehabil* 77(7): 680-7.

Basmajian, J.A. 1985. *Muscles alive. Their functions revealed by electromyography.* 5th ed. Baltimore: Lippincott Williams & Wilkins.

Bassett, R.W., A.O. Browne, B.F. Morrey, and K.N. An. 1990. Glenohumeral muscle force and moment mechanics in a position of shoulder instability. *J Biomech* 23(5): 405-15.

Batt, B.E., J.L. Tanji, and N. Skattum. 1996. Plantar fasciitis: A prospective randomized clinical trial of the tension night splint. *Clin J Sport Med* 6: 158-62.

Bauer, J.A., and R.D. Murray. 1999. Electromyographic patterns of individuals suffering from lateral tennis elbow. *J Electromyogr Kinesiol* 9(4): 245-52.

Baumhauer, J.F., D.M. Alosa, A.F. Renstrom, S. Trevino, and B. Beynnon. 1995. A prospective study of ankle injury risk factors. *Am J Sports Med* 23(5): 564-70.

Bayramoglu, M., R. Toprak, and S. Sozay. 2007. Effects of osteoarthritis and fatigue on proprioception of the knee joint. *Arch Phys Med Rehabil.* 88(3): 346-50.

Baysal, O., Z. Altay, C. Ozcan, K. Ertem, S. Yologlu, and A. Kayhan. 2006. Comparison of three conservative treatment protocols in carpal tunnel syndrome. *Int J Clin Pract* 60(7): 820-8.

Beard, D.J., C.A.F. Dodd, H.R. Trundle, and A. Simpson. 1994. Proprioception enhancement for anterior cruciate ligament deficiency. *J Bone Joint Surg Br* 76B: 654-9.

Beard, D.J., P.J. Kyberd, C.M. Fergusson, and C.A. Dodd.1993. Proprioception after rupture of the anterior cruciate ligament. An objective indication of the need for surgery? *J Bone Joint Surg Br* 75(2): 311-5.

Becker, R., Berth, A., Nehring, M., and Awiszus, F. 2004. Neuromuscular quadriceps dysfunction prior to osteoarthritis of the knee. *J Orthop Res.* Jul;22(4): 768-73.

Beckett, M.E., D.L. Massie, K.D. Bowers, and D.A. Stol. 1992. Incidence of hyperpronation in the ACL injured knee: A clinical perpective. *J Athl Train* 27: 58-62.

Beckman, S.M., and T.S. Buchanan. 1995. Ankle inversion injury and hypermobility: Effect on hip and ankle muscle electromyography onset latency. *Arch Phys Med Rehabil* 76(12): 1138-43.

Bednar, D.A., F.W. Orr, and G.T. Simon. 1995. Observations on the pathomorphology of the thoracolumbar fascia in chronic mechanical back pain. A microscopic study. *Spine* 20(10): 1161-4.

Behm, D.G., A.M. Leonard, W.B. Young, W.A. Bonsey, and S.N. MacKinnon. 2005. Trunk muscle electromyographic activity with unstable and unilateral exercises. *J Strength Cond Res.* 19(1): 193-201

Belling Sørensen, A.K., and U. Jørgensen. 2000. Secondary impingement in the shoulder. An improved terminology in impingement. *Scand J Med Sci Sports* 10(5): 266-78.

Bennett, R.M. 1996. Fibromyalgia and the disability dilemma. A new era in understanding a complex, multidimensional pain syndrome. *Arthritis Rheum* 39(10): 1627-34.

Bennett, S.E., R.J. Schenk, and E.D. Simmons. 2002. Active range of motion utilized in the cervical spine to perform daily functional tasks. *J Spinal Disord Tech* 15(4): 307-11.

Benson, H. 1984. Beyond the relaxation response. New York: Berkeley.

Berg, H.E., G. Berggren, and P.A. Tesch. 1994. Dynamic neck strength training effect on pain and function. *Arch Phys Med Rehabil* 75(6): 661-5.

Berglund, B., E.L. Harju, E. Kosek, and U. Lindblom. 2002. Quantitative and qualitative perceptual analysis of cold dysesthesia and hyperalgesia in fibromyalgia. *Pain* 96(1-2): 177-87.

Bergmark, A. 1989. Stability of the lumbar spine: A study in mechanical engineering. *Acta Orthop Scand Suppl.* 230: 1-54.

Beukeboom, C., T.B. Birmingham, L. Forwell, and D. Ohrling. 2000. Asymmetrical strength changes and injuries in athletes training on a small radius curve indoor track. *Clin J Sport Med* 10(4): 245-50.

Bey, M.J., S.K. Brock, W.N. Beierwaltes, R. Zauel, P.A. Kolowich, and T.R. Lock. 2007. In vivo measurement of subacromial space width during shoulder elevation: Technique and preliminary results in patients following unilateral rotator cuff repair. *Clin Biomech (Bristol, Avon)* 22(7): 767-73.

Beynnon, B.D., B.S. Uh BS R.J. Johnson, J.A. Abate, C.E. Nichols, B.C. Fleming, A.R. Poole, and H. Roos.

2005. Rehabilitation after anterior cruciate ligament reconstruction: A prospective, randomized, double-blind comparison of programs administered over 2 different time intervals. *Am J Sports Med* 33(3): 347-59.

Bigliani, L.U., and W.N. Levine. 1997. Subacromial impingement syndrome. *J Bone Joint Surg Am* 79(12): 1854-68.

Bigliani, L.U., J.B. Ticker, E.L. Flatow, L.J. Soslowsky, and V.C. Mow. 1991. The relationship of acromial architecture to rotator cuff disease. *Clin Sports Med* 10(4): 823-38.

Bisset, L., A. Paungmali, B. Vicenzino, and E. Beller. 2005. A systematic review and meta-analysis of clinical trials on physical interventions for lateral epicondylalgia. *Br J Sports Med* 39(7): 411-22.

Blackburn, J.T., C.J. Hirth, and K.M. Guskiewicz. 2002. EMG comparison of lower leg musculature during functional activities with and without balance shoes. Abstract. *J Athl Train* 37(2): S-97.

Blackburn, J.T., C.J. Hirth, and K.M. Guskiewicz. 2003. Exercise sandals increase lower extremity electromyographic activity during functional activities. *J Athl Train* 38(3): 198-203.

Blackwell, J.R., and K.J. Cole. 1994. Wrist kinematics differ in expert and novice tennis players performing the backhand stroke: Implications for tennis elbow. *J Biomech* 27(5): 509-16.

Blasier, R.B., J.E. Carpenter, and L.J. Huston. 1994. Shoulder proprioception. Effect of joint laxity, joint position, and direction of motion. *Orthop Rev* 23(1): 45-50.

Bloem, B.R., J.H. Allum, M.G. Carpenter, and F. Honegger. 2000. Is lower leg proprioception essential for triggering human automatic postural responses? *Exp Brain Res* 130(3): 375-91.

Bloem, B.R., J.H. Allum, M.G. Carpenter, J.J. Verschuuren, and F. Honegger. 2002. Triggering of balance corrections and compensatory strategies in a patient with total leg proprioceptive loss. *Exp Brain Res* 142(1): 91-107.

Bobath, K., and B. Bobath. 1964. The facilitation of normal postural reactions and movement in treatment of cerebral palsy. *Physiotherapy* 50: 246.

Boden, S.D., P.R. McCowin, D.O. Davis, T.S. Dina, A.S. Mark, and W. Wiesel. 1990. Abnormal magnetic-resonance scans of the cervical spine in asymptomatic subjects. A prospective investigation. *J Bone Joint Surg Am* 72(8): 1178-84.

Bohannon, R.W., P.A. Larkin, A.C. Cook, J. Gear, and J. Singer. 1984. Decrease in timed balance test scores with aging. *Phys Ther* 64(7): 1067-70.

Boline, P.D., K. Kassak, G. Bronfort, C. Nelson, and A.V. Anderson. 1995. Spinal manipulation vs. amitriptyline for the treatment of chronic tension-type headaches: A randomized clinical trial. *J Manipulative Physiol Ther* 18(3): 148-54.

Bonica, J.J. 1991. History of pain concepts and pain therapy. *Mt Sinai J Med* 58(3): 191-202.

Borman, P., R. Celiker, and Z. Hasçelik. 1999. Muscle performance in fibromyalgia syndrome. *Rheumatol Int* 19(1-2): 27-30.

Borsa, P.A., G.C. Dover, K.E. Wilk, and M.M. Reinold. 2006. Glenohumeral range of motion and stiffness in professional baseball pitchers. *Med Sci Sports Exerc* 38(1): 21-6.

Borsa, P.A., K.E. Wilk, J.A. Jacobson, J.S. Scibek, G.C. Dover, M.M. Reinold, and J.R. Andrews. 2005. Correlation of range of motion and glenohumeral translation in professional baseball pitchers. *Am J Sports Med* 33(9): 1392-9.

Borsa, P.A., M.K. Timmons, and E.L. Sauers. 2003. Scapular-positioning patterns during humeral elevation in unimpaired shoulders. *J Athl Train* 38(1): 12-7.

Borstad, J.D. 2006. Resting position variables at the shoulder: Evidence to support a posture-impairment association. *Phys Ther* 86(4): 549-57.

Borstad, J.D., and P.M. Ludewig. 2002. Comparison of scapular kinematics between elevation and lowering of the arm in the scapular plane. *Clin Biomech (Bristol, Avon)* 17(9-10): 650-9.

Borstad, J.D., and P.M. Ludewig. 2005. The effect of long versus short pectoralis minor resting length on scapular kinematics in healthy individuals. *J Orthop Sports Phys Ther* 35(4): 227-38.

Borstad, J.D., and P.M. Ludewig. 2006. Comparison of three stretches for the pectoralis minor muscle. *J Shoulder Elbow Surg* 15(3): 324-30.

Bosco, C., M. Cardinale, O. Tsarpela, and E. Locatelli. 1999. New trends in training science: The use of vibrations for enhancing performance. *New Studies in Athletics* 14(4): 55-62.

Bosco, C., R. Colli, E. Introini, M. Cardinale, M. Lacovelli, J. Tihanyi, S.P. von Diuvillard, and A. Vira. 1999. Adaptive responses of human skeletal muscle to vibration exposure *Clin Physiol* 19(2): 183-7.

Bouche, K., V. Stevens, D. Cambier, J. Caemaert, and L. Danneels. 2006. Comparison of postural control in unilateral stance between healthy controls and lumbar discectomy patients with and without pain. *Eur Spine J* 15(4): 423-32.

Boyd-Clark, L.C., C.A. Briggs, and M.P. Galea. 2002. Muscle spindle distribution, morphology, and density in longus colli and multifidus muscles of the cervical spine. *Spine* 27(7): 694-701.

Braun, B.L., and L.R. Amundson. 1989. Quantitative assessment of head and shoulder posture. *Arch Phys Med Rehabil* 70(4): 322-9.

Briggs, C.A., and B.G. Elliott. 1985. Lateral epicondylitis. A review of structures associated with tennis elbow. *Anat Clin* 7(3): 149-53.

Brindle, T.J., J.A. Nyland, A.J. Nitz, and R. Shapiro. 2007. Scapulothoracic latent muscle reaction timing comparison between trained overhead throwers and untrained control subjects. *Scand J Med Sci Sports* 17(3): 252-9.

Bronfort, G., N. Nilsson, M. Haas, R. Evans, C.H. Goldsmith, W.J. Assendelft, and L.M. Bouter. 2004. Noninvasive physical treatments for chronic/recurrent headache. *Cochrane Database Syst Rev* 3: CD001878.

Bronfort, G., W.J. Assendelft, R. Evans, M. Haas, and L. Bouter. 2001. Efficacy of spinal manipulation for chronic headache: A systematic review. *J Manipulative Physiol Ther* 24(7): 457-66.

Brossmann, J., K.W. Preidler, R.A. Pedowitz, L.M. White, D. Trudell, and D. Resnick. 1996. Shoulder impingement syndrome: Influence of shoulder position on rotator cuff impingement—an anatomic study. *AJR Am J Roentgenol* 167(6): 1511-5.

Browne, A.O., P. Hoffmeyer, S. Tanaka, K.N. An, and B.F. Morrey. 1990. Glenohumeral elevation studied in three dimensions. *J Bone Joint Surg Br* 72(5): 843-5.

Brox, J.I., and J.I. Brevik. 1996. Prognostic factors in patients with rotator tendinosis (stage II impingement syndrome) of the shoulder. *Scand J Prim Health Care* 14(2): 100-5.

Brox, J.I., C. Røe, E. Saugen, and N.K. Vøllestad. 1997. Isometric abduction muscle activation in patients with rotator tendinosis of the shoulder. *Arch Phys Med Rehabil* 78(11): 1260-7.

Brox, J.I., E. Gjengedal, G. Uppheim, A.S. Bøhmer, J.I. Brevik, A.E. Ljunggren, and P.H. Staff. 1999. Arthroscopic surgery versus supervised exercises in patients with rotator cuff disease (stage II impingement syndrome): A prospective, randomized, controlled study in 125 patients with a 2 1/2-year follow-up. *J Shoulder Elbow Surg* 8(2): 102-11.

Brox, J.I., P.H. Staff, A.E. Ljunggren, and J.I. Brevik. 1993. Arthroscopic surgery compared with supervised exercises in patients with rotator cuff disease (stage II impingement syndrome). *BMJ* 307(6909): 899-903.

Brügger, A. 2000. *Lehrbuch der Funktionellen Störungen des Bewegungssystems. [Textbook of the functional disturbances of the movement system].* Zollikon/Benglen, Switzerland: Brügger-Verlag.

Bruhn, S., N. Kullmann, and A. Gollhofer. 2004. The effects of a sensorimotor training and a strength training on postural stabilisation, maximum isometric contraction and jump performance. *Int J Sports Med* 25(1): 56-60.

Brumagne, S., P. Cordo, R. Lysens, S. Verschueren, and S. Swinnen. 2000. The role of paraspinal muscle spindles in lumbosacral position sense in individuals with and without low back pain. *Spine* 25: 989-94.

Brunet, M.E., S.D. Cook, M.R. Brinker, and J.A. Dickinson. 1990. A survey of running injuries in 1505 competitive

and recreational runners. *J Sports Med Phys Fitness* 30: 307-15.

Brunt, D., J.C. Andersen, B. Huntsman, L.B. Reinhert, A.C. Thorell, and J.C. Sterling. 1992. Postural responses to lateral perturbation in healthy subjects and ankle sprain patients. *Med Sci Sports Exerc* 24(2): 171-6.

Buchanan, T.S., A.W. Kim, and D.G. Lloyd. 1996. Selective muscle activation following rapid varus/valgus perturbations at the knee. *Med Sci Sports Exerc* 28(7): 870-6.

Buckelew, S.P., R. Conway, J. Parker, W.E. Deuser, J. Read, T.E. Witty, J.E. Hewett, M. Minor, J.C. Johnson, L. Van Male, M.J. McIntosh, M. Nigh, and D.R. Kay. 1998. Biofeedback/relaxation training and exercise interventions for fibromyalgia: A prospective trial. *Arthritis Care Res* 11(3): 196-209.

Buckelew, S.P., R. Conway, J. Parker, W.E. Deuser, J. Read, T.E. Witty, J.E. Hewett et al. 1998. Biofeedback/relaxation training and exercise interventions for fibromyalgia: A prospective trial. *Arthritis Care Res* 11(3): 196-209.

Buckley, B.D., and T.W. Kaminski. 2003. Hamstring and quadriceps strength ratios in healthy males and females: Implications for ACL injury. Abstract. *J Athl Train* 38(2): S14-15.

Büll, M.L., V. de Freitas, and M. Vitti. 1990. Electromyographic study of the trapezius (pars superior) and serratus anterior (pars inferior) in free movements of the arm. *Anat Anz* 171(2): 125-33.

Bullock, M.P., N.E. Foster, and C.C. Wright. 2005. Shoulder impingement: The effect of sitting posture on shoulder pain and range of motion. *Man Ther* 10(1): 28-37.

Bullock-Saxton, J. 1994. Local sensation changes and altered hip muscle function following severe ankle sprain. *Phys Ther* 74(1): 17-28.

Bullock-Saxton, J., D. Murphy, C. Norris, C. Richardson, and P. Tunnell. 2000. The muscle designation debate: The experts respond. *J Bodyw Mov Ther* 4(4): 225-7.

Bullock-Saxton, J., V. Janda, and M. Bullock. 1993. Reflex activation of gluteal muscles in walking with balance shoes: An approach to restoration of function for chronic low back pain patients. *Spine* 18(6): 704-8.

Bullock-Saxton, J., V. Janda, and M. Bullock. 1994. The influence of ankle sprain injury on muscle activation during hip extension. *Int J Sports Med* 15(6): 330-4.

Bullock-Saxton, J.E. 1995. Sensory changes associated with severe ankle sprain. *Scand J Rehabil Med* 27(3): 161-7.

Burke, J., D.J. Buchberger, M.T. Carey-Loghmani, P.E. Dougherty, D.S. Greco, and J.D. Dishman. 2007. A pilot study comparing two manual therapy interventions for carpal tunnel syndrome. *J Manipulative Physiol Ther* 30(1): 50-61.

Burkhart, S.S., C.D. Morgan, and W.B. Kibler. 2003. The disabled throwing shoulder: Spectrum of pathology part III: The SICK scapula, scapular dyskinesis, the kinetic chain, and rehabilitation. *Arthroscopy* 19(6): 641-61.

Burkhead Jr., W.Z., and C.A. Rockwood Jr. 1992. Treatment of instability of the shoulder with an exercise program. *J Bone Joint Surg Am* 74(6): 890-6.

Burnham, R.S., L. May, E. Nelson, R. Steadward, and D.C. Reid. 1993. Shoulder pain in wheelchair athletes. The role of muscle imbalance. *Am J Sports Med* 21(2): 238-42.

Busch, A., C.L. Schachter, P.M. Peloso, and C. Bombardier. 2002. Exercise for treating fibromyalgia syndrome. *Cochrane Database Syst Rev* 3: CD003786.

Butler, D.S. 1991. *The mobilisation of the nervous system.* Melbourne: Churchill Livingstone.

Byl, N. , and P.L. Sinnot. 1991. Variations in balance and body sway in middle aged adults: Subjects with healthy backs compared with subjects with low back dysfunction. *Spine* 16: 325-30.

Cain, P.R., T.A. Mutschler, F.H. Fu, and S.K. Lee. 1987. Anterior stability of the glenohumeral joint. A dynamic model. *Am J Sports Med* 15(2): 144-8.

Cameron, M., R. Adams, and C. Maher. 2003. Motor control and strength as predictors of hamstring injury in elite players of Australian football. *Phys Ther Sport* 4: 159-66.

Caraffa, A., G. Cerulli, A. Rizzo, V. Buompadre, S. Appoggetti, and M. Fortuna. 1996. An arthroscopic and electromyographic study of painful shoulders in elite gymnasts. *Knee Surg Sports Traumatol Arthrosc* 4(1): 39-42.

Carr, J.H., and R. Shepherd. 1980. Physiotherapy in disorders of the brain. Oxford: Heinemann Medical Books.

Carson, P.A. 1999. The rehabilitation of a competitive swimmer with an asymmetrical breaststroke movement pattern. *Man Ther* 4(2): 100-6.

Carter, A.B., T.W. Kaminski, A.T. Douex Jr, C.A. Knight, and J.G. Richards. 2007. Effects of high volume upper extremity plyometric training on throwing velocity and functional strength ratios of the shoulder rotators in collegiate baseball players. *J Strength Cond Res* 21(1): 208-15.

Carter, A.M., S.J. Kinzey, L.F. Chitwood, and J.L. Cole. 2000. Proprioceptive neuromuscular facilitation decreases muscle activity during the stretch reflex in selected posterior thigh muscles. *J Sport Rehabil* 9: 269-78.

Cavanaugh, J.M., Y. Lu, C. Chen, and S. Kallakuri. 2006. Pain generation in lumbar and cervical facet joints. *J Bone Joint Surg Am* 88(Suppl. no. 2): 63-7.

Cerulli, G., Benoit, D.L., Caraffa, A., and Ponteggia, F. 2001. Proprioceptive training and prevention of anterior cruciate ligament injuries in soccer. J Orthop Sports Phys Ther. 31(11): 655-60.

Chandler, T.J., W.B. Kibler, E.C. Stracener, A.K. Ziegler, and B. Pace. 1992. Shoulder strength, power, and endurance in college tennis players. *Am J Sports Med* 20(4): 455-8.

Chauhan, S.K., T. Peckham, and R. Turner. 2003. Impingement syndrome associated with whiplash injury. *J Bone Joint Surg Br* 85(3): 408-10.

Chen, C., Y. Lu, S. Kallakuri, A. Patwardhan, and J.M. Cavanaugh. 2006. Distribution of A-delta and C-fiber receptors in the cervical facet joint capsule and their response to stretch. *J Bone Joint Surg Am* 88(8): 1807-16.

Chen, S.K., P.T. Simonian, T.L. Wickiewicz, J.C. Otis, and R.F. Warren. 1999. Radiographic evaluation of glenohumeral kinematics: A muscle fatigue model. *J Shoulder Elbow Surg* 8(1): 49-52.

Chester Jr., J.B. 1991. Whiplash, postural control, and the inner ear. *Spine* 16(7): 716-20.

Cheung, J.T., Zhang, M., and An, K.N. 2006. Effect of Achilles tendon loading on plantar fascia tension in the standing foot. *Clin Biomech (Bristol, Avon).* Feb;21(2): 194-203.

Chiu, T.T., E.Y. Law, and T.H. Chiu. 2005. Performance of the craniocervical flexion test in subjects with and without chronic neck pain. *J Orthop Sports Phys Ther* 35(9): 567-71.

Chmielewski, T.L., W.J. Hurd, and L. Snyder-Mackler. 2005. Elucidation of a potentially destabilizing control strategy in ACL deficient non-copers. *J Electromyogr Kinesiol* 15(1): 83-92.

Chmielewski, T.L., W.J. Hurd, K.S. Rudolph, M.J. Axe, and L. Snyder-Mackler. 2005. Perturbation training improves knee kinematics and reduces muscle co-contraction after complete unilateral anterior cruciate ligament rupture. *Phys Ther* 85(8): 740-9.

Cholewicki, J., and S.M. McGill. 1995. Mechanical stability of the in vivo lumbar spine: Implications for injury and chronic low back pain. *Clin Biomech (Bristol, Avon)* 11: 1-15.

Cholewicki, J., K. Juluru, and S.M. McGill. 1999. Intra-abdominal pressure mechanism for stabilizing the lumbar spine. *J Biomech* 32(1): 13-7.

Cholewicki, J., M.M. Panjabi, and A. Khachatryan. 1997. Stabilizing function of trunk flexor-extensor muscles around a neutral spine posture. *Spine* 22(19): 2207-12.

Chu, D., R. LeBlanc, P. D'Ambrosia, R. D'Ambrosia, R.V. Baratta, and M. Solomonow. 2003. Neuromuscular disorder in response to anterior cruciate ligament creep. *Clin Biomech (Bristol, Avon)* 18(3): 222-30.

Cibulka, M.T. 2006. Sternocleidomastoid muscle imbalance in a patient with recurrent headache. *Man Ther* 11(1): 78-82.

Cichanowski, H.R., J.S. Schmitt, R.J. Johnson, and P.E. Niemuth. 2007. Hip strength in collegiate female athletes with patellofemoral pain. *Med Sci Sports Exerc* 39(8): 1227-32.

Clark, G.T., E.M. Green, M.R. Dornan, and V.F. Flack. 1987. Craniocervical dysfunction levels in a patient sample from a temporomandibular joint clinic. *J Am Dent Assoc* 115(2): 251-6.

Clark, V.M., Bruden, A.M. 2005. A 4-week wobble board exercise programme improved muscle onset latency and perceived stability in individuals with a functionally unstable ankle. Physical Therapy in Sport 6(4): 181-187 .

Cleland, J.A., J.D. Childs, M. McRae, J.A. Palmer, and T. Stowell. 2005. Immediate effects of thoracic manipulation in patients with neck pain: A randomized clinical trial. *Man Ther* 10(2): 127-35.

Cockerill, I.M. 1972. The development of ballistic skilled movements. In *Readings in sports psychology,* ed. H.T.A. Whiting. London: Henry Kimpton.

Cohen, L.A. 1961. Role of eye and neck proprioceptive mechanisms in body orientation and motor coordination. *J Neurophysiol* 1: 1-11.

Cohen, L.A., and M.L. Cohen. 1956. Arthrokinetic reflex of the knee. *Am J Physiol* 184(2): 433-7.

Cole, A., P. McClure, and N. Pratt. 1996. Scapular kinmeatics during arm elevation in healthy subjects and patients with shoulder impingement syndrome. Abstract. *J Orthop Sports Phys Ther* 23(1): 68.

Comtet, J.J., G. Herzberg, and I.A. Naasan. 1989. Biomechanical basis of transfers for shoulder paralysis. *Hand Clin* 5(1): 1-14.

Conway, P.J.W., W. Herzog, Y. Zhang, E.M. Hasler, and K. Ladly. 1993. Forces required to cause cavitation during spinal manipulation of the thoracic spine. *Clin Biomech (Bristol, Avon)* 8: 210-4.

Cook, E.E., V.L. Gray, E. Savinar-Nogue, and J. Medeiros. 1987. Shoulder antagonistic strength ratios: A comparison between college-level baseball pitchers and non-pitchers. *J Orthop Sports Phys Ther* 8(9): 451-61.

Cools, A.M., E.E. Witvrouw, G.A. De Clercq, L.A. Danneels, T.M. Willems, D.C. Cambier, and M.L. Voight. 2002. Scapular muscle recruitment pattern: Electromyographic response of the trapezius muscle to sudden shoulder movement before and after a fatiguing exercise. *J Orthop Sports Phys Ther* 32(5): 221-9.

Cools, A.M., E.E. Witvrouw, G.A. Declercq, G.G. Vanderstraeten, and D.C. Cambier. 2004. Evaluation of isokinetic force production and associated muscle activity in the scapular rotators during a protraction-retraction movement in overhead athletes with impingement symptoms. *Br J Sports Med* 38(1): 64-8.

Cools, A.M., E.E. Witvrouw, G.A. Declercq, L.A. Danneels, and D.C. Cambier. 2003. Scapular muscle recruitment patterns: Trapezius muscle latency with and without impingement symptoms. *Am J Sports Med* 31(4): 542-9.

Cools, A.M., E.E. Witvrouw, N.N. Mahieu, L.A. Danneels. 2005. Isokinetic scapular muscle performance in overhead athletes with and without impingement symptoms. *J Athl Train* 40(2): 104-110.

Cools, A.M., G.A. Declercq, D.C. Cambier, N.N. Mahieu, and E.E. Witvrouw. 2007. Trapezius activity and intramuscular balance during isokinetic exercise in overhead athletes with impingement symptoms. *Scand J Med Sci Sports* 17(1): 25-33.

Cools, A.M., V. Dewitte, F. Lanszweert, D. Notebaert, A. Roets, B. Soetens, B. Cagnie, and E.E. Witvrouw. 2007. Rehabilitation of scapular muscle balance: Which exercises to prescribe? *Am J Sports Med* 35(10): 1744-51.

Cooper, D.E., S.J. O'Brien, and R.F. Warren. 1993. Supporting layers of the glenohumeral joint. An anatomic study. *Clin Orthop Relat Res* 289: 144-55.

Cordo, P.J., and L.M. Nashner. 1982. Properties of postural adjustments associated with rapid arm movements. *J Neurophysiol* 47: 287-302.

Cordova, M.L., L.S. Jutte, and J.T. Hopkins. 1999. EMG comparison of selected ankle rehabilitation exercises. *J Sport Rehabil* 8: 209-18.

Cornwall, M.W., and P. Murrell. 1991. Postural sway following inversion sprain of the ankle. *J Am Podiatr Med Assoc* 81(5): 243-7.

Cote, K.P., M.E. Brunet, B.M. Gansneder, and S.J. Shultz. 2005. Effects of pronated and supinated foot postures on static and dynamic postural stability. *J Athl Train* 40(1): 41-6.

Cotton, R.E., and D.F. Rideout. 1964. Tears of the humeral rotator cuff; a radiological and pathological necropsy survey. *J Bone Joint Surg Br* 46: 314-28.

Cowan, S.M., A.G. Schache, P. Brukner, K.L. Bennell, P.W. Hodges, P. Coburn, and K.M. Crossley. 2004. Delayed onset of transversus abdominus in long-standing groin pain. *Med Sci Sports Exerc* 36(12): 2040-5.

Cram, J.R., and G.S. Kasman. 1998. *Introduction to surface electromyography.* Gaithersburg, MD: Aspen.

Crawford, F., and C. Thomson. 2003. Interventions for treating plantar heel pain. *Cochrane Database Syst Rev* 3: CD000416.

Cresswell, A.G., H. Grundstrom, and A. Thorstensson. 1992. Observations on intra-abdominal pressure and patterns of abdominal intra-muscular activity in man. *Acta Physiol Scand* 144(4): 409-18.

Crockett, H.C., L.B. Gross, K.E. Wilk, M.L. Schwartz, J. Reed, J. O'Mara, M.T. Reilly et al. 2002. Osseous adaptation and range of motion at the glenohumeral joint in professional baseball pitchers. *Am J Sports Med* 30(1): 20-6.

Croisier, J.L., B. Forthomme, M.H. Namurois, M. Vanderthommen, and J.M. Crielaard. 2002. Hamstring muscle strain recurrence and strength performance disorders. *Am J Sports Med* 30(2): 199-203.

Crosbie, J., S.L. Kilbreath, L. Hollmann, and S. York. 2007. Scapulohumeral rhythm and associated spinal motion. *Clin Biomech (Bristol, Avon)*.

Crotty, N.M., and J. Smith. 2000. Alterations in scapular position with fatigue: A study in swimmers. *Clin J Sport Med* 10(4): 251-8.

Culham, E., and M. Peat. 1993. Functional anatomy of the shoulder complex. *J Orthop Sports Phys Ther* 18(1): 342-50.

Cummins, C.A., T.M. Messer, and M.F. Schafer. 2004. Infraspinatus muscle atrophy in professional baseball players. *Am J Sports Med* 32(1): 116-20.

Cuoco, A., T.F. Tyler, and M.P. McHugh. 2004. Effect of fatigued scapular stabilizers on shoulder external and internal rotation strength. Abstract. *J Orthop Sports Phys Ther* 34(1): A58.

Curatolo, M., S. Petersen-Felix, L. Arendt-Nielsen, C. Giani, A.M. Zbinden, and B.P. Radanov. 2001. Central hypersensitivity in chronic pain after whiplash injury. *Clin J Pain* 17(4): 306-15.

Dalstra, M. 1997. Biomechanics of the human pelvic bone. In *Movement stability and low back pain,* ed. A. Vleeming, V. Mooney, T. Dorman, C. Snijders, and R. Soteckhart, 91-102. New York: Churchill Licvingstone.

Danneels, L.A., P.L. Coorevits, A.M. Cools, G.G. Vanderstraeten, D.C. Cambier, E.E. Witvrouw, and H.J. De Cuyper. 2002. Differences in electromyographic activity in the multifidus muscle and the iliocostalis lumborum between healthy subjects and patients with sub-acute and chronic low back pain. *Eur Spine J* 11: 13-9.

Davey, N.J., R.M. Lisle, B. Loxton-Edwards, A.V. Nowicky, and A.H. McGregor. 2002. Activation of back muscles during voluntary abduction of the contralateral arm in humans. *Spine* 27(12): 1355-60.

David, G., M.E. Magarey, M.A. Jones, Z. Dvir, K.S. Türker, and M. Sharpe. 2000. EMG and strength correlates of selected shoulder muscles during rotations of the glenohumeral joint. *Clin Biomech (Bristol, Avon)* 15(2): 95-102.

Davies, P.M. 1985. *Steps to follow. A guide to the treatment of adult hemiplegia.* Berlin: Springer-Verlag.

Day, J.W., G.L. Smidt, and T. Lehmann. 1984. Effect of pelvic tilt on standing posture. *Phys Ther* 64(4): 510-6.

de Groot, J.H., W. van Woensel, and F.C. van der Helm. 1999. Effect of different arm loads on the position of the scapula in abduction postures. *Clin Biomech (Bristol, Avon)* 14(5): 309-14.

De Wilde, L., F. Plasschaert, B. Berghs, M. Van Hoecke, K. Verstraete, and R. Verdonk. 2003. Quantified measurement of subacromial impingement. *J Shoulder Elbow Surg* 12(4): 346-9.

DeAndrade, J., C. Grant, and A. Dison. 1965. Joint distension and reflex inhibition of the knee. *J Bone Joint Surg* 47A: 313-22.

Decker, M.J., R.A. Hintermeister, K.J. Faber, and R.J. Hawkins. 1999. Serratus anterior muscle activity during selected rehabilitation exercises. *Am J Sports Med* 27(6): 784-91.

Delacerda, F.G. 1980. The relationship of foot pronation, foot position, and electromyography of the anterior tibialis muscle in three subjects with different histories of shin splints. *J Orthop Sports Phys Ther* 2: 60-4.

Delahunt, E., K. Monaghan, and B. Caulfield. 2006. Altered neuromuscular control and ankle joint kinematics during walking in subjects with functional instability of the ankle joint. *Am J Sports Med* 34(12): 1970-6.

Desmeules, F., C.H. Côté, and P. Frémont. 2003. Therapeutic exercise and orthopedic manual therapy for impingement syndrome: A systematic review. *Clin J Sport Med* 13(3): 176-82.

Desmeules, F., L. Minville, B. Riederer, C.H. Côté, and P. Frémont. 2004. Acromio-humeral distance variation measured by ultrasonography and its association with the outcome of rehabilitation for shoulder impingement syndrome. *Clin J Sport Med* 14(4): 197-205.

Desmeules, J.A., C. Cedraschi, E. Rapiti, E. Baumgartner, A. Finckh, P. Cohen, P. Dayer, and T.L. Vischer. 2003. Neurophysiologic evidence for a central sensitization in patients with fibromyalgia. *Arthritis Rheum* 48(5): 1420-9.

Deutsch, A., D.W. Altchek, E. Schwartz, J.C. Otis, and R.F. Warren. 1996. Radiologic measurement of superior displacement of the humeral head in the impingement syndrome. *J Shoulder Elbow Surg* 5(3): 186-93.

Diederichsen, L., M. Krogsgaard, M. Voigt, and P. Dyhre-Poulsen. 2002. Shoulder reflexes. *J Electromyogr Kinesiol* 12(3): 183-91.

DiGiovanni, B.F., Nawoczenski, D.A., Lintal, M.E., Moore, E.A., Murray, J.C., Wilding, G.E., and Baumhauer, J.F. 2003. Tissue-specific plantar fascia-stretching exercise enhances outcomes in patients with chronic heel pain. A prospective, randomized study. *J Bone Joint Surg Am.* Jul;85-A(7): 1270-7.

DiVeta, J., M.L. Walker, and B. Skibinski. 1990. Relationship between performance of selected scapular muscles and scapular abduction in standing subjects. *Phys Ther* 70(8): 470-6.

Donatelli, R., T.S. Ellenbecker, S.R. Ekedahl, J.S. Wilkes, K. Kocher, and J. Adam. 2000. Assessment of shoulder strength in professional baseball pitchers. *J Orthop Sports Phys Ther* 30(9): 544-51.

Doody, S.G., L. Freedman, and J.C. Waterland. 1970. Shoulder movements during abduction in the scapular plane. *Arch Phys Med Rehabil* 51(10): 595-604.

Drenckhahn, D., and W. Zenekr (eds.) 1994. *Benninghoff anatomy.* Vol. 1. Munich: Urban & Schwarzenberg. 304-7.

Drury, D.G. 2000. Strength and proprioception. *J Orthop Sports Phys Ther* 9(4): 549-61.

Ebaugh, D.D., P.W. McClure, and A.R. Karduna. 2005. Three-dimensional scapulothoracic motion during active and passive arm elevation. *Clin Biomech (Bristol, Avon)* 20(7): 700-9.

Ebaugh, D.D., P.W. McClure, and A.R. Karduna. 2006a. Effects of shoulder muscle fatigue caused by repetitive overhead activities on scapulothoracic and glenohumeral kinematics. *J Electromyogr Kinesiol* 16(3): 224-35.

Ebaugh, D.D., P.W. McClure, and A.R. Karduna. 2006b. Scapulothoracic and glenohumeral kinematics following an external rotation fatigue protocol. *J Orthop Sports Phys Ther* 36(8): 557-71.

Ebenbichler, G.R., L.I. Oddson, J. Kollmitzer, and Z. Erim. 2001. Sensory-motor control of the lower back: Implications for rehabilitation. *Med Sci Sports Exerc* 33(11): 1889-98.

Edgerton, V.R., S.L. Wolf, D.J. Levendowski, and R.R. Roy. 1996. Theoretical basis for patterning EMG amplitudes to assess muscle dysfunction. *Med Sci Sports Exerc* 28(6): 744-51.

Edstrom, L. 1970. Selective atrophy of red muscle fibres in the quadriceps in long-standing knee-joint dysfunction. Injuries to the anterior cruciate ligament. *J Neurol Sci* 11(6): 551-8.

Eils, E., and D. Rosenbaum. 2001. A multi-station proprioceptive exercise program in patients with ankle instability. *Med Sci Sports Exerc* 33(12): 1991-8.

Eklund, G., and K.E. Hagbarth. 1966. Normal variability of tonic vibration reflexes in man. *Exp Neurol* 16(1): 80-92.

Ekstrand, J., and J. Gillquist J. 1982. The frequency of muscle tightness and injuries in soccer players. *Am J Sports Med* 10(2): 75-8.

Ekstrand, J., and J. Gillquist. 1983. Soccer injuries and their mechanisms: A prospective study. *Med Sci Sports Exerc* 15(3): 267-70.

Ekstrand, J., and J. Gillquist. 1983. The avoidability of soccer injuries. *Int J Sports Med* 4(2): 124-8.

Ekstrand, J., J. Gillquist, and S.O. Liljedahl. 1983. Prevention of soccer injuries. Supervision by doctor and physiotherapist. *Am J Sports Med* 11(3): 116-20.

Ekstrom, R.A., G.L. Soderberg, and R.A. Donatelli. 2005. Normalization procedures using maximum voluntary isometric contractions for the serratus anterior and trapezius muscles during surface EMG analysis. *J Electromyogr Kinesiol* 15(4): 418-28.

Ekstrom, R.A., K.M. Bifulco, C.J. Lopau, C.F. Andersen, and J.R. Gough. 2004. Comparing the function of the upper and lower parts of the serratus anterior muscle using surface electromyography. *J Orthop Sports Phys Ther* 34(5): 235-43.

Ekstrom, R.A., R.A. Donatelli, and G.L. Soderberg. 2003. Surface electromyographic analysis of exercises for the trapezius and serratus anterior muscles. *J Orthop Sports Phys Ther* 33(5): 247-58.

Elert, J., S.A. Kendall, B. Larsson, B. Månsson, and B. Gerdle. 2001. Chronic pain and difficulty in relaxing postural muscles in patients with fibromyalgia and chronic whiplash associated disorders. *J Rheumatol* 28(6): 1361-8.

Ellenbecker, T.S., and A.J. Mattalino. 1997. Concentric isokinetic shoulder internal and external rotation strength in professional baseball pitchers. *J Orthop Sports Phys Ther* 25(5): 323-8.

Ellenbecker, T.S., and E.P. Roetert. 2003. Isokinetic profile of elbow flexion and extension strength in elite junior tennis players. *J Orthop Sports Phys Ther* 33(2): 79-84.

Ellenbecker, T.S., E.P Roetert, and S. Riewald. 2006. Isokinetic profile of wrist and forearm strength in elite female junior tennis players. *Br J Sports Med* 40(5): 411-4.

Ellenbecker, T.S., E.P. Roetert, D.S. Bailie, G.J. Davies, and S.W. Brown. 2002. Glenohumeral joint total rotation range of motion in elite tennis players and baseball pitchers. *Med Sci Sports Exerc* 34(12): 2052-6.

Ellenbecker, T.S., E.P. Roetert, P.A. Piorkowski, and D.A. Schulz. 1996. Glenohumeral joint internal and external rotation range of motion in elite junior tennis players. *J Orthop Sports Phys Ther* 24(6): 336-41.

Ellison, J.B., S.J. Rose, and S.A. Sahrmann. 1990. Patterns of hip rotation range of motion: A comparison between healthy subjects and patients with low back pain. *Phys Ther* 70(9): 537-41.

Elvey, R.L. 1986. Treatment of arm pain associated with abnormal brachial plexus tension. *Aust J Physiother* 32: 225-30.

Endo, K., K. Yukata, and N. Yasui. 2004. Influence of age on scapulo-thoracic orientation. *Clin Biomech (Bristol, Avon)* 19(10): 1009-13.

Endo, K., T. Ikata, S. Katoh, and Y. Takeda. 2001. Radiographic assessment of scapular rotational tilt in chronic shoulder impingement syndrome. *J Orthop Sci* 6(1): 3-10.

Enoka, P.M. 1988. Muscle strength and its development. New perspectives. *Sports Med* 6(3): 146-68.

Erak, S., R. Day, and A. Wang. 2004. The role of supinator in the pathogenesis of chronic lateral elbow pain: A biomechanical study. *J Hand Surg [Br]* 29(5): 461-4.

Ervilha, U.F., D. Farina, L. Arendt-Nielsen, and T. Graven-Nielsen. 2005. Experimental muscle pain changes motor control strategies in dynamic contractions. *Exp Brain Res* 164(2): 215-24.

Erzog, W., D. Scheele, and P.J. Conway. 1999. Electromyographic responses of back and limb muscles associated with spinal manipulative therapy. *Spine* 24(2): 146-52.

Etnyre, B.R., and L.D. Abraham. 1986. H-reflex changes during static stretching and two variations of proprioceptive neuromuscular facilitation techniques. *Electroencephalogr Clin Neurophysiol* 63(2): 174-9.

Evans, R., G. Bronfort, B. Nelson, and C.H. Goldsmith. 2002. Two-year follow-up of a randomized clinical trial of spinal manipulation and two types of exercise for patients with chronic neck pain. *Spine* 27(21): 2383-9.

Evetovich, T.K., T.J. Housh, D.J. Housh, G.O. Johnson, D.B. Smith, and K.T. Ebersole. 2001. The effect of concentric isokinetic strength training of the quadriceps femoris on electromyography and muscle strength in the trained and untrained limb. *J Strength Cond Res* 15(4): 439-45.

Ezzo, J., B.G. Haraldsson, A.R. Gross, C.D. Myers, A. Morien, C.H. Goldsmith, G. Bronfort, and P.M. Peloso. Cervical Overview Group. 2007. Massage for mechanical neck disorders: A systematic review. *Spine* 32(3): 353-62.

Faes, M., N. van Elk, J.A. de Lint, H. Degens, J.G. Kooloos, and M.T. Hopman. 2006. A dynamic extensor brace reduces electromyographic activity of wrist extensor muscles in patients with lateral epicondylalgia. *J Orthop Sports Phys Ther* 36(3): 170-8.

Fairbank, S.M., and R.J. Corlett. 2002. The role of the extensor digitorum communis muscle in lateral epicondylitis. *J Hand Surg [Br]* 27(5): 405-9.

Falla, D. 2004. Unravelling the complexity of muscle impairment in chronic neck pain. *Man Ther* 9(3): 125-33.

Falla, D., A. Rainoldi, R. Merletti, and G. Jull. 2003. Myoelectric manifestations of sternocleidomastoid and anterior scalene muscle fatigue in chronic neck pain patients. *Clin Neurophysiol* 114(3): 488-495.

Falla, D., A. Rainoldi, R. Merletti, and G. Jull. 2004. Spatio-temporal evaluation of neck muscle activation during postural perturbations in healthy subjects. *J Electromyogr Kinesiol* 14(4): 463-74.

Falla, D., D. Farina, and T. Graven-Nielsen. 2007. Experimental muscle pain results in reorganization of coordination among trapezius muscle subdivisions during repetitive shoulder flexion. *Exp Brain Res* 178(3): 385-93.

Falla, D., G. Bilenkij, and G. Jull. 2004. Patients with chronic neck pain demonstrate altered patterns of muscle activation during performance of a functional upper limb task. *Spine* 29(13): 1436-40.

Falla, D., G. Jull, A. Rainoldi, and R. Merletti. 2004. Neck flexor muscle fatigue is side specific in patients with unilateral neck pain. *Eur J Pain* 8(1): 71-7.

Falla, D., G. Jull, and P.W. Hodges. 2004. Feedforward activity of the cervical flexor muscles during voluntary arm movements is delayed in chronic neck pain. *Exp Brain Res* 157(1): 43-8.

Falla, D., G. Jull, and P.W. Hodges. 2006. An endurance-strength training regime is effective in reducing myoelectric manifestations of cervical flexor muscle fatigue in females with chronic neck pain. *Clin Neurophysiol* 117(4): 823-37.

Falla, D., G. Jull, P. Dall'Alba, A. Rainoldi, and R. Merletti. 2003. An electromyographic analysis of the deep cervical flexor muscles in performance of craniocervical flexion. *Phys Ther* 83(10): 899-906.

Falla, D., G. Jull, P. Hodges, and B. Vicenzino. 2006. An endurance-strength training regime is effective in reducing myoelectric manifestations of cervical flexor muscle fatigue in females with chronic neck pain. *Clin Neurophysiol* 117(4): 828-37.

Falla, D., G. Jull, S. Edwards, K. Koh, and A. Rainoldi. 2004. Neuromuscular efficiency of the sternocleidomastoid and anterior scalene muscles in patients with chronic neck pain. *Disabil Rehabil* 26(12): 712-7.

Falla, D., G. Jull, T. Russell, B. Vicenzino, and P. Hodges. 2007. Effect of neck exercise on sitting posture in patients with chronic neck pain. *Phys Ther* 87(4): 408-17.

Falla, D., G.A. Jull, and P.W. Hodges. 2004. Patients with neck pain demonstrated reduced electromyographic activity of the deep cervical flexor muscles during performance of the craniocervical flexion test. *Spine* 29: 2108-14.

Falla, D.L., C.D. Campbell, A.E. Fagan, D.C. Thompson, and G.A. Jull. 2003. Relationship between craniocervical flexion range of motion and pressure change during the cranio-cervical flexion test. *Man Ther* 8(2): 92-6.

Falla, D.L., S. Hess, and C. Richardson. 2003. Evaluation of shoulder internal rotator muscle strength in baseball players with physical signs of glenohumeral joint instability. *Br J Sports Med* 37(5): 430-2.

Fann, A.V. 2002. The prevalence of postural asymmetry in people with and without chronic low back pain. *Arch Phys Med Rehabil* 83(12): 1736-8.

Feldenkrais, M. 1972. *Awareness through movement.* New York: Harper & Row.

Fernández-Carnero, J., C. Fernández-de-Las-Peñas, A.I. de la Llave-Rincón, H.Y. Ge, and L. Arendt-Nielsen. 2007. Prevalence of and referred pain from myofascial trigger points in the forearm muscles in patients with lateral epicondylalgia. *Clin J Pain* 23(4): 353-60.

Ferris, D.P., H.J. Huang, P.C. Kao. 2006. Moving the arms to activate the legs. *Exercise & Sport Sciences Reviews* 34(3): 113-20.

Finley, M.A., and R.Y. Lee. 2003. Effect of sitting posture on 3-dimensional scapular kinematics measured by skin-mounted electromagnetic tracking sensors. *Arch Phys Med Rehabil* 84(4): 563-8.

Finsen, L., K. Søgaard, T. Graven-Nielsen, and H. Christensen. 2005. Activity patterns of wrist extensor muscles during wrist extensions and deviations. *Muscle Nerve* 31(2): 242-51.

Fitzgerald, G.K., M.J. Axe, and L. Snyder-Mackler. 2000. The efficacy of perturbation training in nonoperative anterior cruciate ligament rehabilitation programs for physical active individuals. *Phys Ther* 80(2): 128-40.

Fitzgerald, G.K., Piva, S.R., Irrgang, J.J., Bouzubar, F., and Starz, T.W. 2004. Quadriceps activation failure as a moderator of the relationship between quadriceps strength and physical function in individuals with knee osteoarthritis. *Arthritis Rheum.* Feb 15;51(1): 40-8.

Fitzpatrick, R., and D.I. McCloskey. 1994. Proprioceptive, visual and vestibular thresholds for the perception of sway during standing in humans. *J Physiol* 478(Pt. 1): 173-86.

Fitzpatrick, R., D.K. Rogers, and D.I. McCloskey. 1994. Stable human standing with lower-limb muscle afferents providing the only sensory input. *J Physiol* 480(Pt. 2): 395-403.

Fitz-Ritson, D. 1995. Phasic exercises for cervical rehabilitation after "whiplash" trauma. *J Manipulative Physiol Ther* 18(1): 21-4.

Flatow, E.L., L.J. Soslowsky, J.B. Ticker, R.J. Pawluk, M. Hepler, J. Ark, V.C. Mow, and L.U. Bigliani. 1994. Excursion of the rotator cuff under the acromion. Patterns of subacromial contact. *J Sports Med* 22(6): 779-88.

Forman, W.M., and Green, M.A. 1990. The role of intrinsic musculature in the formation of inferior calcaneal exostoses. *Clin Podiatr Med Surg.* Apr;7(2): 217-23. Review.

Frankel, S.A., and I. Hirata Jr. 1971. The scalenus anticus syndrome and competitive swimming. Report of two cases. *JAMA* 215(11): 1796-8.

Fredericson, M., C.L. Cookingham, A.M. Chaudhari, B.C. Dowdell, N. Oestreicher, and S.A. Sahrmann. 2000. Hip abductor weakness in distance runners with iliotibial band syndrome. *Clin J Sport Med* 10(3): 169-75.

Freedman, L., R.R. Munro. 1966. Abduction of the arm in the scapular plane: Scapular and glenohumeral movements. A roentgenographic study. *J Bone Joint Surg Am* 48(8): 1503-10.

Freeman, M.A., and B. Wyke. 1965. Reflex innervation of the ankle joint. *Nature* 207(993): 196.

Freeman, M.A., and B. Wyke. 1966. Articular contributions to limb muscle reflexes. The effects of partial neurectomy of the knee-joint on postural reflexes. *Br J Surg* 53(1): 61-8.

Freeman, M.A., and B. Wyke. 1967a. Articular reflexes at the ankle joint: An electromyographic study of normal and abnormal influences of ankle-joint mechanoreceptors upon reflex activity in the leg muscles. *Br J Surg* 54(12): 990-1001.

Freeman, M.A., and B. Wyke. 1967b. The innervation of the ankle joint. An anatomical and histological study in the cat. *Acta Anat (Basel)* 68(3): 321-33.

Freeman, M.A., and B. Wyke. 1967c. The innervation of the knee joint. An anatomical and histological study in the cat. *J Anat* 101(3): 505-32.

Freeman, M.A., M.R. Dean, and I.W. Hanham. 1965. The etiology and prevention of functional instability of the foot. *J Bone Joint Surg Br* 47(4): 678-85.

Freeman, M.A.R. 1965. Coordination exercises in the treatment of functional instability of the foot. *Physiotherapy* 51(12): 393-5.

Freeman, M.A.R. 1965. Instability of the foot after injuries to the lateral ligament of the ankle. *J Bone Joint Surg* 47B(4): 669-77.

Friberg, O. 1983. Clinical symptoms and biomechanics of the lumbar spine and hip joint in leg length inequality. *Spine* 8: 643-51.

Friden, J., and R.L. Lieber. 1992. The structural and mechanical basis of exercise-induced muscle injury. *Med Sci Sports Exerc* 24: 521.

Friedli, W.G., L. Cohen, M. Hallett, S. Stanhope, and S.R. Simon. 1988. Postural adjustments associated with rapid voluntary arm movements. II. Biomechanical analysis. *J Neurol Neurosurg Psychiatry* 51(2): 232-43.

Friel, K., N. McLean, C. Myers, and M. Caceres. 2006. Ipsilateral hip abductor weakness after inversion ankle sprain. *J Athl Train* 41(1): 74-8.

Fujii, H., S. Kobayashi, T. Sato, K. Shinozaki, and A. Naito. 2007. Co-contraction of the pronator teres and extensor carpi radialis during wrist extension movements in humans. *J Electromyogr Kinesiol* 17(1): 80-9.

Fukushima, H., and M. Hinoki. 1984. Role of the cervical and lumbar proprioceptors during stepping: An electromyographic study of the muscular activities of the lower limbs. *Acta Otolaryngol Suppl* 419: 91-105.

Furto, E.S., J.A. Cleland, J.M. Whitman, and K.A. Olson. 2006. Manual physical therapy interventions and exercise for patients with temporomandibular disorders. *Cranio* 24(4): 283-91.

Furto, E.S., J.A. Cleland, J.M. Whitman, and K.A. Olson. 2006. Manual physical therapy interventions and exercise for patients with temporomandibular disorders. *Cranio* 24(4): 283-91.

Gandevia, S.C., R.D. Herbert, and J.B. Leeper. 1998. Voluntary activation of human elbow flexor muscles during maximal concentric contractions. *J Physiol* 512: 595-602.

Ganong, W.F. 1981. Dynamics of blood and lymph flow. In *Review of medical physiology,* 470-84. California: Lange Medical Publications.

Garces, G.L., D. Medina, L. Milutinovic, P. Garavote, and E. Guerado. 2002. Normative database of isometric cervical strength in a healthy population. *Med Sci Sports Exerc* 34(3): 464-70.

Gardener, W.N. 1996. The pathophysiology of hyperventilation disorders. *Chest* 109: 516-34.

Gardner-Morse, M., and I. Stokes. 1998. The effect of abdominal muscle co-activation on lumbar spine stability. *Spine* 23: 86-92.

Gauffin, H., and H. Tropp. 1992. Altered movement and muscular-activation patterns during the one-legged jump in patients with an old anterior cruciate ligament rupture. *Am J Sports Med* 20(2): 182-92.

Gauffin, H., H. Tropp, and P. Odenrick. 1988. Effect of ankle disk training on postural control in patients with functional instability of the ankle joint. *Int J Sports Med* 9(2): 141-4.

Ge, H.Y., L. Arendt-Nielsen, D. Farina, and P. Madeleine. 2005. Gender-specific differences in electromyographic changes and perceived pain induced by experimental muscle pain during sustained contractions of the upper trapezius muscle. *Muscle Nerve* 32(6): 726-33.

Geraets, J.J., M.E. Goossens, I.J. de Groot , C.P. de Bruijn, R.A. de Bie, G.J. Dinant, G. van der Heijden, and W.J. van den Heuvel. 2005. Effectiveness of a graded exercise therapy program for patients with chronic shoulder complaints. *Aust J Physiother* 51(2): 87-94.

Gerhardt, M.B., J.A. Brown, and E. Giza. 2006. Occult groin injuries: Athletic pubalgia sports hernia and osteitis pubis. In *Practical orthopedics, sports medicine and arthroscopy,* ed. D.A. Johnson and R.A. Pedowitz, 531-44. Baltimore: Lippincott Williams & Wilkins.

Gervais, R.O., G.W. Fitzsimmons, and N.R. Thomas NR. 1989. Masseter and temporalis electromyographic activity in asymptomatic, subclinical, and temporomandibular joint dysfunction patients. *Cranio* 7(1): 52-7.

Ghez, C. 1991. Posture. In *Principles of neural science.* 3rd ed., ed. E.R. Kandel, J.H. Schwartz, and T.M. Jessell, 596-607. New York: Elsevier.

Giangarra, C.E., B. Conroy B, F.W. Jobe, M. Pink, and J. Perry. 1993. Electromyographic and cinematographic analysis of elbow function in tennis players using single- and double-handed backhand strokes. *Am J Sports Med* 21(3): 394-9.

Giannakopoulos, K., A. Beneka, P. Malliou, and G. Godolias. 2004. Isolated vs. complex exercise in strengthening the rotator cuff muscle group. *J Strength Cond Res* 18(1): 144-8.

Gibson, K., A. Growse, L. Korda, E. Wray, and J.C. MacDermid. 2004. The effectiveness of rehabilitation for nonoperative management of shoulder instability: A systematic review. *J Hand Ther* 17(2): 229-42.

Gibson, M.H., G.V. Goebel, T.M. Jordan, S. Kegerreis, and T.W. Worrell. 1995. A reliability study of measurement techniques to determine static scapular position. *J Orthop Sports Phys Ther* 21(2): 100-6.

Gibson, S.J., G.O. Littlejohn, M.M. Gorman, R.D. Helme, and G. Granges. 1994. Altered heat pain thresholds and cerebral event-related potentials following painful CO_2 laser stimulation in subjects with fibromyalgia syndrome. *Pain* 58(2): 185-93.

Giesbrecht, R.J., and M.C. Battié. 2005. A comparison of pressure pain detection thresholds in people with chronic low back pain and volunteers without pain. *Phys Ther* 85(10): 1085-92.

Giesecke, T., R.H. Gracely, M.A. Grant, A. Nachemson, F. Petzke, D.A. Williams, and D.J. Clauw. 2004. Evidence of augmented central pain processing in idiopathic chronic low back pain. *Arthritis Rheum* 50(2): 613-23.

Gifford, P., and P. Tehan. 2003. Patient positioning and spinal locking for lumbar spine rotation manipulation. In *Manual therapy masterclasses: The vertebral column,* ed. K.S. Beeton, 93-102. London: Churchill Livingstone.

Giladi, M., C. Milgrom, M. Stein, H. Kashtan, J. Margulies, R. Chisin, and R. Steinberg. 1985. The low arch, a protective factor in stress fractures. *Orthop Rev* 14: 709-12.

Gill, K.P., and M.J. Callaghan. 1998. The measurement of lumbar proprioception in individuals with and without low back pain. *Spine* 23(3): 371-7.

Ginn, K.A., and M.L. Cohen. 2004. Conservative treatment for shoulder pain: Prognostic indicators of outcome. *Arch Phys Med Rehabil* 85(8): 1231-5.

Ginn, K.A., and M.L. Cohen. 2005. Exercise therapy for shoulder pain aimed at restoring neuromuscular control: A randomized comparative clinical trial. *J Rehabil Med* 37(2): 115-22.

Ginn, K.A., R.D. Herbert, W. Khouw, and R. Lee. 1997. A randomized, controlled clinical trial of a treatment for shoulder pain. *Phys Ther* 77(8): 802-9.

Girometti, R., A. De Candia, M. Sbuelz, F. Toso, C. Zuiani, and M. Bazzocchi. 2006. Supraspinatus tendon US morphology in basketball players: Correlation with main pathologic models of secondary impingement syndrome in young overhead athletes. Preliminary report. *Radiol Med* 111(1): 42-52.

Glousman, R., F. Jobe, J. Tibone, D. Moynes, D. Antonelli, and J. Perry. 1988. Dynamic electromyographic analysis of the throwing shoulder with glenohumeral instability. *J Bone Joint Surg Am* 70(2): 220-6.

Glousman, R.. 1993. Electromyographic analysis and its role in the athletic shoulder. *Clin Orthop Relat Res* 288: 27-34.

Glousman, R.E. 1993. Instability versus impingement syndrome in the throwing athlete. *Orthop Clin North Am* 24(1): 89-99.

Gofton, J.P., and G.E. Trueman. 1971. Studies in osteoarthritis of the hip part 11. Osteoarthritis of the hip and leg length disparity. *Can Med Assoc J* 104: 791-9.

Gogia, P.P., and M.A. Sabbahi. 1994. Electromyographic analysis of neck muscle fatigue in patients with osteoarthritis of the cervical spine. *Spine* 19(5): 502-6.

Goldie, P.A., O.M. Evans, and T.M. Bach. 1994. Postural control following inversion injuries of the ankle. *Arch Phys Med Rehabil* 75(9): 969-75.

Golding, F.C. 1962. The shoulder—the forgotten joint. *Br J Radiol* 35: 149-58.

Goodheart Jr., G.J. 1964. *Applied kinesiology.* Detroit: Privately published.

Gorski, J.M., and L.H. Schwartz. 2003. Shoulder impingement presenting as neck pain. *J Bone Joint Surg Am* 85-A(4): 635-8.

Gosselin, G., H. Rassoulian, and I. Brown. 2004. Effects of neck extensor muscles fatigue on balance. *Clin Biomech (Bristol, Avon)* 19(5): 473-9.

Gossman, M.R., S.A. Sahrmann, and S.J. Rose. 1982. Review of length-associated changes in muscle. Experimental evidence and clinical implications. *Phys Ther* 62(12): 1799-808.

Grabiner, M.D., T.J. Koh, and G.F. Miller. 1986. Fatigue rates of vastus medialis oblique and vastus lateralis during static and dynamic knee extension. *J Orthop Res* 9(3): 391-7.

Grace, T.G., E.R. Sweetser, M.A. Nelson, L.R. Ydens, and B.J. Skipper. 1984. Isokinetic muscle imbalance and knee-joint injuries. A prospective blind study. *J Bone Joint Surg Am* 66(5): 734-40.

Gracely, R.H., F. Petzke, J.M. Wolf, and D.J. Clauw. 2002. Functional magnetic resonance imaging evidence of augmented pain processing in fibromyalgia. *Arthritis Rheum* 46(5): 1333-43.

Gracovetsky, S. 1997. Linking the spinal engine with the legs: A theory of human gait. In *Movement, stability, and low back pain,* ed. A. Vleeming,V. Mooney, T. Dorman, C. Snijders, and R. Stoeckart, 243. Edinburgh: Churchill Livingstone.

Gracovetsky, S., H. Farfan, and C. Helleur. 1985. The abdominal mechanism. *Spine* 10: 317-24.

Graichen, H., H. Bonel, T. Stammberger, K.H. Englmeier, M. Reiser, and F. Eckstein. 1999. Subacromial space width changes during abduction and rotation—a 3-D MR imaging study. *Surg Radiol Anat* 21(1): 59-64.

Graichen, H., H. Bonél, T. Stammberger, K.H. Englmeier, M. Reiser, and F. Eckstein. 2001. Sex-specific differences of subacromial space width during abduction, with and without muscular activity, and correlation with anthropometric variables. *J Shoulder Elbow Surg* 10(2): 129-35.

Graichen, H., H. Bonel, T. Stammberger, M. Haubner, H. Rohrer, K.H. Englmeier, M. Reiser, and F. Eckstein. 1999. Three-dimensional analysis of the width of the subacromial space in healthy subjects and patients with impingement syndrome. *AJR Am J Roentgenol* 172(4): 1081-6.

Graichen, H., S. Hinterwimmer, R. von Eisenhart-Rothe, T. Vogl, K.H. Englmeier, and F. Eckstein. 2005. Effect of abducting and adducting muscle activity on glenohumeral translation, scapular kinematics and subacromial space width in vivo. *J Biomech* 38(4): 755-60.

Graichen, H., T. Stammberger, H. Bonél, E. Wiedemann, K.H. Englmeier, M. Reiser, and F. Eckstein. 2001. Three-dimensional analysis of shoulder girdle and supraspinatus motion patterns in patients with impingement syndrome. *J Orthop Res* 19(6): 1192-8.

Graven-Nielsen, T., H. Lund, L. Arendt-Nielsen, B. Danneskiold-Samsøe, and H. Bliddal. 2002. Inhibition of maximal voluntary contraction force by experimental muscle pain: A centrally mediated mechanism. *Muscle Nerve* 26(5): 708-12.

Graven-Nielsen, T., P. Svensson, and L. Arendt-Nielsen. 1997. Effects of experimental muscle pain on muscle activity and co-ordination during static and dynamic motor function. *Electroencephalogr Clin Neurophysiol* 105(2): 156-64.

Gray, G. 1996. *Chain reaction festival.* Course manual. Wynn Marketing.

Greenfield, B., P.A. Catlin, P.W. Coats, E. Green, J.J. McDonald, and C. North. 1995. Posture in patients with shoulder overuse injuries and healthy individuals. *J Orthop Sports Phys Ther* 21(5): 287-95.

Greenfield, B.H., R. Donatelli, M.J. Wooden, and J. Wilkes. 1990. Isokinetic evaluation of shoulder rotational strength between the plane of scapula and the frontal plane. *Am J Sports Med* 18(2): 124-8.

Gregoric, M., T. Takeya, J.B. Baron, and J.C. Bessineton. 1978. Influence of vibration of neck muscles on balance control in man. *Agressologie* 19(A): 37-8.

Grenier, S., and S.M. McGill. 2007. Quantification of lumbar stability by using 2 different abdominal activation strategies. *Arch Phys Med Rehabil* 1(18): 54-62.

Griegel-Morris, P., K. Larson, K. Mueller-Klaus, and C.A. Oatis. 1992. Incidence of common postural abnormalities in the cervical, shoulder, and thoracic regions and their association with pain in two age groups of healthy subjects. *Phys Ther* 72(6): 425-31.

Grieve, G.P. 1991. *Mobilization of the spine: A primary handbook of clinical method.* 5th ed. Edinburgh: Churchill Livingstone.

Grigg, P. 1994. Peripheral neural mechanisms in proprioception. *J Sport Rehabil* 3: 2-17.

Grimmer, K., and P. Trott. 1998. The association between cervical excursion angles and cervical short flexor muscle endurance. *Aust J Physiother* 44(3): 201-7.

Gronroos, M., and A. Pertovaara. 1993. Capsaicin-induced central facilitation of a nociceptive flexion reflex in humans. *Neurosci Lett* 159(1-2): 215-8.

Gross, A.R., J.L. Hoving, T.A. Haines, C.H. Goldsmith, T. Kay, P. Aker, and G. Bronfort. Cervical Overview Group. 2004. Manipulation and mobilisation for mechanical neck disorders. *Cochrane Database Syst Rev* 1: CD004249.

Gross, A.R., T.M. Kay, C. Kennedy, D. Gasner, L. Hurley, K. Yardley, L. Hendry, and L. McLaughlin. 2002. Clinical practice guideline on the use of manipulation or mobilization in the treatment of adults with mechanical neck disorders. *Man Ther* 7(4): 193-205.

Gruber, M., and A. Gollhofer. 2004. Impact of sensorimotor training on the rate of force development and neural activation. *Eur J Appl Physiol* 92(1-2): 98-105.

Guanche, C., T. Knatt, M. Solomonow, Y. Lu, and R. Baratta. 1995. The synergistic action of the capsule and the shoulder muscles. *Am J Sports Med* 23(3): 301-6.

Guanche, C.A., J. Noble, M. Solomonow, C.S. Wink. 1999. Periarticular neural elements in the shoulder joint. *Orthopedics* 22: 615-17.

Guazzelli Filho, J., J. Furlani, and V. De Freitas. 1991. Electromyographic study of the trapezius muscle in free movements of the arm. *Electromyogr Clin Neurophysiol* 31(2): 93-8.

Guilbaud, G. 1991. Central neurophysiological processing of joint pain on the basis of studies performed in normal animals and in models of experimental arthritis. *Can J Physiol Pharmacol* 69(5): 637-46.

Gummesson, C., I. Atroshi, C. Ekdahl, R. Johnsson, and E. Ornstein. 2003. Chronic upper extremity pain and co-occurring symptoms in a general population. *Arthritis Rheum* 49(5): 697-702.

Gurney, B. 2002. Leg length discrepancy. *Gait Posture* 15: 195-206.

Guskiewicz, K.M., and D.H. Perrin. 1996. Effect of orthotics on postural sway following inversion ankle sprain. *J Orthop Sports Phys Ther* 23(5): 326-31.

Haahr, J.P., and J.H. Andersen. 2006. Exercises may be as efficient as subacromial decompression in patients with subacromial stage II impingement: 4-8-years' follow-up in a prospective, randomized study. *Scand J Rheumatol* 35(3): 224-8.

Haahr, J.P., S. Østergaard, J. Dalsgaard, K. Norup, P. Frost, S. Lausen, E.A. Holm, and J.H. Andersen. 2005. Exercises versus arthroscopic decompression in patients with subacromial impingement: A randomised, controlled study in 90 cases with a one year follow up. *Ann Rheum Dis* 64(5): 760-4.

Hagbarth, K.E., and G. Eklund. 1966. Tonic vibration reflexes (TVR) in spasticity. *Brain Res* 2(2): 201-3.

Hajek, M., V. Janda V, P. Kozak, E. Lukas, and A. Sehr. 1978. Diagnostics and therapy of the thoracic outlet syndromes. *Acta Univ Carol [Med] (Praha)* 24(5-6): 227-87.

Häkkinen, A., K. Häkkinen, P. Hannonen, and M. Alen. 2000. Force production capacity and acute neuromuscular responses to fatiguing loading in women with fibromyalgia are not different from those of healthy women. *J Rheumatol* 27(5): 1277-82.

Häkkinen, A., K. Häkkinen, P. Hannonen, and M. Alen. 2001. Strength training induced adaptations in neuromuscular function of premenopausal women with fibromyalgia: Comparison with healthy women. *Ann Rheum Dis* 60(1): 21-6.

Hale, S.A., Hertel, J., and Olmsted-Kramer, L.C. 2007. The effect of a 4-week comprehensive rehabilitation program on postural control and lower extremity function in individuals with chronic ankle instability. *J Orthop Sports Phys Ther.* Jun;37(6): 303-11.

Hallaçeli, H., and I. Günal. 2002. Normal range of scapular elevation and depression in healthy subjects. *Arch Orthop Trauma Surg* 122(2): 99-101.

Hallaceli, H., M. Manisali, and I. Gunal. 2004. Does scapular elevation accompany glenohumeral abduction in healthy subjects? *Arch Orthop Trauma Surg* 124(6): 378-81.

Hallgren, R.C., P.E. Greenman, and J.J. Rechtien. 1994. Atrophy of suboccipital muscles in patients with chronic pain: A pilot study. *J Am Osteopath Assoc* 94(12): 1032-8.

Hallström, E., and J. Kärrholm. 2006. Shoulder kinematics in 25 patients with impingement and 12 controls. *Clin Orthop Relat Res* 448: 22-7.

Halseth, T., J.W. McChesney, M. DeBeliso, R. Vaughn, and J. Lien. 2004. The effects of kinesiotaping on proprioception at the ankle. *Journal of Sports Science and Medicine* 3(1): 1-7.

Hargrave, M.D., C.R. Carcia, B.M. Gansneder, and S.J. Shultz. 2003. Subtalar pronation does not influence impact forces or rate of loading during a single-leg landing. *J Athl Train* 38(1): 18-23.

Haridas, C., E.P. Zehr, and J.E. Misiaszek. 2005. Postural uncertainty leads to dynamic control of cutaneous reflexes from the foot during human walking. *Brain Res* 1062(1-2): 48-62.

Harris, F.A. 1984. Facilitation techniques and technological adjuncts in therapeutic exercise. In *Therapeutic exercise.* 4th ed., ed. J.V. Basmajian, 110-78. Baltimore: Williams & Wilkins.

Harris, K.D., D.M. Heer, T.C. Roy, D.M. Santos, A.E. Pritchard, R.S. Wainner, and J.M. Whitman. 2003. Reliability of a measurement of deep neck flexor muscle endurance. Abstract. *J Orthop Sports Phys Ther* 33(2): A17.

Hass, C.J., L. Garzarella, D. de Hoyos, and M.L. Pollock. 2000. Single versus multiple sets in long-term recreational weightlifters.*Med Sci Sports Exerc* 32(1): 235-42.

Hassan, B.S., S. Mockett, and M. Doherty. 2001. Static postural sway, proprioception, and maximal voluntary quadriceps contraction in patients with knee osteoarthritis and normal control subjects. *Ann Rheum Dis* 60(6): 612-8.

He, X., U. Proske, H.G. Schaible, and R.F. Schmidt. 1988. Acute inflammation of the knee joint in the cat alters responses of flexor motoneurons to leg movements. *J Neurophysiol* 59(2): 326-40.

Hébert, L.J., H. Moffet, B.J. McFadyen, and C.E. Dionne. 2002. Scapular behavior in shoulder impingement syndrome. *Arch Phys Med Rehabil* 83(1): 60-9.

Hébert, L.J., H. Moffet, M. Dufour, and C. Moisan. 2003. Acromiohumeral distance in a seated position in persons with impingement syndrome. *J Magn Reson Imaging* 18(1): 72-9.

Heikkila, H., and P.G. Astrom. 1996. Cervicocephalic kinesthetic sensibility in patients with whiplash injury. *Scand J Rehabil Med* 28(3): 133-8.

Heikkila, H.V., and B.I. Wenngren. 1998. Cervicocephalic kinesthetic sensibility, active range of cervical motion, and oculomotor function in patients with whiplash injury. *Arch Phys Med Rehabil* 79(9): 1089-94.

Heitkamp, H.C., T. Horstmann, F. Mayer, J. Weller, and H.H. Dickhuth. 2001. Gain in strength and muscular balance after balance training. *Int J Sports Med* 22: 285-90.

Hendriksson, K. 2002. Is fibromyalgia a central pain state? *Journal of Musculoskeletal Pain* 10(1/2): 45-57.

Henke, K.G., M.T. Sharratt, D. Pegelow, and J.A. Dempsey. 1998. Regulation of end-expiratory lung volume during exercise. *J Appl Physiol* 64: 135-46.

Herren-Gerber, R., S. Weiss, L. Arendt-Nielsen, S. Petersen-Felix, G. Di Stefano, B.P. Radanov, and M. Curatolo. 2004. Modulation of central hypersensitivity by nociceptive input in chronic pain after whiplash injury. *Pain Med* 5(4): 366-76.

Hertel, J., M.R. Gay, and C.R. Denegar. 2002. Differences in postural control during single-leg stance among healthy individuals with different foot types. *J Athl Train* 37(2): 129-32.

Herzog, W. 2000. *Clinical biomechanics of spinal manipulation.* New York: Churchill Livingstone.

Herzog, W., D. Scheele, and P.J. Conway. 1999. Electromyographic responses of back and limb muscles associated with spinal manipulative therapy. *Spine* 24: 146-53.

Hess, S.A., C. Richardson, R. Darnell, P. Friis, D. Lisle, P. Myers. 2005. Timing of rotator cuff activation during shoulder external rotation in throwers with and without symptoms of pain. *J Orthop Sports Phys Ther* 35(12): 812-20.

Hettinger, T., and E.A. Muller. 1953. Muscle capacity and muscle training. *Arbeitsphysiologie* 15: 111-26.

Hicks, J.H. 1954. The mechanics of the foot: The plantar aponeurosis and the arch. *J Anat* 88: 25-31.

Hides, J.A., C.A. Richardson, and G.A. Jull. 1994. Multifidus muscle recovery is not automatic after resolution of acute. First-episode low back pain. *Spine* 21(23): 2763-9.

Hides, J.A., M.J. Stokes, M. Saide, G.A. Jull, and D.H. Cooper. 1994. Evidence of lumbar multifidus muscle wasting ipsilateral to symptoms in patients with acute/subacute low back pain. *Spine* 19: 165-72.

Hietkamp, H.C., T. Horstman, F. Mayer, J. Weller, and H.H. Dickhuth. 2001. Gain in strength and muscular balance after balance training. *Int J Sports Med* 22: 285-90.

Hinoki, M., and N. Ushio. 1975. Lumbosacral proprioceptive reflexes in body equilibrium. *Acta Otolaryngol* Suppl. no. 330: 197.

Hintermeister, R.A., G.W. Lange, J.M. Schultheis, M.J. Bey, and R.J. Hawkins. 1998. Electromyographic activity and applied load during shoulder rehabilitation exercises using elastic resistance. *Am J Sports Med* 26(2): 210-20.

Hinterwimmer, S., R. Von Eisenhart-Rothe, M. Siebert, R. Putz, F. Eckstein, T. Vogl, and H. Graichen. 2003. Influence of adducting and abducting muscle forces on the subacromial space width. *Med Sci Sports Exerc* 35(12): 2055-9.

Hinton, R.Y. 1988. Isokinetic evaluation of shoulder rotational strength in high school baseball pitchers. *Am J Sports Med* 16(3): 274-9.

Hodges, P.W. 2003. Core stability exercise in chronic low back pain. *Orthop Clin North Am* 34: 245-54.

Hodges, P.W., A.E. Eriksson, D. Shirley, and S.C. Gandevia. 2005. Intra-abdominal pressure increases stiffness of the lumbar spine. *J Biomech* 38(9): 1873-80.

Hodges, P.W., A.E. Martin Eriksson, D. Shirley, and S.C. Gandevia. 2006. Intra-abdominal pressure increases stiffness of the lumbar spine. *J Biomech* 38: 1873-80.

Hodges, P.W., and C.A. Richardson. 1996. Inefficient muscular stabilization of the lumbar spine associated with low back pain. A motor control evaluation of the transversus abdominus. *Spine* 21(22): 2640-50.

Hodges, P.W., and C.A. Richardson. 1997a. Contraction of the abdominal muscles associated with movement of the lower limb. *Phys Ther* 77(2): 132-42.

Hodges, P.W., and C.A. Richardson. 1997b. Feedforward contraction of transversus abdominus is not influenced by the direction of arm movement. *Exp Brain Res* 114: 362-70.

Hodges, P.W., and C.A. Richardson. 1998. Delayed postural contraction of transversus abdominis in low back pain associated with movement of the lower limb. *J Spinal Disord* 11(1): 46-56.

Hodges, P.W., and C.A. Richardson. 1999. Transversus abdominis and the superficial abdominal muscles are controlled independently in postural task. *Neuroscience* 265: 91-4.

Hodges, P.W., and S.C. Gandevia. 2000a. Activation of the human diaphragm during a repetitive postural task. *J Physiol* 522(Pt. 1): 165-75.

Hodges, P.W., and S.C. Gandevia. 2000b. Changes in intra-abdominal pressure during postural and respiratory activation of the human diaphragm. *J Appl Physiol* 89(3): 967-76.

Hodges, P.W., R. Sapsford, and P.H.M. Pengel. 2007. Postural and respiratory functions of the pelvic floor muscles. *Neurourol Urodyn* 26(3): 362-71.

Hodges, P.W., S.C. Gandevia, and C.A. Richardson. 1997. Contractions of specific abdominal muscles in postural tasks are affected by respiratory maneuvers. *J Appl Physiol* 83(3): 753-60.

Hoffer, J.A., and S. Andreassen. 1981. Regulation of soleus muscle stiffness in premammillary cats: Intrinsic and reflex components. *J Neurophysiol* 45(2): 267-85.

Holm, S., A. Inhahl, and M. Solomonow. 2002. Sensorimotor control of the spine. *J Electromyogr Kinesiol* 12: 219-34.

Holme, E., S.P. Magnusson, K. Becher, T. Bieler, P. Aagaard, and M. Kjaer. 1999. The effect of supervised rehabilitation on strength, postural sway, position sense and re-injury risk after acute ankle ligament sprain. *Scand J Med Sci Sports* 9(2): 104-9.

Hölmich, P., P. Uhrskou, and L. Ulnits. 1999. Effectiveness of active physical training for long-standing adductor-related groin pain in athletes. *Lancet* 353: 439-43.

Holt, L.E., T.M. Travis, and T. Okita. 1970. Comparative study of three stretching techniques. *Percept Mot Skills* 31(2): 611-6.

Hong, C.-Z. 1994. Lidocaine injection versus dry needling to myofascial trigger point; the importance of the local twitch response. *Am J Phys Med Rehabil* 73: 256-63.

Hong, C.Z. 1999. Current research on myofascial trigger points—pathophysiological studies. *Journal of Musculoskeletal Pain* 7(1/2): 121-9.

Hong, C.Z., and D.G. Simons. 1998. Pathophysiologic and electrophysiologic mechanisms of myofascial trigger points. *Arch Phys Med Rehabil* 79(7): 863-72.

Hootman, J., S. Fitzgerald, C. Macera, J. Shannon, and S. Blair. 2004. Lower extremity muscle strength and risk of self-reported hip or knee osteoarthritis. *J Phys Act Health* 1: 321-30.

Hopkins, J.T., and R. Palmieri. 2004. Effects of ankle joint effusion on lower leg function. *Clin J Sport Med* 14(1): 1-7.

Hopkins, J.T., C.D. Ingersoll, M.A. Sandrey, and S.D. Bleggi. 1999. An electromyographic comparison of 4 closed chain exercises. *J Athl Train* 34(4): 353-7.

Horak, F.B., and L.M. Nashner. 1986. Central programming of postural movements: Adaptation to altered support-surface configurations. *J Neurophysiol* 55(6): 1369-81.

Horak, F.B., L.M. Nashner, and H.C. Diener. 1990. Postural strategies associated with somatosensory and vestibular loss. *Exp Brain Res* 82(1): 167-77.

Horal, J. 1969. The clinical appearance of low back disorders in the city of Gothenburg, Sweden. Comparisons of incapacitated probands with matched controls. *Acta Orthop Scand Suppl* 118: 1-109.

Horstmann, T., Martini, F., Knak, J., Mayer, F., Sell S., Zacher, J., and Kusswetter, W. 1994. Isokinetic force-velocity curves in patients following implantation of an individual total hip prosthesis. *Int J Sports Med.* Jan;15 Suppl 1: S64-9.

Horstmann, T., Roecker, K., Vornholt, S., Niess, A.M., Heitkamp, H.C., and Dickuth, H.H. 2002. Deficits in performance in hip osteoarthritis and endoprosthesis patients. *Deutsche Zeitschrift Fur Sportmedizin.* 53(1): 17-21.

Hou, C.R., L.C. Tsai, K.F. Cheng, K.C. Chung, and C.Z. Hong. 2002. Immediate effects of various physical therapeutic modalities on cervical myofascial pain and trigger-point sensitivity. *Arch Phys Med Rehabil* 83(10): 1406-14.

Housh, D.J., and T.J. Housh. 1993. The effects of unilateral velocity-specific concentric strength training. *J Orthop Sports Phys Ther* 17(5): 252-6.

Hruska Jr., R.J. 1999. Influences of dysfunctional respiratory mechanics on orofacial pain. *Dent Clin North Am* 41(2): 211-27.

Hrysomallis, C. 2007. Relationship between balance ability, training and sports injury risk. *Sports Med* 37(6): 547-56.

Hrysomallis, C., and C. Goodman. 2001. A review of resistance exercise and posture realignment. *J Strength Cond Res* 15(3): 385-90.

Hsieh, J.-C., C.-H. Tu, F.-P. Chen, M.-C. Chen, T.-C. Yeh, H.-C. Cheng, Y.T. Wu, R.S. Liu, and L.T. Ho. 2001. Activation of the hypothalamus characterizes the acupuncture stimulation at the analgesic point in human: A positron emission tomography study. *Neurosci Lett* 307(2): 105-8.

Huffman, G.R., J.E. Tibone, M.H. McGarry, B.M. Phipps, Y.S. Lee, and T.Q. Lee. 2006. Path of glenohumeral articulation throughout the rotational range of motion in a thrower's shoulder model. *Am J Sports Med* 34(10): 1662-9.

Hui, K., and J. Lui. 2000. Acupuncture modulates the limbic system and subcortical gray structures of the human brain: Evidence of MRI studies in normal subjects. *Hum Brain Mapp* 9: 13-25.

Hungerford, B., W. Gilleard, and P. Hodges. 2003. Evidence of altered lumbopelvic muscle recruitment in the presence of sacroiliac joint pain. *Spine* 28(14): 1593-600.

Hurley, M.V. 1997. The effects of joint damage on muscle function, proprioception and rehabilitation. *Man Ther* 2(1): 11-7.

Hurley, M.V., and D.J. Newham. 1993. The influence of arthrogenous muscle inhibition on quadriceps rehabilitation of patients with early, unilateral osteoarthritic knees. *Br J Rheumatol* 32: 127–131.

Iams, J. 2005. When reflexes rule: A new paradigm in understanding why some patients don't get well. *Advance for Physical Therapists* 16(3): 41.

Ide, J., S. Maeda, M. Yamaga, K. Morisawa, and K. Takagi. 2003. Shoulder-strengthening exercise with an orthosis for multidirectional shoulder instability: Quantitative evaluation of rotational shoulder strength before and after the exercise program. *J Shoulder Elbow Surg* 12(4): 342-5.

Ihara, H., and A. Nakayama. 1986. Dynamic joint control training for knee ligament injuries. *Am J Sports Med* 14: 309-15.

Ihara, H., and A. Nakayama. 1986. Dynamic joint control training for knee ligament injuries. *Am J Sports Med* 14: 309-15.

Iles, J., M. Stokes, and A. Young. 1990. Reflex actions of knee joint afferents during contractions of the human quadriceps. *Clin Physiol* 10: 489-500.

Illyés, A., and R.M. Kiss. 2006. Kinematic and muscle activity characteristics of multidirectional shoulder joint instability during elevation. *Knee Surg Sports Traumatol Arthrosc* 14(7): 673-85.

Illyés, A., and R.M. Kiss. 2007. Electromyographic analysis in patients with multidirectional shoulder instability during pull, forward punch, elevation and overhead throw. *Knee Surg Sports Traumatol Arthrosc* 15(5): 624-31.

Inman, V.T. 1966. Human locomotion. *Can Med Assoc J* 94(20): 1047-54.

Inman, V.T., H.J. Ralston, F. Todd, and J.C. Lieberman. 1981. *Human walking.* Baltimore: Williams & Wilkins.

Inman, V.T., J.B. Saunders, and L.C. Abbott. 1944. Observations of the function of the shoulder joint. *J Bone Joint Surg* 26(1): 1-30.

Ireland, M.L., J.D. Willson, B.T. Ballantyne, and I.M. Davis. 2003. Hip strength in females with and without patellofemoral pain. *J Orthop Sports Phys Ther* 33(11): 671-6.

Itoi, E., S.R. Newman, D.K. Kuechle, B.F. Morrey, and K.N. An. 1994. Dynamic anterior stabilisers of the shoulder with the arm in abduction. *J Bone Joint Surg Br* 76(5): 834-6.

Jacobs, C., T.L. Uhl, M. Seeley, W. Sterling, and L. Goodrich. 2005. Strength and fatigability of the dominant and nondominant hip abductors. *J Athl Train* 40(3): 203-6.

Jaeger, B., and S.A. Skootsky. 1987. Double blind controlled study of different myofascial trigger point injection techniques. *Pain* Suppl. no. 4: S292.

Janda ,V., and M. VáVrová. 1996. Sensory motor stimulation. In *Rehabilitation of the spine,* ed. C. Liebenson, 319-28. Baltimore: Williams & Wilkins.

Janda V. 1995. Personal communications and course notes.

Janda, V. 1964. Movement patterns in pelvic and thigh region with special reference to pathogenesis of vertebrogenic disturbances. [In Czech.] Thesis, Charles University.

Janda, V. 1978. Muscles, central nervous regulation and back problems. In *Neurobiological mechanisms in manipulative therapy,* ed. I.M. Korr, 27-41. New York: Plenum Press.

Janda, V. 1983. On the concept of postural muscles and posture. *Aust J Physiother* 29: S83-4.

Janda, V. 1984. Gestörte Bewegungsabläufe und Rückenschmerzen. [Disturbed courses of motion and back pain.] *Z Manuelle Med* 22: 74-28.

Janda, V. 1986. Muscle weakness and inhibition (pseudoparesis) in back pain syndromes. In *Modern manual therapy of the vertebral column,* ed. G.P. Grieve**.** 136-139. London: Churchill Livingstone

Janda, V. 1986a. Muscle weakness and inhibition (pseudoparesis) in back syndromes. In *Manual therapy of the vertebral column,* ed. P. Grieve 136-139. New York: Churchill Livingstone.

Janda, V. 1986b. Some aspects of extracranial causes of facial pain. *J Prosthet Dent* 56(4): 484-7.

Janda, V. 1987. Muscles and motor control in low back pain: Assessment and management. In *Physical therapy of the low back,* ed. L.T. Twomey, 253-78. New York: Churchill Livingstone.

Janda, V. 1988. Muscles and cervicogenic pain syndromes. In *Physical therapy of the cervical and thoracic spine,* ed. R. Grand, 153-166. New York: Churchill Livingstone.

Janda, V. 1989a. Differential diagnosis of muscle tone in respect to inhibitory techniques. *Journal of Manual Medicine* 4(3): 96.

Janda, V. 1989b. Impaired muscle function in children and adolescents. *Journal of Manual Medicine* 4(3): 157-60.

Janda, V. 1991. Muscle spasm—A proposed procedure for differential diagnosis. *J Manual Medicine* 6: 136-9.

Janda, V. 1992. Sensorimotor stimulation. [In Czech.] *Rehabilitacia* 3: 14-35.

Janda, V. 1992. Treatment of chronic back pain. *Journal of Manual Medicine* 6(5): 166-8.

Janda, V. 1993. Muscle strength in relation to muscle length, pain, and muscle imbalance. In *Muscle strength.* Vol. 8 of *International perspectives in physical therapy,* ed. K. Harms-Ringdahl, 83-91. Edinburgh: Churchill Livingstone.

Janda, V. 1994. Muscles and motor control in cervicogenic disorders. In *Physical therapy of the cervical and thoracic spine.* 1st ed., ed. R. Grant, 195- 215. Edinburgh: Churchill Livingstone.

Janda, V. 2000. *Manuelle muskelfunktions-diagnostik.* 4th ed. Munich: Urban & Fischer.

Janda, V. 2002. Cervicocervical transits. [In Czech.] *Rehabil Fyz Lek* 9(1): 3-4.

Janda, V., and M. VáVrová. 1996. Sensory motor stimulation. In *Rehabilitation of the spine,* ed. C. Liebenson, 319-28. Baltimore: Williams & Wilkins.

Janda, V., C. Frank, and C. Liebenson. 2007. Evaluation of muscle imbalances. In *Rehabilitation of the spine,* ed. C. Liebenson 203-225. Philadelphia: Lippincott Williams & Wilkins.

Janda, V., M. Vavrova, A. Herbenova, and M. Veverkova. 2007. Sensorimotor stimulation. In *Rehabilitation of the spine.* 2nd ed., ed. C. Liebenson 513-530. Philadelphia: Lippincott Williams & Wilkins.

Janda. V. 2002. Cervicocervical transits. [In Czech.] *Rehabil Fyz Lek* 9(1): 3-4. .

Jaramillo, J., T.W. Worrell, and C.D. Ingersoll. 1994. Hip isometric strength following knee surgery. *J Orthop Sports Phys Ther* 20(3): 160-5.

Järvholm, U., J. Styf, M. Suurkula, and P. Herberts. 1988. Intramuscular pressure and muscle blood flow in supraspinatus. *Eur J Appl Physiol Occup Physiol* 58(3): 219-24.

Jensen, C., and R.H. Westgaard. 1997. Functional subdivision of the upper trapezius muscle during low-level activation. *Eur J Appl Physiol Occup Physiol* 76(4): 335-9.

Jensen, C., L. Finsen, K. Hansen, H. Christensen. 1999. Upper trapezius muscle activity patterns during repetitive manual material handling and work with with a computer mouse. *J Electromyogr Kinesiol* 9(5): 317-25.

Jensen, C., O. Vasseljen, and R.H. Westgaard. 1993. The influence of electrode position on bipolar surface electromyogram recordings of the upper trapezius muscle. *Eur J Appl Physiol Occup Physiol* 67(3): 266-73.

Jerosch, J., J. Steinbeck, H. Clahsen, M. Schmitz-Nahrath, and A. Grosse-Hackmann. 1993. Function of the glenohumeral ligaments in active stabilisation of the shoulder joint. *Knee Surg Sports Traumatol Arthrosc* 1(3-4): 152-8.

Jerosch, J., W.H. Castro, H.U. Sons, and M. Moersler. 1989. Etiology of sub-acromial impingement syndrome—a biomechanical study. [In German.] *Beitr Orthop Traumatol* 36(9): 411-8.

Jobe, F.W. 1989. Impingement problems in the athlete. *Instr Course Lect* 38: 205-9.

Jobe, F.W., and M. Pink. 1993. Classification and treatment of shoulder dysfunction in the overhead athlete. *J Orthop Sports Phys Ther* 18(2): 427-32.

Jobe, F.W., R.S. Kvitne, and C.E. Giangarra. 1989. Shoulder pain in the overhand or throwing athlete. The relationship of anterior instability and rotator cuff impingement. *Orthop Rev* 18(9): 963-75.

Johansson, H., and P. Sojka 1991. Pathophysiological mechanisms involved in genesis and spread of muscular tension in occupational muscle pain and in chronic musculoskeletal pain syndromes: A hypothesis. *Med Hypotheses* 35(3): 196-203.

Johnson, E.G., J.J. Godges, E.B. Lohman, J.A. Stephens, G.J. Zimmerman, and S.P. Anderson. 2003. Disability self-assessment and upper quarter muscle balance between female dental hygienists and non-dental hygienists. *J Dent Hyg* 77(4): 217-23.

Johnson, G., N. Bogduk, A. Nowitzke, and D. House. 1994. Anatomy and actions of the trapezius muscle. [review]. *Clin Biomech (Bristol, Avon)* 9: 44-50.

Johnson, M.A., J. Polgar, D. Weightman, and D. Appleton. 1973. Data on the distribution of fibre types in thirty-six human muscles. An autopsy study. *J Neurol Sci* 18(1): 111-29.

Johnson, M.E., M.L. Mille, K.M. Martinez, and M.W. Rogers. 2002. Age-related changes in hip abductor and adductor muscle strength in women. Abstract. *J Geriatr Phys Ther* 25(3): 24.

Johnston, T.B. 1937. The movements of the shoulder-joint. *Br J Surg* 25: 252-60.

Jones, D.A., O.M. Rutherford, and D.F. Parker. 1989. Physiological changes in skeletal muscle as a result of strength training *Q J Exp Physiol* 1989: 233-56.

Jones, K.D., C.S. Burckhardt, A.A. Deodhar, N.A. Perrin, G.C. Hanson, and R.M. Bennett. 2008. A six-month randomized controlled trial of exercise and pyridostigmine in the treatment of fibromyalgia. *Arthritis Rheum* 58(2): 612-22.

Jones, K.D., C.S. Burckhardt, S.R. Clark, R.M. Bennett, and K.M. Potempa. 2002. A randomized controlled trial of muscle strengthening versus flexibility training in fibromyalgia. *J Rheumatol* 29(5): 1041-8.

Jones, L.H. 1964. Spontaneous release by positioning. *The D.O.* 4: 109.

Jones, P.S., and M.A. Tomski. 2000. Exercise and osteopathic manipulative medicine: The Janda approach. *Physicals Medicine and Rehabilitation: State of the Art Reviews* 14(1): 163-79.

Jönhagen, S., G. Németh, and E. Eriksson. 1994. Hamstring injuries in sprinters. The role of concentric and eccentric hamstring muscle strength and flexibility. *Am J Sports Med* 22(2): 262-6.

Jonsson, P., P. Wahlström, L. Ohberg, and H. Alfredson. 2006. Eccentric training in chronic painful impingement syndrome of the shoulder: Results of a pilot study. *Knee Surg Sports Traumatol Arthrosc* 14(1): 76-81.

Juker, D., S.M. McGill, P. Kropf, and T. Steffen. 1998. Quantitative intramuscular myoelectric activity of lumbar portions of psoas and the abdominal wall during a wide variety of tasks. *Med Sci Sports Exerc* 30(2): 301-10.

Jull, G., C. Barrett, R. Magee, and P. Ho. 1999. Further clinical clarification of the muscle dysfunction in cervical headache. *Cephalalgia* 19(3): 179-85.

Jull, G., D. Falla, J. Treleaven, P. Hodges, and B. Vicenzino. 2007. Retraining cervical joint position sense: The effect of two exercise regimes. *J Orthop Res* 25(3): 404-12.

Jull, G., E. Kristjansson, and P. Dall'Alba. 2004. Impairment in the cervical flexors: A comparison of whiplash and insidious onset neck pain patients. *Man Ther* 9(2): 89-94.

Jull, G., M. Sterling, J. Kenardy, and E. Beller. 2007. Does the presence of sensory hypersensitivity influence outcomes of physical rehabilitation for chronic whiplash? A preliminary RCT. *Pain* 129(1-2): 28-34.

Jull, G., P. Trott, H. Potter, G. Zito, K. Niere, D. Shirley, J. Emberson, I. Marschner, and C. Richardson. 2002. A randomized controlled trial of exercise and manipulative therapy for cervicogenic headache. *Spine* 27(17): 1835-43.

Jull, G.A. 2000. Deep cervical flexor muscle dysfunction in whiplash. *Journal of Musculoskeletal Pain* 8(1/2): 143-54.

Jull, G.A., and V. Janda. 1987. Muscles and motor control in low back pain. In *Physical therapy of the low back.* 1st ed., ed. L.T. Twomey and J.R. Taylor, 253-278. New York: Churchill Livingstone.

Jull, G.A., E. Kristjansson, and P. Dall'Alba. 2004. Impairment in the cervical flexors: A comparision of whiplash and insidious onset neck paitents. *Man Ther* 9: 89-94.

Kabat, H. 1950. Studies on neuromuscular dysfunction XIII. New concepts and techniques of neuromuscular re-education for paralysis. *Perm Found Med Bull* 8: 121-43.

Kaminski, T.W., B.D. Buckley, M.E. Powers, T.J. Hubbard, B.M. Hatzel, and C. Ortiz. 2001. Eversion and inversion strength ratios in subjects with unilateral functional ankle instability. Abstract. *Med Sci Sports Exerc* Suppl. no. 33(5): S135.

Kamkar, A., J.J. Irrgang, and S.L. Whitney. 1993. Non-operative management of secondary shoulder impingement syndrome. *J Orthop Sports Phys Ther* 17(5): 212-24.

Karduna, A.R., P.J. Kerner, and M.D. Lazarus. 2005. Contact forces in the subacromial space: Effects of scapular orientation. *J Shoulder Elbow Surg* 14(4): 393-9.

Karlberg, M., L. Persson, and M. Magnusson. 1995. Impaired postural control in patients with cervico-brachial pain. *Acta Otolaryngol* Suppl. no. 520(Pt. 2): 440-2.

Kase, K., and T. Hashimoto. 1998. Changes in the volume of the peripheral blood flow by using kinesiotaping. Unpublished.

Kase, K., J. Wallis, and T. Kase. 2003. *Clinical therapeutic applications of the kinesio taping method.* 2nd ed. Tokyo: Ken Ikai Co. Ltd

Kashima, K., S. Maeda, S. Higashinaka, N. Watanabe, M. Ogihara, and S. Sakoda. 2006. Relationship between head position and the muscle hardness of the masseter and trapezius muscles: A pilot study. *Cranio* 24(1): 38-42.

Kauffman, T.L., L.M. Nashner, and L.K. Allison. 1997. Balance is a critical parameter in orthopedic rehabilitation. *Orthop Phys Ther Clin N Am* 6(1): 43-78.

Kavcic, N., S. Grenier, and S.M. McGill. 2004. Determining the stabilizing role of individual torso muscles during rehabilitation exercises. *Spine* 29(11): 1254-65.

Kavounoudias, A., R. Roll, and J.P. Roll. 2001. Foot sole and ankle muscle inputs contribute jointly to human erect posture regulation. *J Physiol* 532(Pt3): 869-78.

Kay, T.M., A. Gross, C. Goldsmith, P.L. Santaguida, J. Hoving, and G. Bronfort. Cervical Overview Group. 2005. Exercises for mechanical neck disorders. *Cochrane Database Syst Rev* 3: CD004250.

Keating, J.F., P. Waterworth, J. Shaw-Dunn, and J. Crossan. 1993. The relative strengths of the rotator cuff muscles. A cadaver study. *J Bone Joint Surg Br* 75(1): 137-40.

Kebaetse, M., P. McClure, and N.A. Pratt. 1999. Thoracic position effect on shoulder range of motion, strength, and three-dimensional scapular kinematics. *Arch Phys Med Rehabil* 80(8): 945-50.

Kelley, J.D., S.J. Lombardo, M. Pink, J. Perry, and C.E. Giangarra. 1994. Electromyographic and cinematographic analysis of elbow function in tennis players with lateral epicondylitis. *Am J Sports Med* 22(3): 359-63.

Kelly, B.T., R.J. Williams, F.A. Cordasco, S.I. Backus, J.C. Otis, D.E. Weiland, D.W. Altchek, E.V. Craig, T.L. Wickiewicz, and R.F. Warren. 2005. Differential patterns of muscle activation in patients with symptomatic and asymptomatic rotator cuff tears. *J Shoulder Elbow Surg* 14(2): 165-71.

Kelly, B.T., S.I. Backus, R.F. Warren, and R.J. Williams. 2002. Electromyographic analysis and phase definition of the overhead football throw. *Am J Sports Med* 30(6): 837-44.

Kelsey, B. 1961. Effects of mental practice and physical practice upon muscular endurance. *Res Q* 31(99): 47-54.

Kendall, F.P., E.K. McCreary, and P.G. Provance. 1993. *Muscles. Testing and function.* 4th ed. Baltimore: Williams & Wilkins.

Kenny, R.A., G.B. Traynor, D. Withington, and D.J. Keegan. 1993. Thoracic outlet syndrome: A useful exercise treatment option. *Am J Surg* 165(2): 282-4.

Ker, R.F., M.B. Bennett, S.R. Bibby, R.C. Kester, and R. Alexander. 1987. The spring in the arch of the human foot. *Nature* 325: 147-9.

Kerrigan, D.C., L.W. Lee, J.J. Collins, P.O. Riley, and L.A. Lipsitz. 2001. Reduced hip extension during walking: Healthy elderly and fallers versus young adults. *Arch Phys Med Rehabil* 82(1): 26-30.

Kettunen, J.A., Harilainen, A., Sandelin, J., Schlenzka, D., Hietaniemi, K., Seitsalo, S., Malmivaara, A., and Kujala, U.M. 2007. Knee arthroscopy and exercise versus exercise only for chronic patellofemoral pain syndrome: a randomized controlled trial. *BMC Med.* Dec 13;5: 38.

Kibler, W.B. 1995. Biomechanical analysis of the shoulder during tennis activities. *Clin Sports Med* 14(1): 79-85.

Kibler, W.B. 1998a. Determining the extent of the functional deficit. In *Functional rehabilitation of sports and musculoskeletal injuries,* ed. W.B. Kibler, S.A. Herring, J.M. Press, and P.A. Lee, 16-9. Gaithersburg, MD: Aspen.

Kibler, W.B. 1998b. The role of the scapula in athletic shoulder function. *Am J Sports Med* 26(2): 325-37.

Kibler, W.B. 2006. Scapular involvement in impingement: Signs and symptoms. *Instr Course Lect* 55: 35-43.

Kibler, W.B., and J. McMullen. 2003. Scapular dyskinesis and its relation to shoulder pain. *J Am Acad Orthop Surg* 11(2): 142-51.

Kibler, W.B., C. Goldberg, and T.J. Chandler. 1991. Functional biomechanical deficits in running athletes with plantar fasciitis. *Am J Sports Med* 19(1): 66-71.

Kibler, W.B., T.J. Chandler, and B.K. Pace. 1992. Principles of rehabilitation after chronic tendon injuries. *Clin Sports Med* 11(3): 661-71.

Kibler, W.B., T.J. Chandler, B.P. Livingston, and E.P. Roetert. 1996. Shoulder range of motion in elite tennis players. Effect of age and years of tournament play. *Am J Sports Med* 24(3): 279-85.

Kibler, W.B., T.J. Chandler, R. Shapiro, and M. Conuel. 2007. Muscle activation in coupled scapulohumeral motions in the high performance tennis serve. *Br J Sports Med* 41(11): 745-9.

Kidgell, D.J., Horvath, D.M., Jackson, B.M., and Seymour, P.J. 2007. Effect of six weeks of dura disc and mini-trampoline balance training on postural sway in athletes with functional ankle instability. *J Strength Cond Res.* May;21(2): 466-9.

Kido, T., E. Itoi, N. Konno, A. Sano, M. Urayama, and K. Sato. 2000. The depressor function of biceps on the head of the humerus in shoulders with tears of the rotator cuff. *J Bone Joint Surg Br* 82(3): 416-9.

Kido, T., E. Itoi, S.B. Lee, P.G. Neale, and K.N. An. 2003. Dynamic stabilizing function of the deltoid muscle in shoulders with anterior instability. *Am J Sports Med* 31(3): 399-403.

Kim, A.W., A.M. Rosen, V.A. Brander, and T.S. Buchanan. 1995. Selective muscle activation following electrical stimulation of the collateral ligaments of the human knee joint. *Arch Phys Med Rehabil* 76(8): 750-7.

Kim, S.H., K.I. Ha, H.S. Kim, and S.W. Kim. 2001. Electromyographic activity of the biceps brachii muscle in shoulders with anterior instability. *Arthroscopy* 17(8): 864-8.

King, D. 1995. Student writing contest winner: Glenohumeral joint impingement in swimmers. *J Athl Train* 30(4): 333-7.

Knapik, J.J., C.L. Bauman, B.H. Jones, J.M. Harris, and L. Vaughan. 1991. Preseason strength and flexibility imbalances associated with athletic injuries in female collegiate athletes. *Am J Sports Med* 19(1): 76-81.

Knikou, M., E. Kay, B.D. Schmit. 2007. Parallel facilitatory reflex pathways from the foot and hip to flexors and extensors in the injured human spinal cord. *Exp Neurol* 206(1): 146-58.

Knott, M., and D.E. Voss. 1968. Proprioceptive neuromuscular facilitation. New York: Harper & Row.

Kolář, P. 1999. The sensomotor nature of postural functions. Its fundamental role in rehabilitation of the motor system. *J Orthop Med* 21(2): 40-5.

Kolář, P. 2001. Systematization of muscular dysbalances from the aspect of developmental kinesiology. *Rehabilitation and Physical Medicine* 8(4): 152-64.

Kolář, P. 2007. Facilitation of agonist antagonist coactivation by reflex stimulation methods. In *Rehabilitation of the spine.* 2nd ed., ed. C. Liebenson, 531-65. Philadelphia: Lippincott Williams & Wilkins.

Komi, P.V., and C. Bosco. 1978. Utilization of stored elastic energy in leg extensor muscles by men and women. *Med Sci Sports* 10(4): 261-5.

Konradsen, L., and J.B. Ravn. 1990. Ankle instability caused by prolonged peroneal reaction time. *Acta Orthop Scand* 61(5): 388-90.

Konradsen, L., M. Voigt, and C. Hojsgaard. 1997. Ankle inversion injuries. The role of the dynamic defense mechanism. *Am J Sports Med* 25(1): 54-7.

Korr, I.M. 1979. *The facilitated segment: A factor in injury to the body framework. The collected papers of Irwin M. Korr.* Colorado Springs: American Academy of Osteopathy.

Kosek, E., J. Ekholm, and P. Hansson. 1996. Sensory dysfunction in fibromyalgia patients with implications for pathogenic mechanisms. *Pain* 68(2-3): 375-83.

Kraushaar, B.S., and R.P. Nirschl. 1999. Tendinosis of the elbow (tennis elbow). Clinical features and findings of histological, immunohistochemical, and electron microscopy studies. *J Bone Joint Surg Am* 81(2): 259-78.

Kronberg, M., and L.A. Broström. 1995. Electromyographic recordings in shoulder muscles during eccentric movements. *Clin Orthop Relat Res* 314:143-51.

Kronberg, M., G. Németh, and L.A. Broström. 1990. Muscle activity and coordination in the normal shoulder. An electromyographic study. *Clin Orthop Relat Res* 257: 76-85.

Kronberg, M., L.A. Broström, and G. Németh. 1991. Differences in shoulder muscle activity between patients with generalized joint laxity and normal controls. *Clin Orthop Relat Res* 269: 181-92.

Kronberg, M., P. Larsson, and L.A. Broström. 1997. Characterisation of human deltoid muscle in patients with impingement syndrome. *J Orthop Res* 15(5): 727-33.

Kruse, R.D., and D.K. Mathews. 1958. Bilateral effects of unilateral exercise: Experimental study based on 120 subjects. *Arch Phys Med Rehabil* 39(6): 371-6.

Kugler, A., M. Kruger-Franke, S. Reininger, H.H. Trouillier, and B. Rosemeyer. 1996 Muscular imbalance and shoulder pain in volleyball attackers. *Br J Sports Med* 30(3): 256-9.

Kugler, A., M. Kruger-Franke, S. Reininger, H.H. Trouillier, and B. Rosemeyer. 1996. Muscular imbalance and shoulder pain in volleyball attackers. *Br J Sports Med* 30(3): 256-9.

Kumbhare, D.A., B. Balsor, W.L. Parkinson, P. Harding Bsckin, M. Bedard, A. Papaioannou, and J.D. Adachi. 2005. Measurement of cervical flexor endurance following whiplash. *Disabil Rehabil* 27(14): 801-7.

Kurtz, A.D. 1939. Chronic sprained ankle. *Am J Surg* 44(1): 158-60.

Labriola, J.E., T.Q. Lee, R.E. Debski, and P.J. McMahon. 2005. Stability and instability of the glenohumeral joint: The role of shoulder muscles. *J Shoulder Elbow Surg* 14(1 Suppl. no. S): 32S-38S.

Landis, J., I. Keselman, and C.N. Murphy. 2005. Comparison of electromyographic (EMG) activity of selected forearm muscles during low grade resistance therapeutic exercises in individuals diagnosed with lateral epicondylitis. *Work* 24(1): 85-91.

Lanza, D., Dmowski, B.E., Murillo, P.A., Sarro, C.K., Tribelhorn, P.A., and Norkus, S.A. 2003. Comparison of muscle activity during a single leg stance: stable versus unstable surface (Abstract). J Athl Train. 38(20: S91).

Lardner, R. 2001. Stretching and flexibility: Its importance in rehabilitation. *J Bodyw Mov Ther* 5(4): 254-63.

Larsson, R., H. Cai, Q. Zhang, P.A. Oberg, and S.E. Larsson. 1998. Visualization of chronic neck-shoulder pain: Impaired microcirculation in the upper trapezius muscle in chronic cervico-brachial pain. *Occup Med (Lond)* 48(3): 189-94.

Laudner, K.G., J.B. Myers, M.R. Pasquale, J.P. Bradley, and S.M. Lephart. 2006. Scapular dysfunction in throwers with pathologic internal impingement. *J Orthop Sports Phys Ther* 36(7): 485-94.

Lautenbacher, S., and G.B. Rollman. 1997. Possible deficiencies of pain modulation in fibromyalgia. *Clin J Pain* 13(3): 189-96.

Lawrence, R.C., D.T. Felson, C.G. Helmick, L.M. Arnold, H. Choi, R.A. Deyo, S. Gabriel et al. National Arthritis Data Workgroup. 2008. Estimates of the prevalence of arthritis and other rheumatic conditions in the United States. Part II. *Arthritis Rheum* 58(1): 26-35.

Layton, J.A., C.A. Thigpen, D.A. Padua, W.E. Prentice, and S.G. Karas. 2005. A comparison between swimmers and non-swimmers on posture, range of motion, strength, and scapular motion. Abstract. *J Athl Train* 40(2): S23.

Lear, L.J., and M.T. Gross. 1998. An electromyographical analysis of the scapular stabilizing synergists during a push-up progression. *J Orthop Sports Phys Ther* 28(3): 146-57.

Lederman, E. 1997. *Fundamentals of manual therapy: Physiology, neurology and psychology.* New York: Churchill Livingstone.

Lee, D. 1997. Instability of the sacroiliac joint and the consequences for gait. In *Movement stability and low back pain,* ed. A. Vleeming, V. Mooney, T. Dorman, C. Snijders, and R. Soteckhart, 231-3. New York: Churchill Livingstone.

Lee, D. 1999. *The pelvic girdle.* Edinburgh: Churchill Livingstone.

Lee, H.M. 2000. Rehabilitation of the proximal crossed syndrome in an elderly blind patient: A case report. *J Can Chiropr Assoc* 44(4): 223-9.

Lee, H.M., J.J. Liau, C.K. Cheng, C.M. Tan, and J.T. Shih. 2003. Evaluation of shoulder proprioception following muscle fatigue. *Clin Biomech (Bristol, Avon)* 18(9): 843-7.

Lee, S.B., and K.N. An. 2002. Dynamic glenohumeral stability provided by three heads of the deltoid muscle. *Clin Orthop Relat Res* 400: 40-7.

Lee, S.B., K.J. Kim, S.W. O'Driscoll, B.F. Morrey, and K.N. An. 2000. Dynamic glenohumeral stability provided by the rotator cuff muscles in the mid-range and end-range of motion. A study in cadavera. *J Bone Joint Surg Am* 82(6): 849-57.

Lee, W.A. 1980. Anticipatory control and task muscles during rapid arm flexion. *J Mot Behav* 12: 185- 96.

Leetun, D.T., M.L. Ireland, J.D. Willson, B.T. Ballantyne, and I.M. Davis. 2004. Core stability measures as risk factors for lower extremity injury in athletes. *Med Sci Sports Exerc* 36(6): 926-34.

Leffler, A.S., P. Hansson, and E. Kosek. 2003. Somatosensory perception in patients suffering from long-term trapezius myalgia at the site overlying the most painful part of the muscle and in an area of pain referral. *Eur J Pain* 7(3): 267-76.

Lehman, G.J. 2006. Trunk and hip muscle recruitment patterns during the prone leg extension following a lateral ankle sprain: A prospective case study pre and post injury. *Chiropr Osteopat* 27(14): 4.

Lehman, G.J., and S.M. McGill. 2001. Quantification of the differences in electromyographic activity magnitude between the upper and lower portions of the rectus abdominis muscle during selected trunk exercises. *Phys Ther* 81(5): 1096-101.

Lehman, G.J., D. Lennon, B. Tresidder, B. Rayfield, and M. Poschar. 2004. Muscle recruitment patterns during the prone leg extension. *BMC Musculoskelet Disord* 5: 3.

Leivseth, G., and O. Reikerås. 1994. Changes in muscle fiber cross-sectional area and concentrations of Na,K-ATPase in deltoid muscle in patients with impingement syndrome of the shoulder. *J Orthop Sports Phys Ther* 19(3): 146-9.

Lentell, G.L., L.L. Katzman, and M.R. Walters. 1990. The relationship between muscle function and ankle stability. *J Orthop Sports Phys Ther* 11: 605-11.

Leonard, C.T. 1998. *The neuroscience of human movement.* St. Louis: Mosby.

Lephart, S., and F. Fu, eds. 2000. *Proprioception and neuromuscular control in joint stability.* Champaign, IL: Human Kinetics.

Lephart, S.M., D.M. Pincivero, J.L. Giraldo, and F.H. Fu. 1997. The role of proprioception in the management and rehabilitation of athletic injuries. *Am J Sports Med* 25(1): 130-7.

Lephart, S.M., J.P. Warner, P.A. Borsa, and F.H. Fu. 1994. Proprioception of the shoulder joint in healthy, unstable, and surgically repaired shoulders. *J Shoulder Elbow Surg* 3: 371-80.

Leroux, J.L., P. Codine, E. Thomas, M. Pocholle, D. Mailhe, and F. Blotman. 1994. Isokinetic evaluation of rotational strength in normal shoulders and shoulders with impingement syndrome. *Clin Orthop Relat Res* 304: 108-15.

Letchuman, R., R.E. Gay, R.A. Shelerud, and L.A. VanOstrand. 2005. Are tender points associated with cervical radiculopathy? *Arch Phys Med Rehabil* 86(7): 1333-7.

Levine, D., and M.W. Whittle. 1996. The effects of pelvic movement on lumbar lordosis in the standing position. *J Orthop Sports Phys* 24(3): 130-5.

Lewis, C.L., and S.A. Sahrmann. 2005. Timing of muscle activation during prone hip extension. Abstract. *J Orthop Sports Phys Ther* 35(1): A56.

Lewis, C.L., S.A. Sahrmann, and D.W. Moran. 2007. Anterior hip joint force increases with hip extension, decreased gluteal force, or decreased iliopsoas force. *J Biomech* 40(16): 3725-31.

Lewis, J.S., A. Green, and C. Wright. 2005. Subacromial impingement syndrome: The role of posture and muscle imbalance. *J Shoulder Elbow Surg* 14(4): 385-92.

Lewis, J.S., C. Wright, and A. Green. 2005. Subacromial impingement syndrome: The effect of changing posture on shoulder range of movement. *J Orthop Sports Phys Ther* 35(2): 72-87.

Lewit, K. 1980. Relation of faulty respiration to posture, with clinical implications. *J Am Osteopath Assoc* 8: 525.

Lewit, K. 1986. Postisometric relaxation in combination with other methods of muscular facilitation and inhibition. *Man Med* 2: 101-4.

Lewit, K. 1987. Chain reactions in disturbed function of the motor system. *Man Med* 3: 27-9.

Lewit, K. 1991. *Manipulative therapy in rehabilitation of the locomotor system.* 2nd ed. London: Butterworth.

Lewit, K. 1997. *A course in manual medicine: Unpublished course notes.* Prague.

Lewit, K. 1999. Chain reactions in the locomotor system in light of co-activation patterns based on developmental neurology. *J Orthop Med* 21(1): 52-7.

Lewit, K. 1999. *Manipulative therapy in rehabilitation of the locomotor system.* 3rd ed. Oxford: Butterworth-Heinemann.

Lewit, K. 2000. Relationship between structure and function in the locomotor system. [In Czech.] *Rehabil Fyz Lek* 7(3): 99-101.

Lewit, K. 2001. Rehabilitation of pain disorders of the locomotor system, Part II. [In Czech.] *Rehabil Fyz Lek* 8(4): 130-51.

Lewit, K. 2007. Managing common syndromes and finding the key link. In *Rehabilitation of the spine,* ed. C. Liebenson 776-797. Philadelphia: Lippincott Williams & Wilkins.

Lewit, K., and D.G. Simons. 1984. Myofascial pain: Relief by post-isometric relaxation. *Arch Phys Med Rehabil* 65(8): 452-6.

Lewit, K., M. Berger, G. Hollzmuller, and S. Lechner-scheinleitner. 1997. Breathing movements: The synkinesis of respiration with looking up and down. *Journal of Musculoskeletal Pain* 5: 57-69.

Lewit, K., V. Janda, and M. Veverkova. 1998. Respiratory synkinesis: An EMG investigation. [In Czech.] *Rehabil Fyz Lek* 5(1): 3-7.

Li, Z.M., D.A. Harkness, and R.J. Goitz. 2005. Thumb strength affected by carpal tunnel syndrome. *Clin Orthop Relat Res* 441: 320-6.

Liebenson, C. 2001. Self-treatment of mid-thoracic dysfunction: A key link in the body axis. Part one: Overview and assessment. *J Bodyw Mov Ther* 5(2): 90-8.

Liebenson, C. 2001. Self-treatment of mid-thoracic dysfunction: A key link in the body axis. Part two: Treatment. *J Bodyw Mov Ther* 5(3): 191-5.

Liebenson, C. 2001. Self-treatment of mid-thoracic dysfunction: A key link in the body axis. Part three: Clinical issues. *J Bodyw Mov Ther* 5(4): 264-68.

Liebenson, C. 2001. Sensory-motor training. *J Bodyw Mov Ther* 5(1): 21-7.

Liebenson, C. 2002. Functional reactivation for neck pain patients. *J Bodyw Mov Ther* 6(1): 59-66.

Liebenson, C. 2005. Sensory-motor training—an update. *J Bodyw Mov Ther* 9: 142-47.

Liebenson, C., ed. 1996. *Rehabilitation of the spine. A practitioner's manual.* Baltimore: Williams & Wilkins.

Light, A. 1992. *The initial processing of pain and its descending control: Spinal and trigeminal systems.* New York: Karger.

Lin, J.J., H.K. Lim, and J.L. Yang. 2006. Effect of shoulder tightness on glenohumeral translation, scapular kinematics, and scapulohumeral rhythm in subjects with stiff shoulders. *J Orthop Res* 24(5): 1044-51.

Lin, J.J., W.P. Hanten, S.L. Olson, T.S. Roddey, D.A. Soto-quijano, H.K. Lim, and A.M. Sherwood. 2005. Functional activity characteristics of individuals with shoulder dysfunctions. *J Electromyogr Kinesiol* 15(6): 576-86.

Lin, J.J., Y.T. Wu, S.F. Wang, and S.Y. Chen. 2005. Trapezius muscle imbalance in individuals suffering from frozen shoulder syndrome. *Clin Rheumatol* 24(6): 569-75.

Lindman, R., A. Eriksson, and L.E. Thornell. 1990. Fiber type composition of the human male trapezius muscle: Enzyme-histochemical characteristics. *Am J Anat* 189(3): 236-44.

Linford, C.W., J.T. Hopkins, S.S. Schulthies, B. Freland, D.O. Draper, and I. Hunter. 2006. Effects of neuromuscular training on the reaction time and electromechanical delay of the peroneus longus muscle. *Arch Phys Med Rehabil* 87(3): 395-401.

Liu, J., R.E. Hughes, W.P. Smutz, G. Niebur, and K. Nan-An. 1997. Roles of deltoid and rotator cuff muscles in shoulder elevation. *Clin Biomech (Bristol, Avon)* 12(1): 32-8.

Lloyd, D.G. 2001. Rationale for training programs to reduce anterior cruciate ligament injuries in Australian football. *J Orthop Sports Phys Ther* 31(11): 645-54.

Long W.T., Dorr L.D., Healy B., and Perry J. 1993. Functional recovery of noncemented total hip arthroplasty. *Clin Orthop Relat Res.* Mar;(288): 73-7.

Loudon, J.K., M. Ruhl, and E. Field. 1997. Ability to reproduce head position after whiplash injury. *Spine* 22(8): 865-8.

Lucas, D.B. 1973. Biomechanics of the shoulder joint. *Arch Surg* 107(3): 425-32.

Ludewig, P.M., and T.M. Cook. 2000. Alterations in shoulder kinematics and associated muscle activity in people with symptoms of shoulder impingement. *Phys Ther* 80(3): 276-91.

Ludewig, P.M., and T.M. Cook. 2002. Translations of the humerus in persons with shoulder impingement symptoms. *J Orthop Sports Phys Ther* 32(6): 248-59.

Ludewig, P.M., M.S. Hoff, E.E. Osowski, S.A. Meschke, and P.J. Rundquist. 2004. Relative balance of serratus anterior and upper trapezius muscle activity during push-up exercises. *Am J Sports Med* 32(2): 484-93.

Ludewig, P.M., T.M. Cook, and D.A. Nawoczenski. 1996. Three-dimensional scapular orientation and muscle activity at selected positions of humeral elevation. *J Orthop Sports Phys Ther* 24(2): 57-65.

Lukasiewicz, A.C., P. McClure, L. Michener, N. Pratt, and B. Sennett. 1999. Comparison of 3-dimensional scapular position and orientation between subjects with and without shoulder impingement. *J Orthop Sports Phys Ther* 29(10): 574-83.

Lund, J.P., R. Donga, C.G. Widmer, and C.S. Stohler. 1991. The pain-adaptation model: A discussion of the relationship between chronic musculoskeletal pain and motor activity. *Can J Physiol Pharmacol* 69(5): 683-94.

Lund, S. 1980. Postural effects of neck muscle vibration in man. *Experientia* 36(12): 1398.

Luo, J., B. McNamara, and K. Moran. 2005. The use of vibration training to enhance muscle strength and power. *Sports Med* 35(1): 23-41.

Luoto, S., H. Aalto, S. Taimela, H. Hurri, I. Pyykko, and H. Alaranta. 1998. One-footed and externally disturbed two-footed postural control in patients with chronic low back pain and healthy control subjects. A controlled study with follow-up. *Spine* 23(19): 2081-9.

Luoto, S., S. Taimela, H. Hurri, H. Aalto, I. Pyykko, and H. Alaranta. 1996. Psychomotor speed and postural control in chronic low back pain patients. A controlled follow-up study. *Spine* 21(22): 2621-7.

Ma, Y.-T., Ma, M., and H. Cho. 2005. *Biomedical acupuncture for pain management: An integrative approach.* St. Louis: Elsevier.

Machner, A., H. Merk, R. Becker, K. Rohkohl, H. Wissel, and G. Pap. 2003. Kinesthetic sense of the shoulder in patients with impingement syndrome. *Acta Orthop Scand* 74(1): 85-8.

Mackinnon, S.E., and C.B. Novak. 1994. Clinical commentary: Pathogenesis of cumulative trauma disorder. *J Hand Surg [Am]* 19(5): 873-83.

Mackinnon, S.E., G.A. Patterson, and C.B. Novak. 1996. Thoracic outlet syndrome: A current overview. *Semin Thorac Cardiovasc Surg* 8(2): 176-82.

Madeleine, P., B. Lundager, M. Voigt, and L. Arendt-Nielsen. 1999. Shoulder muscle co-ordination during chronic and acute experimental neck-shoulder pain. An occupational pain study. *Eur J Appl Physiol Occup Physiol* 79(2): 127-40.

Madeleine, P., H. Prietzel, H. Svarrer, and L. Arendt-Nielsen. 2004. Quantitative posturography in altered sensory conditions: A way to assess balance instability in patients with chronic whiplash injury. *Arch Phys Med Rehabil* 85(3): 432-8.

Madeleine, P., P. Vedsted, A.K. Blangsted, G. Sjøgaard, and K. Søgaard. 2006. Effects of electromyographic and mechanomyographic biofeedback on upper trapezius muscle activity during standardized computer work. *Ergonomics* 49(10): 921-33.

Madeleine, P., S.E. Mathiassen, and L. Arendt-Nielsen. 2007. Changes in the degree of motor variability associated with experimental and chronic neck-shoulder pain during a standardised repetitive arm movement. *Exp Brain Res* 185(4): 689-98.

Magarey, M.E., and M.A. Jones. 2003. Dynamic evaluation and early management of altered motor control around the shoulder complex. *Man Ther* 8(4): 195-206.

Magermans, D.J., E.K. Chadwick, H.E. Veeger, and F.C. van der Helm. 2005. Requirements for upper extremity motions during activities of daily living. *Clin Biomech (Bristol, Avon)* 20(6): 591-9.

Majewski M., Bischoff-Ferrari H.A., Gruneberg C., Dick W., and Allum J.H. 2005. Improvements in balance after total hip replacement. *J Bone Joint Surg Br.* Oct;87(10): 1337-43.

Maki, B.E., S.D. Perry, R.G. Norrie, and W.E. McIlroy. 1999. Effect of facilitation of sensation from plantar foot-surface boundaries on postural stabilization in young and older adults *J Gerontol A Biol Sci Med Sci* 54(6): M281-7.

Malliou, P.C., K. Giannakopoulos, A.G. Beneka, A. Gioftsidou, and G. Godolias. 2004. Effective ways of restoring muscular imbalances of the rotator cuff muscle group: A comparative study of various training methods. *Br J Sports Med* 38(6): 766-72.

Mandalidis, D.G., B.S. Mc Glone, R.F. Quigley, D. McInerney, and M. O'Brien. 1999. Digital fluoroscopic assessment of the scapulohumeral rhythm. *Surg Radiol Anat* 21(4): 241-6.

Mann, I.O., M.C. Morrissey, and J.K. Cywinski. 2007. Effect of neuromuscular electrical stimulation on ankle swelling in the early period after ankle sprain. *Phys Ther* 87(1): 53-65.

Mannerkorpi, K., and M.D. Iversen. 2003. Physical exercise in fibromyalgia and related syndromes. *Best Pract Res Clin Rheumatol* 17(4): 629-47.

Mannion, A.F., M. Muntener, S. Taimela, and J. Dvorak. 1999. A randomized clinical trial of three active therapies for chronic low back pain. *Spine* 24(23): 2435-48.

Maquet, D., J.L. Croisier, C. Renard, and J.M. Crielaard. 2002. Muscle performance in patients with fibromyalgia. *Joint Bone Spine* 69(3): 293-9.

Martin, L., A. Nutting, B.R. MacIntosh, S.M. Edworthy, D. Butterwick, and J. Cook. 1996. An exercise program in the treatment of fibromyalgia. *J Rheumatol* 23(6): 1050-3.

Martin, R.M., and D.E. Fish. 2008. Scapular winging: Anatomical review, diagnosis, and treatments. *Curr Rev Musculoskelet Med* 1: 1-11.

Matias, R., and A.G. Pascoal. 2006. The unstable shoulder in arm elevation: A three-dimensional and electromyographic study in subjects with glenohumeral instability. *Clin Biomech (Bristol, Avon)* 21(Suppl. no. 1): S52-8.

Matre, D.A., T. Sinkjaer, P. Svensson, and L. Arendt-Nielsen. 1998. Experimental muscle pain increases the human stretch reflex. *Pain* 75(2-3): 331-9.

Matsusaka, N., S. Yokoyama, T. Tsurusaki, S. Inokuchi, and M. Okita. 2001. Effect of ankle disk training combined with tactile stimulation to the leg and foot on functional instability of the ankle. *Am J Sports Med* 29(1): 25-30.

Mayer, F., D. Axmann, T. Horstmann, F. Martini, J. Fritz, and H.H. Dickhuth. 2001. Reciprocal strength ratio in shoulder abduction/adduction in sports and daily living. *Med Sci Sports Exerc* 33(10): 1765-9.

Mayoux-Benhamou, M.A., M. Revel, C. Vallée, R. Roudier, J.P. Barbet, and F. Bargy. 1994. Longus colli has a postural function on cervical curvature. *Surg Radiol Anat* 16(4): 367-71.

McBride, J.M., P. Cormie, and R. Deane. 2006. Isometric squat force output and muscle activity in stable and unstable conditions. *Journal of Strength and Conditioning Research* 20(4): 915–18.

McCabe, R.A., T.F. Tyler, S.J. Nicholas, P. Malachy, and P. McHugh. 2001. Selective activation of the lower trapezius muscle in patients with shoulder impingement. Abstract. *J Orthop Sports Phys Ther* 31(1): A-45.

McCann, P.D., M.E. Wootten, M.P. Kadaba, and L.U. Bigliani. 1993. A kinematic and electromyographic study of shoulder rehabilitation exercises. *Clin Orthop Relat Res* 288: 179-88.

McCarthy, P.W., J.P. Olsen, and I.H. Smeby. 1997. Effects of contract-relax stretching procedures on active range of motion of the cervical spine in the transverse plane. *Clin Biomech (Bristol, Avon)* 12(2): 136-8.

McClinton, S.M., S.E. Bunch, K.M. Kettmann, and J.M. Padgett. 2005. Muscle firing patterns during hip abduction: A preliminary investigation. Abstract. *J Orthop Sports Phys Ther* 35(1): A29-30.

McClure, P., J. Balaicuis, D. Heiland, M.E. Broersma, C.K. Thorndike, and A. Wood. 2007. A randomized controlled comparison of stretching procedures for posterior shoulder tightness. *J Orthop Sports Phys Ther* 37(3): 108-14.

McClure, P.W., J. Bialker, N. Neff, G. Williams, and A. Karduna. 2004. Shoulder function and 3-dimensional kinematics in people with shoulder impingement syndrome before and after a 6-week exercise program. *Phys Ther* 84(9): 832-48.

McClure, P.W., L.A. Michener, and A.R. Karduna. 2006. Shoulder function and 3-dimensional scapular kinematics in people with and without shoulder impingement syndrome. *Phys Ther* 86(8): 1075-90.

McClure, P.W., L.A. Michener, B.J. Sennett, and A.R. Karduna. 2001. Direct 3-dimensional measurement of scapular kinematics during dynamic movements in vivo. *J Shoulder Elbow Surg* 10(3): 269-77.

McGill, S.M. 1991. Electromyographic activity of the abdominal and low back musculature during the generation of isometric and dynamic axial trunk torque: Implications for lumbar mechanics. *J Orthop Res* 91-103.

McGill, S.M. 1992. A myoelectrically based dynamic three-dimenstional model to predict loads on lumbar spine tissues during lateral bending. *J Biomech* 25: 395-414.

McGill, S.M. 1996. A revised anatomical model of the abdominal musculature for torso flexion efforts. *J Biomech* 29(7): 973-7.

McGill, S.M. 1998. Low back exercise. Evidence for improving exercise regimes. *Phys Ther* 78(7): 754-65.

McGill, S.M. 2002. *Low back disorders: Evidence-based prevention and rehabilitation.* Champaign, IL: Human Kinetics.

McGill, S.M., and R.W. Norman. 1994. Reassessment of the role of intra-abdominal pressure in spinal compression. *Ergonomics* 30: 1565-88.

McGill, S.M., R.L. Hughson, and K. Parks. 2000. Changes in lumbar lordosis modify the role of the extensor muscles. *Clin Biomech (Bristol, Avon)* 15(1): 777-80.

McGuine, T.A., J.J. Green, T.B. Best, and G. Leverson. 2000. Balance as a predictor of ankle injuries in high school basketball players. *Clin J Sport Med* 10: 239-44.

McHugh, M.P., Tyler, T.F., Mirabella, M.R., Mullaney, M.J., and Nicholas, S.J. 2007. The Effectiveness of a Balance Training Intervention in Reducing the Incidence of Noncontact Ankle Sprains in High School Football Players. *American Journal of Sports Medicine.* 35(8): 1289-94.

McKeon, P.O., and J. Hertel. 2007. Diminished plantar cutaneous sensation and postural control. *Percept Mot Skills* 104(1): 56-66.

McKinney, L.A. 1989. Early mobilisation and outcome in acute sprains of the neck. *BMJ* 299(6706): 1006-8.

McLain, R.F. 1994. Mechanoreceptor endings in human cervical facet joints. *Spine* 19(5): 495-501.

McMahon, P.J., F.W. Jobe, M.M. Pink, J.R. Brault, and J. Perry. 1996. Comparative electromyographic analysis of shoulder muscles during planar motions: Anterior glenohumeral instability versus normal. *J Shoulder Elbow Surg* 5(2 Pt. 1): 118-23.

McMahon, P.J., R.E. Debski, W.O. Thompson, J.J. Warner, F.H. Fu, and S.L. Woo. 1995. Shoulder muscle forces and tendon excursions during glenohumeral abduction in the scapular plane. *J Shoulder Elbow Surg* 4(3): 199-208.

McMaster, W.C., A. Roberts, and T. Stoddard. 1998. A correlation between shoulder laxity and interfering pain in competitive swimmers. *Am J Sports Med* 26(1): 83-6.

McMaster, W.C., and J. Troup. 1993. A survey of interfering shoulder pain in United States competitive swimmers. *Am J Sports Med* 21(1): 67-70.

McMaster, W.C., S.C. Long, and V.J. Caiozzo. 1991. Isokinetic torque imbalances in the rotator cuff of the elite water polo player. *Am J Sports Med* 19(1): 72-5.

McMaster, W.C., S.C. Long, and V.J. Caiozzo. 1992. Shoulder torque changes in the swimming athlete. *Am J Sports Med* 20(3): 323-7.

McMullen, J., and T.L. Uhl. 2000. A kinetic chain approach for shoulder rehabilitation. *J Athl Train* 35(3): 329-37.

McNair, P.J., and R.N. Marshall. 1994. Landing characteristics in subjects with normal and anterior cruciate ligament deficient knee joints. *Arch Phys Med Rehabil* 75(5): 584-9.

McNeely, M.L., S. Armijo Olivo, and D.J. Magee. 2006. A systematic review of the effectiveness of physical therapy interventions for temporomandibular disorders. *Phys Ther* 86(5): 710-25.

McNeill, T., D. Warwick, G. Andersson, and A. Schultz. 1980. Trunk strengths in attempted flexion, extension, and lateral bending in healthy subjects and patients with low-back disorders. *Spine* 5(6): 529-38.

McPartland, J.M., R.R. Brodeur, and R.C. Hallgren. 1997. Chronic neck pain, standing balance, and suboccipital muscle atrophy—a pilot study. *J Manipulative Physiol Ther* 20(1): 24-9.

McQuade, K.J., and A.M. Murthi. 2004. Anterior glenohumeral force/translation behavior with and without rotator cuff contraction during clinical stability testing. *Clin Biomech (Bristol, Avon)* 19(1): 10-5.

McQuade, K.J., and G.L. Smidt. 1998. Dynamic scapulohumeral rhythm: The effects of external resistance during elevation of the arm in the scapular plane. *J Orthop Sports Phys Ther* 27(2): 125-33.

McQuade, K.J., J. Dawson, and G.L. Smidt. 1998. Scapulothoracic muscle fatigue associated with alterations in scapulohumeral rhythm kinematics during maximum resistive shoulder elevation. *J Orthop Sports Phys Ther* 28(2): 74-80.

McVey, E.D., R.M. Palmieri, C.L. Docherty, S.M. Zinder, and C.D. Ingersoll. 2005. Arthrogenic muscle inhibition in the leg muscles of subjects exhibiting functional ankle instability. *Foot Ankle Int* 26(12): 1055-61.

Medlicott, M.S., and S.R. Harris. 2006. A systematic review of the effectiveness of exercise, manual therapy, electrotherapy, relaxation training, and biofeedback in the management of temporomandibular disorder. *Phys Ther* 86(7): 955-73.

Meister, K., and J.R. Andrews. 1993. Classification and treatment of rotator cuff injuries in the overhand athlete. *J Orthop Sports Phys Ther* 18(2): 413-21.

Melzack, R., D.M. Stillwell, and E.J. Fox. 1977. Trigger points and acupuncture points for pain: Correlations and implications. *Pain* 3: 3-23.

Menachem, A., O. Kaplan, and S. Dekel. 1993. Levator scapulae syndrome: An anatomic-clinical study. *Bull Hosp Jt Dis* 53(1): 21-4.

Mencher, D.M. 2002. Proprioceptive retraining of chronic ankle instability. In *The unstable ankle,* ed. M. Nyska and G. Mann, 193-200. Champaign, IL: Human Kinetics.

Mengshoel, A.M., O. Førre, and H.B. Komnaes. 1990. Muscle strength and aerobic capacity in primary fibromyalgia. *Clin Exp Rheumatol* 8(5): 475-9.

Mense, S., and D.G. Simons. 2001. *Muscle pain: Understanding its nature, diagnosis, and treatment. Pain associated with increased muscle tension.* Baltimore: Lippincott Williams & Wilkins

Meyer, P.F., L.I. Oddsson, and C.J. De Luca. 2004. The role of plantar cutaneous sensation in unperturbed stance. *Exp Brain Res* 156(4): 505-12.

Meythaler, J.M., N.M. Reddy, and M. Mitz. 1986. Serratus anterior disruption: A complication of rheumatoid arthritis. *Arch Phys Med Rehabil* 67(10): 770-2.

Michaud, M., A.B. Arsenault, D. Gravel, G. Tremblay, and T.G. Simard. 1987. Muscular compensatory mechanism in the presence of a tendinitis of the supraspinatus. *Am J Phys Med* 66(3): 109-20.

Michener, L.A., M.K. Walsworth, and E.N. Burnet. 2004. Effectiveness of rehabilitation for patients with subacromial impingement syndrome: A systematic review. *J Hand Ther* 17(2): 152-64.

Michener, L.A., N.D. Boardman, P.E. Pidcoe, and A.M. Frith. 2005. Scapular muscle tests in subjects with shoulder pain and functional loss: Reliability and construct validity. *Phys Ther* 85(11): 1128-38.

Michener, L.A., P.W. McClure, and A.R. Karduna. 2003. Anatomical and biomechanical mechanisms of subacromial impingement syndrome. *Clin Biomech (Bristol, Avon)* 18(5): 369-79.

Michlovitz, S.L. 2004. Conservative interventions for carpal tunnel syndrome. *J Orthop Sports Phys Ther* 34(10): 589-600.

Mientjes, M.I., and J.S. Frank. 1999. Balance in chronic low back pain patients compared to healthy people under various conditions in upright standing. *Clin Biomech (Bristol, Avon)* 14(10): 710-6.

Miglietta, O.E. 1962. Evaluation of cold in spasticity. *Am J Phys Med* 41: 148-51.

Mihata, T., Y. Lee, M.H. McGarry, M. Abe, and T.Q. Lee. 2004. Excessive humeral external rotation results in increased shoulder laxity. *Am J Sports Med* 32(5): 1278-85.

Mikesky, A.E., J.E. Edwards, J.K. Wigglesworth, and S. Kunkel. 1995. Eccentric and concentric strength of the shoulder and arm musculature in collegiate baseball pitchers. *Am J Sports Med* 23(5): 638-42.

Mima, T., K. Terada, M. Maekawa, T. Nagamine, A. Ikeda, and H. Shibasaki. 1996. Somatosensory evoked potentials following proprioceptive stimulation of finger in man. *Exp Brain Res* 111(2): 233-45.

Miniaci, A., and P.J. Fowler. 1993. Impingement in the athlete. *Clin Sports Med* 12(1): 91-111.

Mirzabeigi, E., C. Jordan, J.K. Gronley, L. Neal, N.L. Rockowitz, and J. Perry. 1999. Isolation of the vastus medialis oblique muscle during exercise. *Am J Sports Med* 27: 50-3.

Mitchell Jr., F., P.S. Moran, and N.A. Pruzzo. 1979. An evaluation of osteopathic muscle energy procedures. Valley Park, MO: Author.

Mochizuki, G., T.D. Ivanova, and S.J. Garland. 2004. Postural muscle activity during bilateral and unilateral arm movements at different speeds. *Exp Brain Res* 155(3): 352-61.

Moghtaderi, A., S. Izadi, and N. Sharafadinzadeh. 2005. An evaluation of gender, body mass index, wrist circumference and wrist ratio as independent risk factors for carpal tunnel syndrome. *Acta Neurol Scand* 112(6): 375-9.

Mok, N.W., S.G. Brauer, and P.W. Hodges. 2004. Hip strategy for balance control in quiet standing is reduced in people with low back pain. *Spine* 29(6): E107-12.

Moller, B.N., B. Krebs, C. Tidemand-Dal, and K. Aaris. 1986. Isometric contractions in the patellofemoral pain syndrome. An electromyographic study. *Arch Orthop Trauma Surg* 105(1): 24-7.

Monaghan, K., E. Delahunt, and B. Caulfield. 2006. Ankle function during gait in patients with chronic ankle instability compared to controls. *Clin Biomech (Bristol, Avon)* 21(2): 168-74.

Montgomery III, W.H., M. Pink, and J. Perry. 1994. Electromyographic analysis of hip and knee musculature during running. *Am J Sports Med* 22(2): 272-8.

Mooney, V., R. Pozos, A. Vleeming, J. Gulick, and D. Swenski. 2001. Exercise treatment for sacroiliac pain. *Orthopedics* 24(1): 29-32.

Moore, J.C. 1975. Excitation overflow: An electromyographic investigation. *Arch Phys Med Rehabil* 56(3): 115-20.

Moore, J.R., and G. Wade. 1989. Prevention of anterior cruciate injuries. *Strength and Conditioning Journal* 11(3): 35-40.

Moore, M.A., and C.G. Kukulka. 1991. Depression of Hoffmann reflexes following voluntary contraction and implications for proprioceptive neuromuscular facilitation therapy. *Phys Ther* 71(4): 321-9.

Moore, M.A., and R.S. Hutton. 1980. Electromyographic investigation of muscle stretching techniques. *Med Sci Sports Exerc* 12(5): 322-9.

Moore, M.K. 2004. Upper crossed syndrome and its relationship to cervicogenic headache. *J Manipulative Physiol Ther* 27(6): 414-20.

Moraes, G.F., C.D. Faria, and L.F. Teixeira-Salmela. 2008. Scapular muscle recruitment patterns and isokinetic strength ratios of the shoulder rotator muscles in individuals with and without impingement syndrome. *J Shoulder Elbow Surg* 17(1 Suppl.): 48S-53S.

Moritani, T., and H.A. deVries.1979. Neural factors versus hypertrophy in the time course of muscle strength gain. *Am J Phys Med* 58(3): 115-30.

Mork, P.J., and R.H. Westgaard. 2006. Low-amplitude trapezius activity in work and leisure and the relation to shoulder and neck pain. *J Appl Physiol* 100(4): 1142-9.

Morris, A.D., G.J. Kemp, and S.P. Frostick. 2004. Shoulder electromyography in multidirectional instability. *J Shoulder Elbow Surg* 13(1): 24-9.

Morris, C.E., P.E. Greenman, M.I. Bullock, J.V. Basmajian, and A. Kobesova. 2006. Vladimir Janda, MD, DSc: Tribute to a master of rehabilitation. *Spine* 31(9): 1060-4.

Morris, J.M., D.M. Lucas, and B. Bresler. 1961. Role of the trunk in the stability of the spine. *J Bone Joint Surg Am* 43: 327-51.

Morris, M., F.W. Jobe, J. Perry, M. Pink, and B.S. Healy. 1989. Electromyographic analysis of elbow function in tennis players. *Am J Sports Med* 17(2): 241-7.

Morrison, D.S., A.D. Frogameni, and P. Woodworth. 1997. Non-operative treatment of subacromial impingement syndrome. *J Bone Joint Surg Am* 79(5): 732-7.

Morrison, D.S., B.S. Greenbaum, and A. Einhorn. 2000. Shoulder impingement. *Orthop Clin North Am* 31(2): 285-93.

Morrissey, M.C. 1989. Reflex inhibition of thigh muscles in knee injury. Causes and treatment. *Sports Med* 7(4): 263-76.

Morrissey, M.C., Z.L. Hudson, W.I. Drechsler, F.J. Coutts, P.R. Knight, and J.B. King. 2000. Effects of open versus closed kinetic chain training on knee laxity in the early period after anterior cruciate ligament reconstruction *Knee Surg Sports Traumatol Arthrosc* 8(6): 343-8.

Morscher, E. 1977. Etiology and pathophysiology of leg length discrepancies. In *Progress in Orthopaedic Surgery Vol. 1. Leg Length Discrepancy. The Injured Knee*, ed. D.S. Hungerford, 9-19. New York: Springer.

Moseley Jr, J.B., F.W. Jobe, M. Pink, J. Perry, and J. Tibone. 1992. EMG analysis of the scapular muscles during a shoulder rehabilitation program. *Am J Sports Med* 20(2): 128-34.

Moseley, G.L. 2004. Impaired trunk muscle function in sub-acute neck pain: Etiologic in the subsequent development of low back pain? *Man Ther* 9(3): 157-63.

Moseley, G.L., and P.W. Hodges. 2005. Are the changes in postural control associated with low back pain caused by pain interference? *Clin J Pain* 21(4): 323-9.

Mottram, S.L. 1997. Dynamic stability of the scapula. *Man Ther* 2(3): 123-31.

Mountz, J.M., L.A. Bradley, J.G. Modell, R.W. Alexander, M. Triana-Alexander, L.A. Aaron, K.E. Stewart, G.S. Alarcón, and J.D. Mountz. 1995. Fibromyalgia in women. Abnormalities of regional cerebral blood flow in the thalamus and the caudate nucleus are associated with low pain threshold levels. *Arthritis Rheum* 38(7): 926-38.

Muller, E.A. 1970. Influence of training and of inactivity on muscle strength. *Arch Phys Med Rehabil* 51(8): 449-62.

Muller, M., D. Tsui, R. Schnurr, L. Biddulph-Deisroth, J. Hard, and J.C. MacDermid. 2004. Effectiveness of hand therapy interventions in primary management of carpal tunnel syndrome: A systematic review. *J Hand Ther* 17(2): 210-28.

Murphy, D.R., D. Byfield, P. McCarthy, K. Humphreys, A.A. Gregory, and R. Rochon. 2006. Interexaminer reliability of the hip extension test for suspected impaired motor control of the lumbar spine. *J Manipulative Physiol Ther* 29(5): 374-7.

Murray H. 2000. Kinesiotaping, muscle strength, and range of motion after ACL repair. *J Orthop Sports Phys Ther* 30: A-14.

Murray, H., and L. Husk. 2001. The effects of kinesio taping on proprioception in the ankle and in the knee. *J Orthop Sports Phys Ther* 31: A-37.

Myers, J.B., J.H. Hwang, M.R. Pasquale, M.W. Rodosky, Y.Y. Ju, and S.M. Lephart. 2003. Shoulder muscle coactivation alterations in patients with subacromial impingement. Abstract. *Med Sci Sports Exerc* 35(5): S346.

Myers, J.B., K.G. Laudner, M.R. Pasquale, J.P. Bradley, and S.M. Lephart. 2005. Scapular position and orientation in throwing athletes. *Am J Sports Med* 33(2): 263-71.

Myers, J.B., K.G. Laudner, M.R. Pasquale, J.P. Bradley, and S.M. Lephart. 2006. Glenohumeral range of motion deficits and posterior shoulder tightness in throwers with pathologic internal impingement. *Am J Sports Med* 34(3): 385-91.

Myers, J.B., K.M. Guskiewicz, R.A. Schneider, and W.E. Prentice. 1999. Proprioception and neuromuscular control of the shoulder after muscle fatigue. *J Athl Train* 34(4): 362-7.

Myers, J.B., Y.Y. Ju, J.H. Hwang, P.J. McMahon, M.W. Rodosky, and S.M. Lephart. 2004. Reflexive muscle activation alterations in shoulders with anterior glenohumeral instability. *Am J Sports Med* 32(4): 1013-21.

Myers, R.L., Padua, D.A., Prentice, W.E., and Petschauer, M.A. 2003. Balance sandals increase gluteus medius and gluteus medius and gluteus maximus muscle activation amplitude during closed kinetic chain exercise (Abstract). J Athl Train. 38(2): S94.

Myers, T. 2001. *Anatomy trains.* Edinburgh: Churchill Livingstone.

Myklebust, G., Engebresten, L., Br, I.H., Skj, A., Olsen, O.E., and Bahr, R. 2003. Prevention of ACL injuries in female team handball players: a prospective intervention study. (Abstract). Med Sci Sports Exerc. 35(5): S156.

Nadler, S.F., G.A. Malanga, J.H. Feinberg, M. Prybicien, T.P. Stitik, and M. DePrince. 2001. Relationship between hip muscle imbalance and occurrence of low back pain in collegiate athletes: A prospective study. *Am J Phys Med Rehabil* 80(8): 572-7.

Nadler, S.F., G.A. Malanga, L.A. Bartoli, J.H. Feinberg, M. Prybicien, and M. Deprince. 2002. Hip muscle imbalance and low back pain in athletes: Influence of core strengthening. *Med Sci Sports Exerc* 34(1): 9-16.

Nadler, S.F., G.A. Malanga, M. DePrince, T.P. Stitik, and J.H. Feinberg. 2000. The relationship between lower extremity injury, low back pain, and hip muscle strength in male and female collegiate athletes. *Clin J Sport Med* 10(2): 89-97.

Nakagawa, S., M. Yoneda, K. Hayashida, S. Wakitani, and K. Okamura. 2001. Greater tuberosity notch: An important indicator of articular-side partial rotator cuff tears in the shoulders of throwing athletes. *Am J Sports Med* 29(6): 762-70.

Nakajima, T., M. Sakamoto, T. Tazoe, T. Endoh, and T. Komiyama. 2006. Location specificity of plantar cutaneous reflexes involving lower limb muscles in humans. *Exp Brain Res* 175(3): 514-25.

Nallegowda, M., Singh, U., Bhan, S., Wadhwa, S., Handa, G., and Dwivedi, S.N. 2003. Balance and gait in total hip replacement: a pilot study. *Am J Phys Med Rehabil.* Sep;82(9): 669-77.

Nashner, L.M. 1989. Sensory, neuromuscular, and biomechanical contributions to human balance. In *Balance. Proceedings of the APTA Forum,* ed P. Duncan, 5-12. Alexandria, VA: American Physical Therapy Association.

Naughton, J., R. Adams, and C. Maher. 2005. Upper-body wobbleboard training effects on the post-dislocation shoulder. *Phys Ther Sport* 6(1): 31-7.

Nederhand, M.J., M.J. Ijzerman, H.J. Hermens, C.T. Baten, and G. Zilvold. 2000. Cervical muscle dysfunction in the chronic whiplash associated disorder grade II (WAD-II). *Spine* 25(15): 1938-43.

Neer II, C.S. 1972. Anterior acromioplasty for the chronic impingement syndrome in the shoulder: A preliminary report. *J Bone Joint Surg Am* 54(1): 41-50.

Newcomer, K.L., E.R. Lasdowski, B. Yu, J.C. Johnson, and K.N. An. 2000. Differences in repositioning error among patients with low back pain compared with control subjects. *Spine* 25: 2488-93.

Newcomer, K.L., T.D. Jacobson, D.A. Gabriel, D.R. Larson, R.H. Brey, and K.N. An. 2002. Muscle activation patterns in subjects with and without low back pain. *Arch Phys Med Rehabil* 83(6): 816-21.

Ng, G.Y., and H.L. Chan. 2004. The immediate effects of tension of counterforce forearm brace on neuromuscular performance of wrist extensor muscles in subjects with lateral humeral epicondylosis. *J Orthop Sports Phys Ther* 34(2): 72-8.

Ng, G.Y., and P.C. Lam. 2002. A study of antagonist/agonist isokinetic work ratios of shoulder rotators in men who play badminton. *J Orthop Sports Phys Ther* 32(8): 399-404.

Nicholas, J.A., A.M. Strizak, and G. Veras. 1976. A study of thigh muscle weakness in different pathological states of the lower extremity. *Am J Sports Med* 4(6): 241-8.

Nicolakis, P., B. Erdogmus, A. Kopf, A. Djaber-Ansari, E. Piehslinger, and V. Fialka-Moser. 2000. Exercise therapy for craniomandibular disorders. *Arch Phys Med Rehabil* 81(9): 1137-42.

Nicolakis, P., B. Erdogmus, A. Kopf, G. Ebenbichler, J. Kollmitzer, E. Piehslinger, and V. Fialka-Moser. 2001. Effectiveness of exercise therapy in patients with internal derangement of the temporomandibular joint. *J Oral Rehabil* 28(12): 1158-64.

Nicolakis, P., B. Erdogmus, A. Kopf, M. Nicolakis, E. Piehslinger, and V. Fialka-Moser. 2002. Effectiveness of exercise therapy in patients with myofascial pain dysfunction syndrome. *J Oral Rehabil* 29(4): 362-8.

Nicolakis, P., E.C. Burak, J. Kollmitzer, A. Kopf, E. Piehslinger, G.F. Wiesinger, and V. Fialka-Moser. 2001. An investigation of the effectiveness of exercise and manual therapy in treating symptoms of TMJ osteoarthritis. *Cranio* 19(1): 26-32.

Nies, N., and P.L. Sinnott. 1991. Variations in balance and body sway in middle-aged adults. Subjects with healthy backs compared with subjects with low-back dysfunction. *Spine* 16(3): 325-30.

Nijs, J., N. Roussel, K. Vermeulen, and G. Souvereyns. 2005. Scapular positioning in patients with shoulder pain: A study examining the reliability and clinical importance of 3 clinical tests. *Arch Phys Med Rehabil* 86(7): 1349-55.

Nilsen, K.B., R.H. Westgaard, L.J. Stovner, G. Helde, M. Rø, and T.H. Sand. 2006. Pain induced by low-grade stress in patients with fibromyalgia and chronic shoulder/neck pain, relation to surface electromyography. *Eur J Pain* 10(7): 615-27.

Nirschl, R.P., and E.S. Ashman. 2003. Elbow tendinopathy: Tennis elbow. *Clin Sports Med* 22(4): 813-36.

Nishioka, G.J., and M.T. Montgomery. 1988. Masticatory muscle hyperactivity in temporomandibular disorders: Is it an extrapyramidally expressed disorder? *J Am Dent Assoc* 116(4): 514-20.

Nitz, A.J., and D. Peck. 1986. Comparison of muscle spindle contractions in large and small human epaxial muscles acting in parallel combinations. *Am Surg* 52: 273-7.

Noffal, G.J. 2003. Isokinetic eccentric-to-concentric strength ratios of the shoulder rotator muscles in throwers and nonthrowers. *Am J Sports Med* 31(4): 537-41.

Nørregaard, J., P.M. Bülow, P. Vestergaard-Poulsen, C. Thomsen, and B. Danneskiold-Samøe. 1995. Muscle strength, voluntary activation and cross-sectional muscle area in patients with fibromyalgia. *Br J Rheumatol* 34(10): 925-31.

Nourbakhsh, M.R., and A.M. Arab. 2002. Relationship between mechanical factors and incidence of low back pain. *J Orthop Sports Phys Ther* 32(9): 447-60.

Nouwen, A., P.F. Van Akkerveeken, and J.M. Versloot. 1987. Patterns of muscular activity during movement in patients with chronic low-back pain. *Spine* 12(8): 777-82.

Novak, C.B. 2004. Upper extremity work-related musculoskeletal disorders: A treatment perspective. *J Orthop Sports Phys Ther* 34(10): 628-37.

Novak, C.B., E.D. Collins, and S.E. Mackinnon. 1995. Outcome following conservative management of thoracic outlet syndrome. *J Hand Surg [Am]* 20(4): 542-8.

Nuber, G.W., F.W. Jobe, J. Perry, D.R. Moynes, and D. Antonelli. 1986. Fine wire electromyography analysis of muscles of the shoulder during swimming. *Am J Sports Med* 14(1): 7-11.

Nurse, M.A., and B.M. Nigg. 2001. The effect of changes in foot sensation on plantar pressure and muscle activity. *Clin Biomech (Bristol, Avon)* 16(9): 719-27.

O'Brien, S.J., M.J. Pagnani, R.A. Panariello, H.M. O'Flynn, and S. Fealy. 1994. Anterior instability of the shoulder. In *The Athlete's Shoulder*, ed. J.R. Andrews and K.E. Wilks, 117-201. New York: Churchill Livingstone.

O'Connell, A.L. 1971. Effect of sensory deprivation on postural reflexes. *Electromyography* 11: 5.

O'Connor, B.L., and J.A. Vilensky. 2003. Peripheral and central nervous system mechanisms of joint protection. *Am J Orthop* 7: 330-336.

O'Connor, B.L., D.M. Visco, K.D. Brandt, S.L. Myers, and L.A. Kalasinski. 1992. Neurogenic acceleration of osteoarthrosis. The effects of previous neurectomy of the articular nerves on the development of osteoarthrosis after transection of the anterior cruciate ligament in dogs. *J Bone Joint Surg Am* 74(3): 367-76.

O'Connor, B.L., M.J. Palmoski, and K.D. Brandt. 1985. Neurogenic acceleration of degenerative joint lesions. *J Bone Joint Surg Am* 67(4): 562-72.

O'Connor, D., S. Marshall, and N. Massy-Westropp. 2003. Non-surgical treatment (other than steroid injection) for carpal tunnel syndrome. *Cochrane Database Syst Rev* 1: CD003219.

O'Leary, S., D. Falla, G. Jull, and B. Vicenzino. 2007. Muscle specificity in tests of cervical flexor muscle performance. *J Electromyogr Kinesiol* 17(1): 35-40.

O'Sullivan, P., L. Towmey, G. Allison 1997. Altered pattern of abdominal muscle activation in patients with chronic low back pain. *Aust J Physiother* 43: 91-8.

O'Sullivan, P.B. 2005. Lumbar segmental "instability": Clinical presentation and specific stabilizing exercise management. *Man Ther* 5(1): 2-12.

Oberg, B., J. Ekstrand, M. Moller, and J. Gillquist. 1984. Muscle strength and flexibility in different positions of soccer players. *Int J Sports Med* 5(4): 213-6.

Ochi, M., J. Iwasa, Y. Uchio, N. Adachi, and K. Kawasaki. 2002. Induction of somatosensory evoked potentials by mechanical stimulation in reconstructed anterior cruciate ligaments. *J Bone Joint Surg Br* 84(5): 761-6.

Oddsson, L.I., T. Persson, A.G. Cresswell, and A. Thorstensson. 1999. Interaction between voluntary and postural motor commands during perturbed lifting. *Spine* 24(6): 545-52.

Odom, C.J., A.B. Taylor, C.E. Hurd, and C.R. Denegar. 2001. Measurement of scapular asymmetry and assessment of shoulder dysfunction using the lateral scapular slide test: A reliability and validity study. *Phys Ther* 81(2): 799-809.

Ogston, J.B., and P.M. Ludewig. 2007. Differences in 3-dimensional shoulder kinematics between persons with multidirectional instability and asymptomatic controls. *Am J Sports Med* 35(8): 1361-70.

Okada, S., K. Hirakawa, Y. Takada, and H. Kinoshita. 2001. Age-related differences in postural control in humans in response to a sudden deceleration generated by postural disturbance. *Eur J Appl Physiol* 85(1-2): 10-8.

Olson, L.E., A.L. Millar, J. Dunker, J. Hicks, and D. Glanz. 2006. Reliability of a clinical test for deep cervical flexor endurance. *J Manipulative Physiol Ther* 29(2): 134-8.

Orchard, J., J. Marsden, S. Lord, and D. Garlick. 1997. Preseason hamstring muscle weakness associated with hamstring muscle injury in Australian footballers. *Am J Sports Med* 25(1): 81-5.

Osborne, M.D., Chou, L.S., Laskowski, E.R., Smith, J., and Kaufman, K.R. 2001. The effect of ankle disk training on muscle reaction time in subjects with a history of ankle sprain. *Am J Sports Med.* Sep-Oct;29(5): 627-32.

Osternig, L.R., R. Robertson, R. Troxel, and P. Hansen. 1987. Muscle activation during proprioceptive neuromuscular facilitation (PNF) stretching techniques. *Am J Phys Med* 66(5): 298-307.

Osternig, L.R., R.N. Robertson, R.K. Troxel, and P. Hansen. 1990. Differential responses to proprioceptive neuromuscular facilitation (PNF) stretch techniques. *Med Sci Sports Exer* 22(1): 106-11.

Otis, J.C., C.C. Jiang, T.L. Wickiewicz, M.G. Peterson, R.F. Warren, and T.J. Santner. 1994. Changes in the moment arms of the rotator cuff and deltoid muscles with abduction and rotation. *J Bone Joint Surg Am* 76(5): 667-76.

Page, P. 2001. Incidence of anterior knee pain in ACL reconstruction: A retrospective multi-case analysis. Abstract. *J Athl Train* Suppl. no. 36(2): S13.

Page, P. 2004. Janda's sensorimotor training program. Abstract presented at the annual meeting of the American Physical Therapy Association, Chicago.

Page, P. 2006. Sensorimotor training: A "global" approach for balance training. *J Bodyw Mov Ther* 10: 77-84.

Page, P., and C. Frank. 2003. Function over structure. *Advance for Directors in Rehabilitation* January: 27-30.

Page, P., and G. Stewart. 1999. Shoulder taping in the management of impingement of the athlete. *Med Sci Sports Exerc* 31(5): S208.

Page, P., and G. Stewart. 2000. Hamstring strength imbalances in athletes with chronic sacroiliac dysfunction. Abstract. *J Orthop Sports Phys Ther* 30(1): A-48.

Page, P., O. Ross, M. Rogers, and N. Rogers. 2004. Muscle activity of the upper extremity during oscillation exercise using the Thera-Band Flexbar. Abstract. *Hand Prints* 21(5): 7.

Paine, R.M., and M. Voight. 1993. The role of the scapula. *J Orthop Sports Phys Ther* 18(1): 386-91.

Palmerud, G., H. Sporrong, P. Herberts, and R. Kadefors. 1998. Consequences of trapezius relaxation on the distribution of shoulder muscle forces: An electromyographic study. *J Electromyogr Kinesiol* 8(3): 185-93.

Palmerud, G., R. Kadefors, H. Sporrong, U. Järvholm, P. Herberts, C. Högfors, and B. Peterson. 1995. Voluntary redistribution of muscle activity in human shoulder muscles. *Ergonomics* 38(4): 806-15.

Panjabi, M. 1992b. The stabilizing system of the spine. Part II: Neutral spine and instability hypothesis. *Spine* 5(4): 390-7.

Panjabi, M.M. 1992a. The stabilizing system of the spine. Part I. Function, dysfunction, adaptation, and enhancement. *J Spinal Disord* 5(4): 383-9.

Panjabi, M.M. 1992b. The stabilizing system of the spine. Part II. Neutral zone and instability hypothesis. *J Spinal Disord* 5(4): 390-7.

Panjabi, M.M. 1994. Lumbar spine instability: A biomechanical challenge. *Curr Orthop* 8: 100-5.

Pappas, G.P., S.S. Blemker, C.F. Beaulieu, T.R. McAdams, S.T. Whalen, and G.E. Gold. 2006. In vivo anatomy of the Neer and Hawkins sign positions for shoulder impingement. *J Shoulder Elbow Surg* 15(1): 40-9.

Parkhurst, T.M., and C.N. Burnett. 1994. Injury and proprioception in the lower back. *J Orthop Sports Phys Ther* 19(5): 282-95.

Pascoal, A.G., F.F. van der Helm, P. Pezarat Correia, and I. Carita. 2000. Effects of different arm external loads on the scapulo-humeral rhythm. *Clin Biomech (Bristol, Avon)* 15(Suppl. no. 1): S21-4.

Pavlu, D., and D. Panek. 2007. EMG Analysis of Muscle Fatigue by Sensorimotor Training—A Contribution to Evidence Based Physiotherapy. *Proceedings of the 9th Annual TRAC Meeting. Budapest, Hungary*. 16-17.

Pavlu, D., and K. Novosadova. 2001. Contribution to the objectivization of the method of sensorimotor training stimulation according to Janda and Vavrova with regard to evidence-based-practice. *Rehabilitation Physical Medicine* 8(4): 178-81.

Pavlu, D., S. Petak- Kreuger, and V. Janda. 2007. Brugger methods for postural correction. In *Rehabilitation of the spine*. 2nd ed., ed. C. Liebenson, 353-68. Philadelphia: Lippincott Williams & Wilkins.

Payne, K.A., K. Berg, W. Richard, and R.W. Latin. 1997. Ankle injuries and ankle strength, flexibility, and proprioception in college basketball players. *J Athl Train* 32(3): 221-5.

Payne, L.Z., X.H. Deng, E.V. Craig, P.A. Torzilli, and R.F. Warren. 1997. The combined dynamic and static contributions to subacromial impingement. A biomechanical analysis. *Am J Sports Med* 25(6): 801-8.

Pearson, N.D., and R.P. Walmsley. 1995. Trial into the effects of repeated neck retractions in normal subjects. *Spine* 20(11): 1245-50.

Peat, M. 1986. Functional anatomy of the shoulder complex. *Phys Ther* 66(12): 1855-65.

Perri, M.A., and D. Halford. 2004. Pain and faulty breathing: A pilot study. *J Bodyw Mov Ther* 8: 297-306.

Perrin, P.P., M.C. Bene, C.A. Perrin, and D. Durupt. 1997. Ankle trauma significantly impairs posture control. A study in basketball players and controls. *Int J Sports Med* 18: 387-92.

Perry, J. 1978. Normal upper extremity kinesiology. *Phys Ther* 58(3): 265-78.

Perry, J. 1983. Anatomy and biomechanics of the shoulder in throwing, swimming, gymnastics, and tennis. *Clin Sports Med* 2(2): 247-70.

Perry, J. 1992. *Gait analysis: Normal and pathological function*. Thorofare, NJ: Slack.

Persson, A.L., G.A. Hansson, J. Kalliomäki, and B.H. Sjölund. 2003. Increases in local pressure pain thresholds after muscle exertion in women with chronic shoulder pain. *Arch Phys Med Rehabil* 84(10): 1515-22.

Petersen Kendall, F., E. Kendall Mccreary, P. Geise Provance, and I. Russell. 1996. Neurochemical pathogenesis of fibromyalgia syndrome. *Journal of Musculoskeletal Pain* 4(1/2): 61-92.

Petersson, C.J., and I. Redlund-Johnell. 1984. The subacromial space in normal shoulder radiographs. *Acta Orthop Scand* 55(1): 57-8.

Piazzini, D.B., I. Aprile, P.E. Ferrara, C. Bertolini, P. Tonali, L. Maggi, A. Rabini, S. Piantelli, and L. Padua. 2007. A systematic review of conservative treatment of carpal tunnel syndrome. *Clin Rehabil* 21(4): 299-314.

Pienimäki, T.T., P.T. Siira, and H. Vanharanta. 2002. Chronic medial and lateral epicondylitis: A comparison of pain, disability, and function. *Arch Phys Med Rehabil* 83(3): 317-21.

Pieper, H.G., G. Quack, and H. Krahl. 1993. Impingement of the rotator cuff in athletes caused by instability of the shoulder joint. *Knee Surg Sports Traumatol Arthrosc* 1(2): 97-9.

Pierce, M.N., and W.A. Lee. 1990. Muscle firing order during active prone hip extension. *J Orthop Sports Phys Ther* 12(1): 2-9.

Pink, M. 1981. Contralateral effects of upper extremity proprioceptive neuromuscular facilitation patterns. *Phys Ther* 61(8): 1158-62.

Pink, M., F.W. Jobe, J. Perry, A. Browne, M.L. Scovazzo, and J. Kerrigan. 1993. The painful shoulder during the butterfly stroke. An electromyographic and cinematographic analysis of twelve muscles. *Clin Orthop Relat Res* 288: 60-72.

Pintsaar, A., J. Brynhildsen, and H. Tropp. 1996. Postural corrections after standardised perturbations of single limb stance: Effect of training and orthotic devices in patients with ankle instability. *Br J Sports Med* 30(2): 151-5.

Pitman, M.I., N. Nainzadeh, D. Menche, R. Gasalberti, and E.K. Song. 1992. The intraoperative evaluation of the neurosensory function of the anterior cruciate ligament in humans using somatosensory evoked potentials. *Arthroscopy* 8(4): 442-7.

Piva, S.R., E.A. Goodnite, and J.D. Childs. 2005. Strength around the hip and flexibility of soft tissues in individuals with and without patellofemoral pain syndrome. *J Orthop Sports Phys Ther* 35(12): 793-801.

Poppen, N.K., and P.S. Walker. 1976. Normal and abnormal motion of the shoulder. *J Bone Joint Surg Am* 58(2): 195-201.

Poppen, N.K., and P.S. Walker. 1978. Forces at the glenohumeral joint in abduction. *Clin Orthop Relat Res* 135:165-70.

Porterfield, J.A., and C. DeRosa. 1998. *Mechanical low back pain: Perspectives in functional anatomy.* Philadelphia: Saunders.

Pötzl, W., L. Thorwesten, C. Götze, S. Garmann, and J. Steinbeck. 2004. Proprioception of the shoulder joint after surgical repair for instability: A long-term follow-up study. *Am J Sports Med* 32(2): 425-30.

Powers, C.M. 2003. The influence of altered lower extremity kinematics on patellofemoral joint dysfunction: A theoretical perspective *J Orthop Sports Phys Ther*. 33: 639-646.

Prentice, W.E. 1983. A comparison of static stretching and PNF stretching for improving hip joint flexibility. *Athletic Training* 18: 56-9.

Prichasuk, S., and Subhadrabandhu, T. 1994. The relationship of pes planus and calcaneal spur to plantar heel pain. *Clin Orthop Relat Res.* Sep;(306):192-6.

Professional Staff Association of Rancho Los Amigos Medical Center. 1989. *Observational gait analysis handbook.* Downey, CA: Rancho Los Amigos Medical CenterProvinciali, L., M. Baroni, L. Illuminati, and M.G. Ceravolo. 1996. Multimodal treatment to prevent the late whiplash syndrome. *Scand J Rehabil Med* 28(2): 105-11.

Prushansky, T., R. Gepstein, C. Gordon, and Z. Dvir. 2005. Cervical muscles weakness in chronic whiplash patients.*Clin Biomech (Bristol, Avon)* 20(8): 794-8.

Radebold, A., J. Cholewicki, G.K. Polzhofer, and H.S. Greene. 2001. Impaired postural control of the lumbar spine is associated with delayed muscle response times in patients with chronic idiopathic low back pain. *Spine* 26(7): 724-30.

Radebold, A., J. Cholewicki, M.M. Panjabi, and T.C. Patel. 2000. Muscle response pattern to sudden trunk loading in healthy individuals and in patients with chronic low back pain. *Spine* 25(8): 947-54.

Rainoldi, A., M. Gazzoni, and R. Casale. 2008. Surface EMG signal alterations in carpal tunnel syndrome: A pilot study. *Eur J Appl Physiol* 103(2): 233-42.

Ramsi, M., K.A. Swanik, C.G. Mattacola, and C.B. Swanic. 2001. Isometric shoulder rotator strength characteristics of high school swimmers throughout a competitive swim season. Abstract. *J Athl Train* Suppl. no. 36(2): S53.

Randlov, A., M. Ostergaard, C. Manniche, P. Kryger, A. Jordan, S. Heegaard, and B. Holm. 1998. Intensive dynamic training for females with chronic neck/shoulder pain. A randomized controlled trial. *Clin Rehabil* 12(3): 200-10.

Rawlings, E.I., I.L. Rawlings, C.S. Chen, and M.D. Yilk. 1972. The facilitating effects of mental rehearsal in the acquisition of rotary pursuit tracking. *Psychon Sci* 26: 71-3.

Ray, C.A., and A.L. Mark. 1995. Sympathetic nerve activity to nonactive muscle of the exercising and nonexercising limb. *Med Sci Sports Exerc* 27(2): 183-7.

Reardon, K., Galea, M., Dennett, X., Choong, P., and Byrne, E. 2001. Quadriceps muscle wasting persists 5 months after total hip arthroplasty for osteoarthritis of the hip: a pilot study. *Intern Med J.* Jan-Feb;31(1): 7-14.

Reddy, A.S., K.J. Mohr, M.M. Pink, and F.W. Jobe. 2000. Electromyographic analysis of the deltoid and rotator cuff muscles in persons with subacromial impingement. *J Shoulder Elbow Surg* 9(6): 519-23.

Reischl, F., C.M. Powers, S. Rao, and J. Perry. 1999. Relationship between foot pronation and rotation of the tibia and femur during walking. *Foot Ankle Int* 20: 513-20.

Revel, M., C. Andre-Deshays, and M. Minguet. 1991. Cervicocephalic kinesthetic sensibility in patients with cervical pain. *Arch Phys Med Rehabil* 72(5): 288-91.

Revel, M., M. Minguet, P. Gregoy, J. Vaillant, and J.L. Manuel. 1994. Changes in cervicocephalic kinesthesia after a proprioceptive rehabilitation program in patients with neck pain: A randomized controlled study. *Arch Phys Med Rehabil* 75(8): 895-9.

Reynolds, M.D. 1983. The development of the concept of fibrositis. *J Hist Med Allied Sci* 38: 5-35.

Richardson, A.B., F.W. Jobe, and H.R. Collins. 1980. The shoulder in competitive swimming. *Am J Sports Med* 8(3): 159-63.

Richardson, C., G. Jull, P. Hodges, and J. Hides. 1999. *Therapeutic exercise for spinal segmental stabilization in low back pain.* London: Churchill Livingstone.

Richardson, C.A., and G.A. Jull. 1995. Muscle control-pain control. What exercises would you prescribe? *Man Ther* 1: 2-10.

Richardson, C.A., C.J. Snidjers, J.A. Hides, L. Damen, M.S. Pas, and J. Storm. 2002. The relation between the transversus abdominis muscles, sacroiliac joint mechanics, and low back pain. *Spine*:27(4): 399-405.

Richardson, C.A., G.A. Jull, P.A. Hodges, and J.A. Hides. 1999. *Therapeutic exercise for spinal segmental stabilization in the low back: Scientific basis and clinical approach.* Edinburgh: Churchill Livingstone.

Richardson, C.A., P. Hodges, and J. Hides. 2004. *Therapeutic exercise for lumbopelvic stabilization. A motor control approach for the treatment and prevention of low back pain.* Edinburgh: Churchill Livingstone.

Riddle, D.L., Pulisic, M., Pidcoe, P., and Johnson, R.E. 2003. Risk factors for Plantar fasciitis: a matched case-control study. *J Bone Joint Surg Am.* May;85-A(5): 872-7.

Riemann, B.L., and S.M. Lephart. 2002a. The sensorimotor system, part I. The physiologic basis of functional joint stability. *J Athl Train* 37(1): 71-9.

Riemann, B.L., and S.M. Lephart. 2002b. The sensorimotor system, part II. The role of proprioception in motor control and functional joint stability. *J Athl Train* 37(1): 80-4.

Riemann, B.L., J.B. Myers, and S.M. Lephart. 2002. Sensorimotor system measurement techniques. *J Athl Train* 37(1): 85-98.

Risberg, M.A., I. Holm, G. Myklebust, and L. Engebretsen. 2007. Neuromuscular training versus strength training during first 6 months after anterior cruciate ligament reconstruction: A randomized clinical trial. *Phys Ther* 87(6): 737-50.

Robbins, S.E., and A.M. Hanna. 1987. Running related injury prevention through barefoot adaptations. 19: 148-56.

Robinson, R.L., and R.J. Nee. 2007. Analysis of hip strength in females seeking physical therapy treatment for unilateral patellofemoral pain syndrome. *J Orthop Sports Phys Ther* 37(5): 232-8.

Rocabado, M., B.E. Johnston Jr, and M.G. Blakney. 1982. Physical therapy and dentistry: An overview. *J Craniomandibular Pract* 1(1): 46-9.

Rock, C.M., and S. Petak-Krueger. 2000. *Thera-Band Grund Übungen.* [In German.] Zürich: Dr. Brügger Institut.

Røe, C., J.I. Brox, A.S. Bøhmer, and N.K. Vøllestad. 2000. Muscle activation after supervised exercises in patients with rotator tendinosis. *Arch Phys Med Rehabil* 81(1): 67-72.

Røe, C., J.I. Brox, E. Saugen, and N.K. Vøllestad. 2000. Muscle activation in the contralateral passive shoulder during isometric shoulder abduction in patients with unilateral shoulder pain. *J Electromyogr Kinesiol* 10(2): 69-77.

Rogers, N., M. Rogers, and P. Page. 2006. Quantification of a sensorimotor training progression: A pilot study. Abstract. *J Orthop Sports Phys Ther* 36(1): A53-4.

Rojas, M., M.A. Mañanas, B. Muller, and J. Chaler. 2007. Activation of forearm muscles for wrist extension in patients affected by lateral epicondylitis. *Conf Proc IEEE Eng Med Biol Soc* 2007: 4858-61.

Roll, R., A. Kavounoudias, and J.P. Roll. 2002. Cutaneous afferents from human plantar sole contribute to body posture awareness. *Neuroreport* 13(15): 1957-61.

Rooks, D.S., S. Gautam, M. Romeling, M.I. Cross, D. Stratigakis, B. Evans, D.L. Goldenberg, M.D. Iversen, and J.N. Katz. 2007. Group exercise, education, and combination self-management in women with fibromyalgia: A randomized trial. *Arch Intern Med* 167(20): 2192-200.

Root, M.C., W.P. Orion, and J.H. Weed. 1977. *Normal and abnormal function of the foot.* Los Angeles: Clinical Biomechanics.

Rosenfeld, M., A. Seferiadis, J. Carlsson, and R. Gunnarsson. 2003. Active intervention in patients with whiplash-associated disorders improves long-term prognosis: A randomized controlled clinical trial. *Spine* 28(22): 2491-8.

Rosenfeld, M., R. Gunnarsson, and P. Borenstein. 2000. Early intervention in whiplash-associated disorders: A comparison of two treatment protocols. *Spine* 25(14): 1782-7.

Ross, S.F., T.B. Michell, and K.M. Guskiewicz. 2005. Effect of coordination training with and without exercise sandals on static postural stability of individuals with functional ankle instability and individuals with stable ankles. Abstract. *J Orthop Sports Phys Ther* 35(5): A-22.

Rothbart, B.A. 2002. Medial column foot systems. An innovative tool for improving posture. *J Bodyw Mov Ther* 6: 37-46.

Rothbart, B.A. 2005. Tactile therapy shifts patients towards equilibrium. *Biomechanics* 12(10): 61-8.

Rothermel, S.A., S.A. Hale, J. Hertel, and C.R. Denegar. 2004. Effect of active foot positioning on the outcome of a balance training program. *Phys Ther Sport* 5: 98-103.

Rothwell, J.C., M.M. Traub, B.L. Day, J.A. Obeso, P.K. Thomas, and C.D. Marsden. 1982. Manual performance in a de-afferented man. *Brain* 105: 515-42.

Roy, J.S., H. Moffet, L.J. Hébert, G. St-Vincent, and B.J. McFadyen. 2007. The reliability of three-dimensional scapular attitudes in healthy people and people with shoulder impingement syndrome. *BMC Musculoskelet Disord* 8: 49.

Roy, S.H., C.J. De Luca, and D.A. Casavant. 1989. Lumbar muscle fatigue and chronic lower back pain. *Spine* 14(9): 992-1001.

Rozmaryn, L.M., S. Dovelle, E.R. Rothman, K. Gorman, K.M. Olvey, and J.J. Bartko. 1998. Nerve and tendon gliding exercises and the conservative management of carpal tunnel syndrome. *J Hand Ther* 11(3): 171-9.

Rupp, S., K. Berninger, and T. Hopf. 1995. Shoulder problems in high level swimmers—impingement, anterior instability, muscular imbalance? *Int J Sports Med* 16(8): 557-62.

Ruwe, P.A., M. Pink, F.W. Jobe, J. Perry, and M.L. Scovazzo. 1994. The normal and the painful shoulders during the breaststroke. Electromyographic and cinematographic analysis of twelve muscles. *Am J Sports Med* 22(6): 789-96.

Ryan, J. 1995. Use of posterior night splints in the treatment of plantar fasciitis. *American Family Physician* 52(3): 893-6.

Ryan, L. 1994. Mechanical stability, muscle strength, and proprioception in the functionally unstable ankle. *Australian J Phys Ther* 40: 41-7.

Ryu, R.K., J. McCormick, F.W. Jobe, D.R. Moynes, and D.J. Antonelli. 1988. An electromyographic analysis of shoulder function in tennis players. *Am J Sports Med* 16(5): 481-5.

Sady, S.P., M. Wortman, and D. Blanke. 1982. Flexibility training: Ballistic, static or proprioceptive neuromuscular facilitation? *Arch Phys Med Rehabil* 63(6): 261-3.

Saha, A.K. 1971. Dynamic stability of the glenohumeral joint. *Acta Orthop Scand* 42(6): 491-505.

Sahrmann, S.A. 2001. *Diagnosis and treatment of movement impairment syndromes.* St Louis: Mosby.

Sahrmann, S.A. 2002. Does postural assessment contribute to patient care? *J Orthop Sports Phys Ther* 32(8): 376-79.

Sale, D.G. 1988. Neural adaptation to resistance training. *Med Sci Sports Exerc* Suppl. no. 20(5): S135-45.

Salter, M. 2002. The neurobiology of central sensitization. *Journal of Musculoskeletal Pain* 10(1/2): 22-33.

Santilli, V., M.A. Frascarelli, M. Paoloni, F. Frascarelli, F. Camerota, L. De Natale, and F. De Santis. 2005. Peroneus longus muscle activation pattern during gait cycle in athletes affected by functional ankle instability: A surface electromyographic study. *Am J Sports Med* 33(8): 1183-7.

Santos, M.J., W.D. Belangero, and G.L. Almeida. 2007. The effect of joint instability on latency and recruitment order of the shoulder muscles. *J Electromyogr Kinesiol* 17(2): 167-75.

Sapega, A.A., T.C. Quedenfeld, R.A. Moyer, and R.A. Butler. 1981. Biophysical factors in range of motion exercise. *Phys Sportsmed* 9(12): 57-65.

Sapsford, R.R., P.W. Hodges, C.A. Richardson, D.H. Cooper, S.J. Markwell, and G.A. Jull. 2001. Co-activation of the abdominal and pelvic floor muscles during voluntary exercises. *Neurourol Urodyn* 20(1): 31-42.

Sarig-Bahat, H. 2003. Evidence for exercise therapy in mechanical neck disorders. *Man Ther* 8(1): 10-20.

Sarrafian, S.K. 1983. Gross and functional anatomy of the shoulder. *Clin Orthop Relat Res* 173: 11-9.

Sayenko, D.G., A.H. Vette, K. Kamibayashi, T. Nakajima, M. Akai, and K. Nakazawa. 2007. Facilitation of the soleus stretch reflex induced by electrical excitation of plantar cutaneous afferents located around the heel. *Neurosci Lett* 415(3): 294-8.

Schade, H.B. 1919. Eiträge zur umgrenzung und klärung einer lehre von erkältung. *Z Gesamte Exp Med* 7: 275-374.

Schaible, H.G., and R.F. Schmidt. 1985. Effects of an experimental arthritis on the sensory properties of fine articular afferent units. *J Neurophysiol* 54(5): 1109-22.

Schenkman, M., and V.R.D. Cartaya. 1987. Kinesiology of the shoulder complex. *J Orthop Sports Phys Ther* 8(9): 438-50.

Schieppati, M., A. Nardone, and M. Schmid. 2003. Neck muscle fatigue affects postural control in man. *Neuroscience* 121(2): 277-85.

Schmid, C., and U. Geiger. 1999. *Rehatrain.* Munich: Urban & Fischer.

Schmitt, L., and L. Snyder-Mackler. 1999. Role of scapular stabilizers in etiology and treatment of impingement syndrome. *J Orthop Sports Phys Ther* 29(1): 31-8.

Schnabel, M., R. Ferrari, T. Vassiliou, and G. Kaluza. 2004. Randomised, controlled outcome study of active mobilisation compared with collar therapy for whiplash injury. *Emerg Med J* 21(3): 306-10.

Schneider, M.J. 1995. Tender points/fibromyalgia vs. trigger points/myofascial pain syndrome: A need for clarity in terminology and differential diagnosis. *J Manipulative Physiol Ther* 18(6): 398-406.

Schoensee, S.K., G. Jensen, G. Nicholson, M. Gossman, and C. Katholi. 1995. The effect of mobilization on cervical headaches. *J Orthop Sports Phys Ther* 21(4): 184-96.

Schulte, E., L.A. Kallenberg, H. Christensen, C. Disselhorst-Klug, H.J. Hermens, G. Rau, and K. Søgaard. 2006. Comparison of the electromyographic activity in the upper trapezius and biceps brachii muscle in subjects with muscular disorders: A pilot study. *Eur J Appl Physiol* 96(2): 185-93.

Schulthies, S.S., M.D. Ricard, K.J. Alexander, and J.W. Myrer. 1998. An electromyographic investigation of 4 elastic tubing closed kinetic chain exercises after anterior cruciate ligament reconstruction. *J Athl Train* 33(4): 328-35.

Schulz, C.U., H. Anetzberger, and C. Glaser. 2005. Coracoid tip position on frontal radiographs of the shoulder: A predictor of common shoulder pathologies? *Br J Radiol* 78(935): 1005-8.

Scovazzo, M.L., A. Browne, M. Pink, F.W. Jobe, and J. Kerrigan. 1991. The painful shoulder during freestyle swimming. An electromyographic cinematographic analysis of twelve muscles. *Am J Sports Med* 19(6): 577-82.

Selkowitz, D.M., C. Chaney, S.J. Stuckey, and G. Vlad. 2007. The effects of scapular taping on the surface electromyographic signal amplitude of shoulder girdle muscles during upper extremity elevation in individuals with suspected shoulder impingement syndrome. *J Orthop Sports Phys Ther* 37(11): 694-702.

Senbursa, G., G. Baltaci, and A. Atay. 2007. Comparison of conservative treatment with and without manual physical therapy for patients with shoulder impingement syndrome: A prospective, randomized clinical trial. *Knee Surg Sports Traumatol Arthrosc* 15(7): 915-21.

Seradge, H., W. Parker, C. Baer, K. Mayfield, and L. Schall. 2002. Conservative treatment of carpal tunnel syndrome: An outcome study of adjunct exercises. *J Okla State Med Assoc* 95(1): 7-14.

Sessle, B.J., and J.W. Hu. 1991. Mechanisms of pain arising from articular tissues. *Can J Physiol Pharmacol* 69(5): 617-26.

Shacklock, M. 2005. *Clinical neurodynamics.* London: Elsevier Butterworth-Heinemann.

Shah, N.N., and P. Diamantopoulos. 2004. Position of the humeral head and rotator cuff tear: An anatomical observation in cadavers. *Acta Orthop Scand* 75(6): 746-9.

Shakespeare, D.T., M. Stokes, K.P. Sherman, and A. Young. 1985. Reflex inhibition of the quadriceps after meniscectomy: Lack of association with pain. *Clin Physiol* 5(2): 137-44.

Sharkey, N.A., and R.A. Marder. 1995. The rotator cuff opposes superior translation of the humeral head. *Am J Sports Med* 23(3): 270-5.

Sharkey, N.A., R.A. Marder, and P.B. Hanson. 1994. The entire rotator cuff contributes to elevation of the arm. *J Orthop Res* 12(5): 699-708.

Sherrington, C. 1906. *The integrative action of the nervous system.* New Haven, CT: Yale University Press.

Sherrington, C.S. 1907. On reciprocal innervation of antagonistic muscles. *Proc R Soc Lond B Biol Sci* 79B: 337.

Sherry, M.A., and T.M. Best. 2004. A comparison of 2 rehabilitation programs in the treatment of acute hamstring strains. *J Orthop Sports Phys Ther* 34(3): 116-25.

Sheth, P., B. Yu, E.R. Laskowski, and K.N. An. 1997. Ankle disk training influences reaction times of selected muscles in a simulated ankle sprain. *Am J Sports Med* 25(4): 538-43.

Shields, R.K., S. Madhaven, and K. Cole. 2005. Sustained muscle activity minimally influences dynamic position sense of the ankle. *J Orthop Sports Phys Ther* 35(7): 443-51.

Shih, C.H., Du, Y.K., Lin, Y.H., and Wu, C.C. 1994. Muscular recovery around the hip joint after total hip arthroplasty. *Clin Orthop Relat Res.* May;(302): 115-20.

Shima, N., K. Ishida, K. Katayama, Y. Morotome, Y. Sato, and M. Miyamura. 2002. Cross education of muscular strength during unilateral resistance training and detraining. *Eur J Appl Physiol* 86(4): 287-94.

Shirley, D., P.W. Hodges, A.E. Eriksson, and S.C. Gandevia. 2003. Spinal stiffness changes throughout the respiratory cycle. *J Appl Physiol* 95(4): 1467-75.

Shumway-Cook, A., and F. Horak. 1989. Vestibular rehabilitation: An exercise approach to managing symptoms of vestibular dysfunction. *Semin Hear* 10: 199.

Shumway-Cook, A., and M. Woollacott. 2000. Attentional demands and postural control: The effect of sensory context. *J Gerontol A Biol Sci Med Sci* 55(1): 10-16.

Shumway-Cook, A., and M.H. Woollacott. 1995. *Motor control: Theory and practical applications.* Baltimore: Williams & Wilkins.

Shumway-Cook, A., M. Woollacott, K.A. Kerns, and M. Baldwin. 1997. The effects of two types of congitive tasks on postural stability in older adults with and without a history of falls. *J Gerontol A Biol Sci Med Sci* 52(4): 232-40.

Silverman, J.L., A.A. Rodriquez, and J.C. Agre. 1991. Quantitative cervical flexor strength in healthy subjects and in subjects with mechanical neck pain. *Arch Phys Med Rehabil* 72(9): 679-81.

Silvestri, P.G., C.G. Mattacoloa, J.A. Madaleno, D.L. Johnson, and T.L. Uhl. 2003. Relationship between mechanical foot position and postural sway. Abstract. *J Athl Train* 3: S52-53.

Simard, T.G., J.V. Basmajian, and V. Janda. 1968. Effects of ischemia on trained motor units. *Am J Phys Med* 47(2): 64-71.

Simms, R.W. 1996. Is there muscle pathology in fibromyalgia syndrome? *Rheum Dis Clin North Am* 22(2): 245-66.

Simons, D.G. 1996. Clinical and etiological update of myofascial pain from trigger points. *Journal of Musculoskeletal Pain* 1(2): 93-121.

Simons, D.G., J.G. Travell, and L.S. Simons. 1999. *Upper half of body.* Vol. 1 of *Travell and Simons' myofascial pain and dysfunction: The trigger point manual.* 2nd ed. Philadelphia: Lippincott Williams & Wilkins.

Sims K.J., Richardson C.A., and Brauer S.G.2002. Investigation of hip abductor activation in subjects with clinical unilateral hip osteoarthritis. *Ann Rheum Dis.* Aug;61(8): 687-92.

Singh, M., and P.V. Karpovich. 1967. Effect of eccentric training of agonists on antagonistic muscles. *J Appl Physiol* 23(5): 742-5.

Sirota, S.C., G.A. Malanga, J.J. Eischen, and E.R. Laskowski. 1997. An eccentric- and concentric-strength profile of shoulder external and internal rotator muscles in professional baseball pitchers. *Am J Sports Med* 25(1): 59-64.

Sjostrom, H., J.H. Allum, M.G. Carpenter, A.L. Adkin, F. Honegger, and T. Ettlin. 2003. Trunk sway measures of postural stability during clinical balance tests in patients with chronic whiplash injury symptoms. *Spine* 28(15): 1725-34.

Slemenda, C., D.K. Heilman, K.D. Brandt, B.P. Katz, S.A. Mazzuca, E.M. Braunstein, and D. Byrd. 1998. Reduced quadriceps strength relative to body weight: A risk factor for knee osteoarthritis in women? *Arthritis Rheum* 41: 1951-9.

Slemenda, C., K.D. Brandt, D.K. Heilman, S. Mazzuca, E.M. Braunstein, B.P. Katz, and F.D. Wolinsky. 1997. Quadriceps weakness and osteoarthritis of the knee. *Ann Intern Med* 127(2): 97-104.

Smith, J., B.R. Kotajarvi, D.J. Padgett, and J.J. Eischen. 2002. Effect of scapular protraction and retraction on isometric shoulder elevation strength. *Arch Phys Med Rehabil* 83(3): 367-70.

Smith, J., C.T. Dietrich, B.R. Kotajarvi, and K.R. Kaufman. 2006. The effect of scapular protraction on isometric shoulder rotation strength in normal subjects. *J Shoulder Elbow Surg* 15(3): 339-43.

Smith, J., D.J. Padgett, D.L. Dahm, K.R. Kaufman, S.P. Harrington, D.A. Morrow, and S.E. Irby. 2004. Electromyographic activity in the immobilized shoulder girdle musculature during contralateral upper limb movements. *J Shoulder Elbow Surg* 13(6): 583-8.

Smith, J., D.J. Padgett, K.R. Kaufman, S.P. Harrington, K.N. An, and S.E. Irby. 2004. Comparing the function of the upper and lower parts of the serratus anterior muscle using surface electromyography. *J Orthop Sports Phys Ther* 34(5): 235-43.

Smith, J., J.E. Szczerba, B.L. Arnold, D.E. Martin, and D.H. Perrin. 1997. Role of hyperpronation as a possible risk factor for anterior cruciate ligament injuries. *J Athl Train* 32: 25-8.

Smith, M., M.W. Coppieters, and P.W. Hodges. 2005. Effect of experimentally induced low back pain on postural sway with breathing. *Exp Brain Res* 166(1): 109-17.

Smith, M..D., A. Russell, and P.W. Hodges. 2006. Disorders of breathing and continence have a stronger association with back pain than obesity and physical activity. *Aust J Physiother* 52(1): 11-6.

Smith, M.D., A. Russell, and P.W. Hodges. 2000. Changes in intra-abdominal pressure during postural and respiratory activation of the human diaphragm. *J Appl Physiol* 89(3): 967-76.

Smith, R.L., and J. Brunolli. 1989. Shoulder kinesthesia after anterior glenohumeral joint dislocation. *Phys Ther* 69(2): 106-12.

Snijders, C.J., A. Vleeming, and R. Stoeckart. 1993. Transfer of lumbosacral load to iliac bones and legs. Part 1: Biomechanics of self-bracing of the sacroiliac joints and its significance for treatment and exercise. *Clin Biomech* 8: 285-94.

Sobush, D.C., G.G. Simoneau, K.E. Dietz, J.A. Levene, R.E. Grossman, and W.B. Smith. 1996. The lennie test for measuring scapular position in healthy young adult females: A reliability and validity study. *J Orthop Sports Phys Ther* 23(1): 39-50.

Soderberg, G.L., and L.M. Knutson. 2000. A guide for use and interpretation of kinesiologic electromyographic data. *Phys Ther* 80(5): 485-98.

Sokk, J., H. Gapeyeva, J. Ereline, I. Kolts, and M. Pääsuke. 2007. Shoulder muscle strength and fatigability in patients with frozen shoulder syndrome: The effect of 4-week individualized rehabilitation. *Electromyogr Clin Neurophysiol* 47(4-5): 205-13.

Solem-Bertoft, E., K.A. Thuomas, and C.E. Westerberg. 1993. The influence of scapular retraction and protraction on the width of the subacromial space. An MRI study. *Clin Orthop Relat Res* 296: 99-103.

Solomonow, M., B.H. Zhou, M. Harris, Y. Lu, and R.V. Baratta. 1998. The ligamento-muscular stabilizing system of the spine. *Spine* 23(23): 2552-62.

Solomonow, M., R. Baratta, B.H. Zhou, H. Shoji, W. Bose, C. Beck, and R. D'Ambrosia. 1987. The synergistic action of the anterior cruciate ligament and thigh muscles in maintaining joint stability. *Am J Sports Med* 15(3): 207-13.

Sommer, H.M. 1988. Patellar chondropathy and apicitis, and muscle imbalances of the lower extremities in competitive sports. *Sports Med* 5(6): 386-94.

Spitzer, W.O., M.L. Skovron, L.R. Salmi, J.D. Cassidy, J. Duranceau, S. Suissa, and E. Zeiss. 1995. Scientific monograph of the Quebec Task Force on whiplash-associated disorders: Redefining "whiplash" and its management. *Spine* Suppl. no. 20(8): 1S-73S.

Sporrong, H., G. Palmerud, and P. Herberts. 1996. Hand grip increases shoulder muscle activity. An EMG analysis with static hand contractions in 9 subjects. *Acta Orthop Scand* 67(5): 485-90.

Standaert, C.J., and S.A. Herring. 2007. Expert opinion and controversies in musculoskeletal and sports medicine: Core stabilization as a treatment for low back pain. *Arch Phys Med Rehabil* 88(12): 1734-6.

Starkey, C. 1999. *Therapeutic modalities.* 2nd ed. Philadelphia: Davis.

Stasinopoulos, D., and M.I. Johnson. 2005. Effectiveness of extracorporeal shock wave therapy for tennis elbow (lateral epicondylitis). *Br J Sports Med* 39(3): 132-6.

Stasinopoulos, D., and M.I. Johnson. 2006. "Lateral elbow tendinopathy" is the most appropriate diagnostic term for the condition commonly referred to as lateral epicondylitis. *Med Hypotheses* 67(6): 1400-2.

Staud, R. 2002. Evidence of involvement of central neural mechanisms in generating fibromyalgia pain. *Curr Rheumatol Rep* 4(4): 299-305.

Staud, R., M.E. Robinson, and D.D. Price. 2005. Isometric exercise has opposite effects on central pain mechanisms in fibromyalgia patients compared to normal controls. *Pain* 118(1-2): 176-84.

Steenbrink, F., J.H. de Groot, H.E. Veeger, C.G. Meskers, M.A. van de Sande, and P.M. Rozing. 2006. Pathological muscle activation patterns in patients with massive rotator cuff tears, with and without subacromial anesthetics. *Man Ther* 11(3): 231-7.

Steinbeck, J., J. Bruntrup, O. Greshake, W. Potzl, T. Filler, and U. Liljenqvist. 2003. Neurohistological examination of the inferior glenohumeral ligament of the shoulder. *J Orthop Res* 21: 250-55.

Sterling, M., G. Jull, and A. Wright. 2001. The effect of musculoskeletal pain on motor activity and control. *J Pain* 2(3): 135-45.

Sterling, M., G. Jull, B. Vicenzino, J. Kenardy, and R. Darnell. 2003. Development of motor system dysfunction following whiplash injury. *Pain* 103(1-2): 65-73.

Sterling, M., J. Treleaven, and G. Jull. 2002. Responses to a clinical test of mechanical provocation of nerve tissue in whiplash associated disorder. *Man Ther* 7(2): 89-94.

Sterling, M., J. Treleaven, S. Edwards, and G. Jull. 2002. Pressure pain thresholds in chronic whiplash associated disorder: Further evidence of altered central pain processing. *Journal of Musculoskeletal Pain* 10(3): 69-81.

Stocker, D., M. Pink, and F.W. Jobe. 1995. Comparison of shoulder injury in collegiate- and master's-level swimmers. *Clin J Sport Med* 5(1): 4-8.

Stokdijk, M., P.H. Eilers, J. Nagels, and P.M. Rozing. 2003. External rotation in the glenohumeral joint during elevation of the arm. *Clin Biomech (Bristol, Avon)* 18(4): 296-302.

Stokes, M., and A. Young. 1984. The contribution of reflex inhibition of arthrogenenous muscle weakness. *Clin Sci* 67: 7-14.

Strizak, A.M., G.W. Gleim, A. Sapega, and J.A. Nicholas. 1983.. Hand and forearm strength and its relation to tennis. *Am J Sports Med* 11(4): 234-9.

Struijs, P.A., G.M. Kerkhoffs, W.J. Assendelft, and C.N. van Dijk. 2004. Conservative treatment of lateral epicondylitis: Brace versus physical therapy or a combination of both—a randomized clinical trial. *Am J Sports Med* 32(2): 462-9.

Struijs, P.A., I.B. Korthals-de Bos, M.W. van Tulder, C.N. van Dijk, L.M. Bouter, and W.J. Assendelft. 2006. Cost effectiveness of brace, physiotherapy, or both for treatment of tennis elbow. *Br J Sports Med* 40(7): 637-43.

Stubbs, M., M. Harris, M. Solomonow, B. Zhou, Y. Lu, and R.V. Baratta. 1998. Ligamento-muscular protective reflex in the lumbar spine of the feline. *J Electromyogr Kinesiol* 8(4): 197-204.

Su, K.P., M.P. Johnson, E.J. Gracely, and A.R. Karduna. 2004. Scapular rotation in swimmers with and without impingement syndrome: Practice effects. *Med Sci Sports Exerc* 36(7): 1117-23.

Sullivan, S.J., S. Seguin, D. Seaborne, and J. Goldberg.1993. Reduction of H-reflex amplitude during the application of effleurage to the triceps surae in neurologically healthy subjects. *Physiother Theory and Pract* 9: 25-31.

Suter, E., and G. McMorland. 2002. Decrease in elbow flexor inhibition after cervical spine manipulation in patients with chronic neck pain. *Clin Biomech (Bristol, Avon)* 17(7): 541-4.

Swaney, M.R., and R.A. Hess. 2003. The effects of core stabilization on balance and posture in female collegiate swimmers. Abstract. *J Athl Train* 38(2): S-95.

Szeto, G.P., L.M. Straker, and P.B. O'Sullivan. 2005. A comparison of symptomatic and asymptomatic office workers performing monotonous keyboard work—1: Neck and shoulder muscle recruitment patterns. *Man Ther* 10(4): 270-80.

Szeto, G.P., L.M. Straker, and P.B. O'Sullivan. 2005. EMG median frequency changes in the neck-shoulder stabilizers of symptomatic office workers when challenged by different physical stressors. *J Electromyogr Kinesiol* 15(6): 544-55.

Taimela, S., K. Osterman, H. Alaranta, A. Soukka, and U.M. Kujala. 1993. Long psychomotor reaction time in patients with chronic low-back pain: Preliminary report. *Arch Phys Med Rehabil* 74(11): 1161-4.

Taimela, S., M. Kankaanpaa, and S. Luoto. 1999. The effect of lumbar fatigue on the ability to sense a change in lumbar position. A controlled study. *Spine* 24(13): 1322-7.

Takala, E.P., I. Korhonen, and E. Viikari-Juntura. 1997. Postural sway and stepping response among working population: Reproducibility, long-term stability, and associations with symptoms of the low back. *Clin Biomech* 12(7-8): 429-437.

Takeda, Y., S. Kashiwaguchi, K. Endo, T. Matsuura, and T. Sasa. 2002. The most effective exercise for strengthening the supraspinatus muscle: Evaluation by magnetic resonance imaging. *Am J Sports Med* 30(3): 374-81.

Taskiran, E., Z. Dinedurga, A. Yagis, B. Uludag, C. Ertekin, and V. Lök. 1998. Effect of the vastus medialis obliquus on the patellofemoral joint. *Knee Surg Sports Traumatol Arthrosc* 6(3): 173-80.

Tata, G.E., L. Ng, and J.F. Kramer. 1993. Shoulder antagonistic strength ratios during concentric and eccentric muscle actions in the scapular plane. *J Orthop Sports Phys Ther* 18(6): 654-60.

Taylor, D.C., D.E. Brooks, and J.B. Ryan. 1997. Viscoelastic characteristics of muscle: Passive stretching versus muscular contractions. *Med Sci Sports Exerc* 29(12): 1619-24.

Taylor, D.C., J. Dalton, A.V. Seaber, and W.E. Garrett. 1990. The viscoelastic properties of muscle tendon units. *Am J Sports Med* 18: 303-4.

Taylor, D.C., J.D. Dalton, A.V. Seaber, and W.E. Garrett. 1990. Viscoelastic properties of muscle-tendon units. The biomechanical effects of stretching. *Am J Sports Med* 18(3): 300-9.

Thein, L.A. 1989. Impingement syndrome and its conservative management. *J Orthop Sports Phys Ther* 11(5): 183-91.

Theodoridis, D., and S. Ruston. 2002. The effect of shoulder movements on thoracic spine 3D motion. *Clin Biomech (Bristol, Avon)* 17(5): 418-21.

Thigpen, C.A., D.A. Padua, N. Morgan, C. Kreps, and S.G. Karas. 2006. Scapular kinematics during supraspinatus rehabilitation exercise: A comparison of full-can versus empty-can techniques. *Am J Sports Med* 34(4): 644-52.

Tibone, J.E., J. Fechter, and J.T. Kao. 1997. Evaluation of a proprioception pathway in patients with stable and unstable shoulders with somatosensory cortical evoked potentials. *J Shoulder Elbow Surg* 6(5): 440-3.

Tittel, K. 2000. *Describing functional anatomy in humans.* 13th ed. Munich: Urban & Fischer.

Travell, J.G., and D.G. Simons. 1983. *Myofascial pain and dysfunction: The trigger point manual.* Baltimore: Williams & Wilkins.

Travell, J.G., and D.G. Simons. 1992a. *Myofascial pain and dysfunction: The trigger point manual.* Baltimore: Williams & Wilkins.

Travell, J.G., and D.G. Simons. 1992b. *The lower extremities.* Vol. 2 of *Myofascial pain and dysfunction: The trigger point manual.* Baltimore: Williams & Wilkins.

Treleaven, J., G. Jull, and M. Sterling. 2003. Dizziness and unsteadiness following whiplash injury: Characteristic features and relationship with cervical joint position error. *J Rehabil Med* 35(1): 36-43.

Treleaven, J., G. Jull, and N. Lowchoy. 2005. Standing balance in persistent whiplash: A comparison between subjects with and without dizziness. *J Rehabil Med* 37(4): 224-9.

Tropp, H. 1986. Pronator muscle weakness in functional instability of the ankle joint. *Int J Sports Med* 7: 291-4.

Tropp, H. 2002. Commentary: Functional ankle instability revisited. *J Athl Train* 37(4): 512-15.

Tropp, H., and P. Odenrick. 1988. Postural control in single-limb stance. *J Orthop Res* 6(6): 833-9.

Tropp, H., C. Askling, and J. Gillquist. 1985. Prevention of ankle sprains. *Am J Sports Med* 13(4): 259-62.

Tropp, H., J. Ekstrand, and J. Gillquist. 1984a. Factors affecting stabilometry recordings of single limb stance. *Am J Sports Med* 12(3): 185-8.

Tropp, H., J. Ekstrand, and J. Gillquist. 1984b. Stabilometry in functional instability of the ankle and its value in predicting injury. *Med Sci Sports Exerc* 16(1): 64-6.

Tropp, H., P. Odenrick, and J. Gillquist. 1985. Stabilometry recordings in functional and mechanical instability of the ankle joint. *Int J Sports Med* 6(3): 180-2.

Troy Blackburn, J., C.J. Hirth, and K.M. Guskiewicz. 2003. Exercise sandals increase lower extremity electromyographic activity during functional activities. *J Athl Train* 38(3): 198-203.

Trudelle-Jackson, E., Emerson, R., and Smith, S. 2002. Outcomes of total hip arthroplasty: a study of

patients one year postsurgery. *J Orthop Sports Phys Ther.* Jun;32(6): 260-7.

Tsai, L.C., B. Yu, V.S. Mercer, and M.T. Gross. 2006. Comparison of different structural foot types for measures of standing postural control. *J Orthop Sports Phys Ther* 36(12): 942-53.

Tsai, N.T., P.W. McClure, and A.R. Karduna. 2003. Effects of muscle fatigue on 3-dimensional scapular kinematics. *Arch Phys Med Rehabil* 84(7): 1000-5.

Tsuda, E., Y. Okamura, H. Otsuka, T. Komatsu, and S. Tokuya. 2001. Direct evidence of anterior cruciate ligament-hamstring reflex arc in humans. *Am J Sports Med* 29(1): 83-7.

Tunnell, P.W. 1996. Muscle length assessment of tightness-prone muscles. *J Bodyw Mov Ther* 1(1): 21-7.

Tunnell, P.W. 1996. Protocol for visual assessment. *J Bodyw Mov Ther* 2(1): 21-6.

Tuzun, C., I. Yorulmaz, A. Cindas, and S. Vatan. 1999. Low back pain and posture. *Clin Rheumatol* 18(4): 308-12.

Tyler, T., S. Nicholas, R. Campbell, S. Donellan, and M.P. McCugh. 2002. The effectiveness of a preseason exercise program to prevent adductor muscle strains in professional ice hockey players. *Am J Sports Med* 30: 680-3.

Tyler, T.F., R.C. Nahow, S.J. Nicholas, and M.P. McHugh. 2005. Quantifying shoulder rotation weakness in patients with shoulder impingement. *J Shoulder Elbow Surg* 14(6): 570-4.

Tyler, T.F., S.J. Nicholas, M.J. Mullaney, and M.P. McHugh. 2006. The role of hip muscle function in the treatment of patellofemoral pain syndrome. *Am J Sports Med* 34(4): 630-6.

Tyler, T.F., S.J. Nicholas, R.J. Campbell, and M.P. McHugh. 2001. The association of hip strength and flexibility with the incidence of adductor muscle strains in professional ice hockey players. *Am J Sports Med* 29(2): 124-8.

Tyler, T.F., S.J. Nicholas, T. Roy, and G.W. Gleim. 2000. Quantification of posterior capsule tightness and motion loss in patients with shoulder impingement. *Am J Sports Med* 28(5): 668-73.

Tyler, T.F., T. Roy, S.J. Nicholas, and G.W. Gleim. 1999. Reliability and validity of a new method of measuring posterior shoulder tightness. *J Orthop Sports Phys Ther* 29(5): 262-69; discussion: 270-74.

Uh, B.S., B.D. Beynnon, B.V. Helie, D.M. Alosa, and P.A. Renstrom. 2000. The benefit of a single-leg strength training program for the muscles around the untrained ankle. *Am J Sports Med* 28(4): 568-73.

Uhlig, Y., B.R. Weber, D. Grob, and M. Muntener. 1995. Fiber composition and fiber transformations in neck muscles of patients with dysfunction of the cervical spine. *J Orthop Res* 13(2): 240-9.

Umphred, D.A. 2001. The limbic system: Influence over motor control and learning. In *Neurological rehabilitation.* 4th ed., ed. D.A. Umphred, 148-77. St. Louis: Mosby.

Umphred, D.A., N. Byl, R.T. Lazaro, and M. Roller. 2001. Interventions for neurological disabilities. In *Neurological rehabilitation*. 4th ed., ed. D.A. Umphred, 56-134. St. Louis: Mosby.

Vacek, J., M. Vererkova, V. Janda, V. Besvodova, and P. Dvorakova. 2000. The painful coccyx and its influence on the movement pattern for hip extension. *J Orthop Med* 22(2): 42-4.

Valeriani, M., D. Restuccia, V. DiLazzaro, F. Franceschi, C. Fabbriciani, and P. Tonali. 1996. Central nervous system modifications in patients with lesion of the anterior cruciate ligament of the knee. *Brain* 119(Pt. 5): 1751-62.

Valkeinen, H., A. Häkkinen, P. Hannonen, K. Häkkinen, and M. Alén. 2006. Acute heavy-resistance exercise-induced pain and neuromuscular fatigue in elderly women with fibromyalgia and in healthy controls: Effects of strength training. *Arthritis Rheum* 54(4): 1334-9.

Valkeinen, H., K. Häkkinen, A. Pakarinen, P. Hannonen, A. Häkkinen, O. Airaksinen, L. Niemitukia, W.J. Kraemer, and M. Alén. 2005. Muscle hypertrophy, strength development, and serum hormones during strength training in elderly women with fibromyalgia. *Scand J Rheumatol* 34(4): 309-14.

Valkeinen, H., M. Alen, P. Hannonen, A. Häkkinen, O. Airaksinen, and K. Häkkinen. 2004. Changes in knee extension and flexion force, EMG and functional capacity during strength training in older females with fibromyalgia and healthy controls. *Rheumatology (Oxford)* 43(2): 225-8.

Valmassey, R.L. 1996. Clinical biomechanics of the lower extremity. St. Louis: Mosby.

Van Buskirk, R.L. 1990. Nociceptive reflexes and the somatic dysfunction: A model. *J Am Osteopath Assoc* 909: 785-9.

van der Helm, F.C. 1994. Analysis of the kinematic and dynamic behavior of the shoulder mechanism. *J Biomech* 27(5): 527-50.

van der Wees, P.J., Lenssen, A.F., Hendriks, E.J., Stomp, D.J., Dekker, J., and de Bie, R.A. 2006. Effectiveness of exercise therapy and manual mobilisation in ankle sprain and functional instability: a systematic review. *Aust J Physiother.* 52(1): 27-37.

van der Windt, D.A., B.W. Koes, A.J. Boeke, W. Devillé, B.A. De Jong, and L.M. Bouter. 1996. Shoulder disorders in general practice: Prognostic indicators of outcome. *Br J Gen Pract* 46(410): 519-23.

van der Windt, D.A., B.W. Koes, B.A. de Jong, and L.M. Bouter. 1995. Shoulder disorders in general practice: Incidence, patient characteristics, and management. *Ann Rheum Dis* 54(12): 959-64.

Van Dillen, L.R., M.K. McDonnell, D.A. Fleming, and S.A. Sahrmann. 2000. Effect of knee and hip position on hip extension range of motion in individuals with and without low back pain. *J Orthop Sports Phys Ther* 30(6): 307-16.

van Elk, N., M. Faes, H. Degens, J.G. Kooloos, J.A. de Lint, and M.T. Hopman. 2004. The application of an external wrist extension force reduces electromyographic activity of wrist extensor muscles during gripping. *J Orthop Sports Phys Ther* 34(5): 228-34.

van Ettekoven, H., and C. Lucas. 2006. Efficacy of physiotherapy including a craniocervical training programme for tension-type headache; a randomized clinical trial. *Cephalalgia* 26(8): 983-91.

Vangsness Jr, C.T., M. Ennis, J.G. Taylor, and R. Atkinson. 1995. Neural anatomy of the glenohumeral ligaments, labrum, and subacromial bursa. *Arthroscopy* 11(2): 180-4.

Vasara, A.I., J.S. Jurvelin, L. Peterson, and I. Kiviranta. 2005. Arthroscopic cartilage indentation and cartilage lesions of anterior cruciate ligament-deficient knees. *Am J Sports Med* 33(3): 408-14.

Vasseljen Jr., O., B.M. Johansen, and R.H. Westgaard. 1995. The effect of pain reduction on perceived tension and EMG-recorded trapezius muscle activity in workers with shoulder and neck pain. *Scand J Rehabil Med* 27(4): 243-52.

Vassiliou, T., G. Kaluza, C. Putzke, H. Wulf, and M. Schnabel. 2006. Physical therapy and active exercises—an adequate treatment for prevention of late whiplash syndrome? Randomized controlled trial in 200 patients. *Pain* 124(1-2): 69-76.

Vecchio, P., R. Kavanagh, B.L. Hazleman, and R.H. King. 1995. Shoulder pain in a community-based rheumatology clinic. *Br J Rheumatol* 34(5): 440-2.

Veeger, H.E., and F.C. van der Helm. 2007. Shoulder function: The perfect compromise between mobility and stability. *J Biomech* 40(10): 2119-29.

Vera-Garcia, F.J., S.G. Grenier, and S.M. McGill. 2000. Abdominal muscle response during curl-ups on both stable and labile surfaces. *Phys Ther* 80(6): 564-9.

Verhagen, E.A., van Tulder, M., van der Beek, A.J., Bouter, L.M., and van Mechelen, W. 2005. An economic evaluation of a proprioceptive balance board training programme for the prevention of ankle sprains in volleyball. *Br J Sports Med.* Feb;39(2): 111-5.

Vernon, H., K. Humphreys, and C. Hagino. 2007. Chronic mechanical neck pain in adults treated by manual therapy: A systematic review of change scores in randomized clinical trials. *J Manipulative Physiol Ther* 30(3): 215-27.

Vicenzino, B., J. Brooksbank, J. Minto, S. Offord, and A. Paungmali. 2003. Initial effects of elbow taping on pain-free grip strength and pressure pain threshold. *J Orthop Sports Phys Ther* 33(7): 400-7.

Viitasalo, J.T., and M. Kvist. 1983. Some biomechanical aspects of the foot and ankle in athletes with and without shin splints. *Am J Sports Med* 11: 125-30.

Vilensky, J.A., B.L. O'Connor, J.D. Fortin, G.J. Merkel, A.M. Jimenez, B.A. Scofield, and J.B. Kleiner. 2002.

Histologic analysis of neural elements in the human sacroiliac joint. *Spine* 27(11): 1202-7.

Vleeming, A., A.L. Pool-Goudzwaard, R. Stoeckart, J.P. van Wingerden, and C.J. Snijders. 1995. The posterior layer of the thoracolumbar fascia. Its function in load transfer from spine to legs. *Spine* 20(7): 753-8.

Vleeming, A., C. Stoeckart, and C. Snijders. 1989. The sacrotuberous ligament: A conceptual approach to its dynamic role in stabilizing the sacroiliac joint. *Clin Biomech* 4: 201-3.

Vleeming, A., C.J. Snijders, R. Stoeckart, and J.M.A. Mens. 1997. The role of the sacroiliac joints in coupling between the spine, pelvis, legs, and arms. In *Movement, stability, and low back pain*, ed. A. Vleeming, V. Mooney, T. Dorman, C. Snijders, and R. Stoeckart, 53. Edinburgh: Churchill Livingstone.

Voerman, G.E., M.M. Vollenbroek-Hutten, and H.J. Hermens. 2007. Upper trapezius muscle activation patterns in neck-shoulder pain patients and healthy controls. *Eur J Appl Physiol* 102(1): 1-9.

Vogt, L., and W. Banzer. 1997. Dynamic testing of the motor stereotype in prone hip extension from neutral position. *Clin Biomech (Bristol, Avon)* 12(2): 122-7.

Vogt, L., K. Pfeifer, and W. Banzer. 2003. Neuromuscular control of walking with chronic low-back pain. *Man Ther* 8(1): 21-8.

Voight, M.L., and B.C. Thomson. 2000. The role of the scapula in the rehabilitation of shoulder injuries. *J Athl Train* 35(3): 364-72.

Voight, M.L., and D.L. Wieder. 1991. Comparative reflex response times of vastus medialis obliquus and vastus lateralis in normal subjects and subjects with extensor mechanism dysfunction. An electromyographic study. *Am J Sports Med* 19(2): 131-7.

Vojta, V., and A. Peters. 1997. *Das Vojta-Prinzip. Muskelspiele in Reflexfortbewegung und motorischer Ontogenese. [The Vojta principle. Muscle activity in reflex progressive movement and motor development.]* 2nd ed. Berlin: Springer-Verlag.

Vojta, V., and A. Peters. 2007. *Das Vojta-Prinzip. Muskelspiele in Reflexfortbewegung und motorischer Ontogenese. [The Vojta principle. Muscle activity in reflex progressive movement and motor development.]* Berlin: Spinger-Verlag.

von Eisenhart-Rothe, R., F.A. Matsen III, F. Eckstein, T. Vogl, and H. Graichen. 2005. Pathomechanics in atraumatic shoulder instability: Scapular positioning correlates with humeral head centering. *Clin Orthop Relat Res* 433: 82-9.

von Porat, A., E.M. Roos, and H. Roos. 2004. High prevalence of osteoarthritis 14 years after an anterior cruciate ligament tear in male soccer players: A study of radiographic and patient relevant outcomes. *Ann Rheum Dis* 63(3): 269-73.

Voss, D. 1982. Everything is there before you discover it. *Phys Ther* 62(11): 1617-24.

Vuilerme, N., B. Anziani, and P. Rougier. 2007. Trunk extensor muscles fatigue affects undisturbed postural control in young healthy adults. *Clin Biomech (Bristol, Avon)* 22(5): 489-94.

Waddington, G., and R. Adams. 2003. Ankle disc training improves lower limb movement sensitivity in active walkers over 65 years old. Abstract presented at the World Congress of Physical Therapy, Barcelona.

Waddington, G., and R. Adams. 2003b. Football boot insoles and sensitivity to extent of ankle inversion movement. *Br J Sports Med* 37(2): 170-4.

Wadsworth, D.J., and J.E. Bullock-Saxton. 1997. Recruitment patterns of the scapular rotator muscles in freestyle swimmers with subacromial impingement. *Int J Sports Med* 18(8): 618-24.

Waling, K., B. Järvholm, and G. Sundelin. 2002. Effects of training on female trapezius myalgia: An intervention study with a 3-year follow-up period. *Spine* 27(8): 789-96.

Waling, K., G. Sundelin, C. Ahlgren, and B. Järvholm. 2000. Perceived pain before and after three exercise programs—a controlled clinical trial of women with work-related trapezius myalgia. *Pain* 85(1-2): 201-7.

Walker, M.L., J.M. Rothstein, S.D. Finucane, and R.L. Lamb. 1987. Relationships between lumbar lordosis, pelvic tilt, and abdominal muscle performance. *Phys Ther* 67(4): 512-6.

Wallin, D., B. Ekblom, R. Grahn, and T. Nordenborg. 1985. Improvement of muscle flexibility. A comparison between two techniques. *Am J Sports Med* 13(4): 263-8.

Walloe, L., and J. Wesche. 1988. Time course and magnitude of blood flow changes in human quadriceps muscles during and following rhythmic exercise. *J Physiol* 405: 257-73.

Walsh, M.T. 1994. Therapist management of thoracic outlet syndrome. *J Hand Ther* 7(2): 131-44.

Walther, D.S. 1988. *Applied kinesiology synopsis*. Pueblo, CO: Systems DC.

Walther, D.S. 2000. *Applied kinesiology synopsis*. 2nd ed. Pueblo, CO: Systems DC.

Walther, M., A. Werner, and T. Stahlschmidt. 2004. The subacromial impingement syndrome or the shoulder treated by conventional physiotherapy, self-training, and a shoulder brace. *J Shoulder Elbow Surg* 30(4): 417-23.

Wang, C.H., P. McClure, N.E. Pratt, and R. Nobilini. 1999. Stretching and strengthening exercises: Their effect on three-dimensional scapular kinematics. *Arch Phys Med Rehabil* 80(8): 923-9.

Wang, H.K., A. Macfarlane, and T. Cochrane. 2000. Isokinetic performance and shoulder mobility in elite volleyball athletes from the United Kingdom. *Br J Sports Med* 34(1): 39-43.

Wang, H.K., and T. Cochrane. 2001. Mobility impairment, muscle imbalance, muscle weakness, scapular asymmetry and shoulder injury in elite volleyball athletes. *J Sports Med Phys Fitness* 41(3): 403-10.

Wang, S.S., L.M. Jenkins, V.C. Taylor, and E.J. Trudelle-Jackson. 2005. Can physical therapy intervention improve muscle balance between the upper and lower trapezius? An electromyographic study. Abstract. *J Orthop Sports Phys Ther* 35(1): A32.

Wang, S.S., S.L. Whitney, R.G. Burdett, and J.E. Janosky. 1993. Lower extremity muscular flexibility in long distance runners. *J Orthop Sports Phys Ther* 17(2): 102-7.

Wannier, T., C. Bastiaanse, G. Colombo, and V. Dietz. 2001. Arm to leg coordination in humans during walking, creeping and swimming activities. *Exp Brain Res* 141(3): 375-9.

Ward, S.R., E.R. Hentzen, L.H. Smallwood, R.K. Eastlack, K.A. Burns, D.C. Fithian, J. Friden, and R.L. Lieber. 2006. Rotator cuff muscle architecture: Implications for glenohumeral stability. *Clin Orthop Relat Res* 448: 157-63.

Warner, J.J., L.J. Micheli, L.E. Arslanian, J. Kennedy, and R. Kennedy. 1990. Patterns of flexibility, laxity, and strength in normal shoulders and shoulders with instability and impingement. *Am J Sports Med* 18(4): 366-75.

Warner, J.J., L.J. Micheli, L.E. Arslanian, J. Kennedy, and R. Kennedy. 1992. Scapulothoracic motion in normal shoulders and shoulders with glenohumeral instability and impingement syndrome. A study using Moiré topographic analysis. *Clin Orthop Relat Res* 285: 191-9.

Watanabe, I., and J. Okubo. 1981. The role of the plantar mechanoreceptors in equilibrium control. *Ann NY Acad Sci* 374: 855-64.

Watelain E., Dujardin F., Babier F., Dubois D., and Allard P. 2001. Pelvic and lower limb compensatory actions of subjects in an early stage of hip osteoarthritis. *Arch Phys Med Rehabil.* Dec; 82(12): 1705-11.

Watson, D.H., and P.H. Trott. 1993. Cervical headache: An investigation of natural head posture and upper cervical flexor muscle performance. *Cephalalgia* 13(4): 272-84.

Wegener, L., C. Kisner, and D. Nichols. 1997. Static and dynamic balance responses in persons with bilateral knee osteoarthritis. *J Orthop Sports Phys Ther* 25(1): 13-8.

Weiner, D.S., and I. Macnab. 1970. Superior migration of the humeral head. A radiological aid in the diagnosis of tears of the rotator cuff. *J Bone Joint Surg Br* 52(3): 524-7.

Weldon III, E.J., and A.B. Richardson. 2001. Upper extremity overuse injuries in swimming. A discussion of swimmer's shoulder. *Clin Sports Med* 20(3): 423-38.

Werner, C.M., P. Favre, and C. Gerber. 2007. The role of the subscapularis in preventing anterior glenohumeral subluxation in the abducted, externally rotated position of the arm. *Clin Biomech (Bristol, Avon)* 22(5): 495-501.

Wester, J.U., S.M. Jepersen, K.D. Nielsen, and L. Neumann. 1996. Wobble board training after partial

sprains of lateral ligaments of the ankle: A prospective randomized study. *J Orthop Sports Phys Ther* 23(5): 332-6.

Westgaard, R.H., O. Vasseljen, and K.A. Holte. 2001. Trapezius muscle activity as a risk indicator for shoulder and neck pain in female service workers with low biomechanical exposure. *Ergonomics* 44(3): 339-53.

Whitcomb, L.J., M.J. Kelley, and C.I. Leiper. 1995. A comparison of torque production during dynamic strength testing of shoulder abduction in the coronal plane and the plane of the scapula. *J Orthop Sports Phys Ther* 21(4): 227-32.

Wiedenbauer, M.M., and O.A. Mortensen. 1952. An electromyographic study of the trapezius muscle. *Am J Phys Med* 31(5): 363-72.

Wikstrom, E.A., M.D. Tillman, T.L. Chmielewski, J.H. Cauraugh, and P.A. Borsa. 2007. Dynamic postural stability deficits in subjects with self-reported ankle instability. *Med Sci Sports Exerc* 39(3): 397-402.

Wilder, D., A. Aleksiev, M. Magnusson, K. Pope, K. Spratt, and V. Goel. 1996. Muscular response to sudden load: A tool to evaluate fatigue and rehabilitation. *Spine* 21: 2638-9.

Wilk, K.E., C.A. Arrigo, and J.R. Andrews. 1997. Current concepts: The stabilizing structures of the glenohumeral joint. *J Orthop Sports Phys Ther* 25(6): 364-79.

Wilk, K.E., J.R. Andrews, C.A. Arrigo, M.A. Keirns, and D.J. Erber. 1993. The strength characteristics of internal and external rotator muscles in professional baseball pitchers. *Am J Sports Med* 21(1): 61-6.

Wilk, K.E., K. Meister, and J.R. Andrews. 2002. Current concepts in the rehabilitation of the overhead throwing athlete. *Am J Sports Med* 30(1): 136-51.

Wilkerson, G.B., and A.J. Nitz. 1994. Dynamic ankle instability: Mechanical and neuromuscular relationships. *J Sport Rehabil* 3: 43-57.

Wilkerson, G.B., J.J. Pinerola, and R.W. Caturano. 1997. Invertor vs. evertor peak torque and power deficiencies associated with lateral ankle ligament injury. *J Orthop Sports Phys Ther* 26(2): 78-86.

Williams, G.N., L. Snyder-Mackler, P.J. Barrance, and T.S. Buchanan. 2005. Quadriceps femoris function after ACL injury; a differential response in copers versus non-copers. *J Biomech* 38: 685-93.

Witvrouw, E., J. Bellemans, R. Lysens, L. Danneels, and D. Cambier. 2001. Intrinsic risk factors for the development of patellar tendinitis in an athletic population. A two-year prospective study. *Am J Sports Med* 29(2): 190-5.

Witvrouw, E., L. Danneels, P. Asselman, T. D'Have, and D. Cambier. 2003. Muscle flexibility as a risk factor for developing muscle injuries in male professional soccer players. A prospective study. *Am J Sports Med* 31(1): 41-6.

Wojtys, E.M., and L.J. Huston. 1994. Neuromuscular performance in normal and anterior cruciate ligament-deficient lower extremities. *Am J Sports Med* 22(1): 89-104.

Wojtys, E.M., L.J. Huston, P.D. Taylor, and S.D. Bastian. 1996. Neuromuscular adaptations in isokinetic, isotonic, and agility training programs. *Am J Sports Med* 24(2): 187-92.

Wolfe, F., H.A. Smythe, M.B. Yunus, R.M. Bennett, C. Bombardier, D.L. Goldenberg, P. Tugwell et al. 1990. The American College of Rheumatology 1990 criteria for the classification of fibromyalgia. Report of the Multicenter Criteria Committee. *Arthritis Rheum* 33(2): 160-72.

Woodley, B.L., R.J. Newsham-West, and G.D. Baxter. 2007. Chronic tendinopathy: Effectiveness of eccentric exercise. *Br J Sports Med* 41(4): 188-98.

Woolacott, M.H. 1986. Aging and postural control: Changes in sensory organization and muscular coordination. *Int J Aging Hum Dev* 23(2): 97-114.

Woolf, C. 1987. Physiological, inflammatory and neuropathic pain. *Adv Tech Stand Neurosurg* 15: 39-62.

Woolf, C.J. 1983. Evidence for a central component of post-injury pain hypersensitivity. *Nature* 306(5944): 686-8.

Worrell, T.W., D.H. Perrin, B.M. Gansneder, and J.H. Gieck. 1991. Comparison of isokinetic strength and flexibility measures between hamstring injured and noninjured athletes. *J Orthop Sports Phys Ther* 13(3): 118-25.

Wright, A. 1995. Hypoalgesia post-manipulative therapy: A review of a potential neurophysiological mechanism. *Man Ther* 1: 16.

Wuelker, N., H. Schmotzer, K. Thren, and M. Korell. 1994. Translation of the glenohumeral joint with simulated active elevation. *Clin Orthop Relat Res* 309: 193-200.

Wuelker, N., M. Korell, and K. Thren. 1998. Dynamic glenohumeral joint stability. *J Shoulder Elbow Surg* 7(1): 43-52.

Wyke, B. 1967. The neurology of joints. *Ann R Coll Surg Engl* 41(1): 25-50.

Wyke, B.K., and P. Polacek. 1975. Articular neurology: The present position. *J Bone Joint Surg Br* 57-B(3): 401.

Xue, Q., and G. Huang. 1998. Dynamic stability of glenohumeral joint during scapular plane elevation. *Chin Med J (Engl)* 111(5): 447-9.

Yahia, L., S. Rhalmi, N. Newman, and M. Isler. 1992. Sensory innervation of human thoracolumbar fascia. An immunohistochemical study. *Acta Orthop Scand* 63(2): 195-7.

Yamaguchi, K., J.S. Sher, W.K. Andersen, R. Garretson, J.W. Uribe, K. Hechtman, and R.J. Neviaser. 2000. Glenohumeral motion in patients with rotator cuff tears: A comparison of asymptomatic and symptomatic shoulders. *J Shoulder Elbow Surg* 9(1): 6-11.

Yanai, T., F.K. Fuss, and T. Fukunaga. 2006. In vivo measurements of subacromial impingement: Substantial compression develops in abduction with large internal rotation. *Clin Biomech (Bristol, Avon)* 21(7): 692-700.

Yang, J.F., and D.A. Winter. 1983. Electromyography reliability in maximal and submaximal isometric contractions. *Arch Phys Med Rehabil* 64(9): 417-20.

Yildiz, Y., T. Aydin, U. Sekir, M.Z. Kiralp, B. Hazneci, and T.A. Kalyon. 2006. Shoulder terminal range eccentric antagonist/concentric agonist strength ratios in overhead athletes. *Scand J Med Sci Sports* 16(3): 174-80.

Ylinen, J., E.P. Takala, M. Nykänen, A. Häkkinen, E. Mälkiä, T. Pohjolainen, S.L. Karppi, H. Kautiainen, and O. Airaksinen. 2003. Active neck muscle training in the treatment of chronic neck pain in women: A randomized controlled trial. *JAMA* 289(19): 2509-16.

Ylinen, J., H. Kautiainen, K. Wirén, and A. Häkkinen. 2007. Stretching exercises vs manual therapy in treatment of chronic neck pain: A randomized, controlled crossover trial. *J Rehabil Med* 39(2): 126-32.

Ylinen, J., P. Salo, M. Nykänen, H. Kautiainen, and A. Häkkinen. 2004. Decreased isometric neck strength in women with chronic neck pain and the repeatability of neck strength measurements. *Arch Phys Med Rehabil* 85(8): 1303-8.

Yue, G., and K.J. Cole. 1993. Strength increases from the motor programme: Comparison of training with maximal voluntary contraction and imagined muscle contraction *J Neurophysiol* 67(5): 1114-23.

Zätterstrom, R., T. Friden, A. Lindstrand, and U. Moritz. 1994. The effect of physiotherapy on standing balance in chronic anterior cruciate ligament insufficiency. *Am J Sports Med* 22(4): 531-6.

Zepa, I., K. Hurmerinta, O. Kovero, M. Nissinen, M. Kononen, and J. Huggare. 2000. Associations between thoracic kyphosis, head posture, and craniofacial morphology in young adults. *Acta Odontol Scand* 58(6): 237-42.

Zepa, I., K. Hurmerinta, O. Kovero, M. Nissinen, M. Kononen, and J. Huggare. 2003. Trunk asymmetry and facial symmetry in young adults. *Acta Odontol Scand* 61(3): 149-53.

Zhang, Q., and G.Y.F. Ng. 2007. EMG analysis of vastus medialis obliquus/vastus lateralis activities in subjects with patellofemoral pain syndrome before and after a home exercise program. *J Phys Ther Sci* 19(2): 131-7.

Zidar, J., E. Bäckman, A. Bengtsson, and K.G. Henriksson. 1990. Quantitative EMG and muscle tension in painful muscles in fibromyalgia. *Pain* 40(3): 249-54.

Zito, G., G. Jull, and I. Story. 2006. Clinical tests of musculoskeletal dysfunction in the diagnosis of cervicogenic headache. *Man Ther* 11(2): 118-29.

Zusman, M. 1986. Spinal manipulative therapy: Some proposed mechanisms and a new hypothesis. *Aust J Physiother* 32: 89-99.

INDEX

Note: The italicized *f* and *t* following page numbers refer to figures and tables, respectively.

ABOUT THE AUTHORS

Phil Page, MS, PT, ATC, CSCS, trained under the guidance of Dr. Vladimir Janda and has taught the Janda approach at national and international workshops. A certified kinesiotaping practitioner, Page is currently working toward his doctorate in kinesiology at Louisiana State University in Baton Rouge, where his research focuses on EMG and muscle imbalance. He is also director of clinical education and research for Thera-Band products.

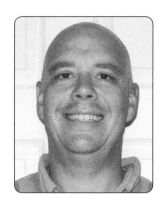

Page and his wife, Angela, live in Baton Rouge with their four children. In his free time, he enjoys spending time with his family, fishing, and cooking.

Clare C. Frank, DPT, is an orthopedic clinical specialist in private practice in Los Angeles. She serves on the clinical faculty for Kaiser Permanente Movement Science Fellowship in Los Angeles. She also serves as a guest lecturer at the local universities and teaches throughout the United States and internationally.

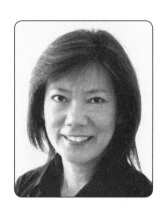

Frank studied under and taught with Dr. Vladimir Janda. She is a certified instructor of the Janda approach to musculoskeletal pain syndromes, a certified kinesiotaping practitioner, and a certified instructor of Kolar's approach to dynamic neuromuscular stabilization.

Frank is board certified in orthopedic physical therapy and a fellow of the American Academy of Orthopedic Manual Physical Therapy.

Robert Lardner, PT, was born in Nigeria in 1961. His first career was as a professional ballet and modern dancer after studying at the Rambert Academy outside London, England. He graduated from the department of physical therapy, Lund's University, Sweden in 1991. He studied with Professors Janda, Lewit and Kolář from the Czech Republic, who are pioneers of functional rehabilitation and manual medicine.

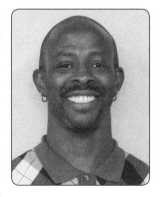

Lardner worked in several inpatient and outpatient rehabilitation facilities in Sweden prior to moving to the United States in 1992. He was a staff physical therapist at McNeal Hospital, Clearing Industrial Clinic, and a physical therapy supervisor at Mercy Hospital. He also was in charge of physical therapy services at a number of private outpatient and sports clinics.

Lardner is currently in private practice in Chicago and teaches various rehabilitation seminars throughout the United States and Europe.

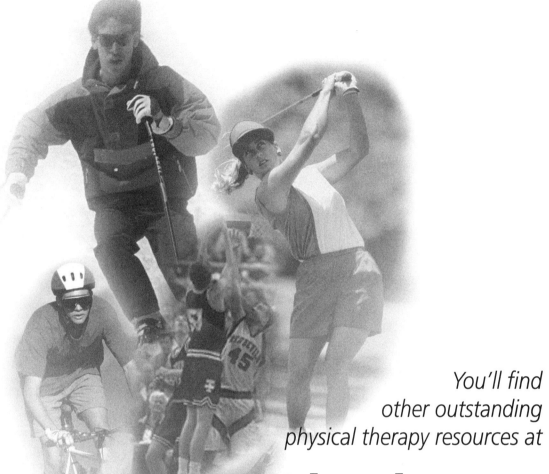